MO

POCKET GUIDE TO Fetal

Monitoring

A MULTIDISCIPLINARY APPROACH

NINTH EDITION

LISA A. MILLER, CNM, JD

Founder, Perinatal Risk Management and Education Services
Portland, Oregon

DAVID A. MILLER, MD

Professor of Obstetrics, Gynecology, and Pediatrics
Keck School of Medicine
University of Southern California
Chief, Division of Maternal Fetal Medicine
Children's Hospital Los Angeles
Director, CHLA-USC Fetal Maternal Center
Los Angeles, California

REBECCA L. CYPHER, MSN, PNNP

Perinatal Nurse Practitioner
Founder, Cypher Maternal Fetal Solutions LLC
Gig Harbor, Washington

ELSEVIER

ELSEVIER

3251 Riverport Lane
St. Louis, MO 63043

MOSBY'S® POCKET GUIDE TO FETAL MONITORING:
A MULTIDISCIPLINARY APPROACH, NINTH EDITION   ISBN: 978-0-323-64260-6

Notice

Practitioners and researchers must always rely on their own experience and knowledge in evaluating
and using any information, methods, compounds or experiments described herein. Because of rapid
advances in the medical sciences, in particular, independent verification of diagnoses and drug dosages
should be made. To the fullest extent of the law, no responsibility is assumed by Elsevier, authors, editors
or contributors for any injury and/or damage to persons or property as a matter of products liability,
negligence or otherwise, or from any use or operation of any methods, products, instructions, or ideas
contained in the material herein.

Library of Congress Control Number: 2020949257

Senior Content Strategist: Sandy Clark
Director, Content Development: Ellen Wurm-Cutter
Senior Content Development Specialist: Kathleen Nahm
Publishing Services Manager: Shereen Jameel
Senior Project Manager: Kamatchi Madhavan
Design Direction: Ryan Cook/Bridget Hoette

Printed in India

Last digit is the print number: 9   8   7   6   5   4   3

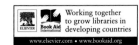

JANICE DENNY GIBBS, MSN, RNC-INPT OB, C-EFM
Louisville, Kentucky

ELISABETH HOWARD, PhD, CNM, FACNM
Associate Professor of Obstetrics and Gynecology, Clinician Educator
Director, Midwifery
Women and Infants Hospital
Department of Obstetrics and Gynecology
Warren Alpert Medical School
Brown University
Providence, Rhode Island

JAMES M. KELLEY, JD
Elk & Elk
Mayfield Heights, Ohio

PAULA WELLDE, MSN, RNC-OB, C-EFM
Perinatal Safety Nurse
Elliot Hospital
Manchester, New Hampshire

ACKNOWLEDGMENTS

Clinical Computer Systems, Inc.
Elgin, Illinois

GE Medical Systems Information Technologies
Milwaukee, Wisconsin

Hill-Rom Company, Inc.
Batesville, Indiana

Huntleigh Healthcare Ltd.
Cardiff, United Kingdom

Philips Medizin Systemes
Böblingen, Germany

We are proud to continue nursing, midwifery, and physician collaboration in this new ninth edition of *Mosby's® Pocket Guide to Fetal Monitoring: A Multidisciplinary Approach,* consistent with the inter- and intradisciplinary approach all of us bring to teaching this subject matter. Diligently revised, this new edition continues to emphasize standardized terminology and an evidence-based approach to interpretation and management. This text remains a key resource for the most clinically useful information for clincians of all levels on every aspect of fetal monitoring, including intermittent auscultation, assessment and management of uterine activity, and the crucial role of both communication and documentation in risk management related to fetal monitoring. Whether your practice is office-based, in a birth center, in a hospital serving the community, or in an academic tertiary care center, this text provides a relevant and easily understood reference for daily clinical practice as well as clinician orientation and ongoing education.

DESCRIPTION

Primarily an oxygen monitor, the electronic fetal monitor is a tool used to prevent fetal injury resulting from interruption of fetal oxygenation, whether used during labor or in the antepartum period. Key to this goal is standardization and simplification of clinical practices related to interpretation and management of fetal monitoring. This book provides clinicians with the tools needed to understand both the strengths and the weaknesses of both electronic fetal monitoring (EFM) and intermittent auscultation; as well as apply a collaborative approach to clinical practice that is evidence- and consensus-based. After a brief overview of the history of fetal monitoring, the text provides core clinical information on the physiologic basis for monitoring, reviews the newest instrumentation for uterine and fetal heart rate (FHR) monitoring, including the newer abdominal "patch" technology, and identifies key factors in the evaluation of uterine activity. In keeping with maintaining the legal standard of care in the United States, the National Institute of Child Health and Human Development (NICHD) definitions are presented and reviewed, and a standardized approach to interpretation and management is clearly outlined. The influence of gestational age on FHR is examined, along with the evaluation of fetal status outside the obstetric unit and in the antenatal setting. Documentation and risk management issues are delineated, including issues of informed consent in choice of monitoring modality. An overview of fetal monitoring in Europe provides clinicians with a look at fetal monitoring outside the United States. Patient safety, communication, and clinical collaboration are the cornerstones of each chapter, and suggestions for practice improvement make this edition an invaluable resource for the busy clinician.

FEATURES

This book has a number of distinctive features:

- Content is organized in a manner that allows clinicians to build on key fundamental concepts and progress logically to advanced principles, making the text suitable for novices needing basic information as well as experienced practitioners seeking greater insight into clinical practice issues.
- Critical information is highlighted using illustrations, tables, and illustrative fetal monitor tracings.
- FHR characteristics are explained and the supporting level of evidence is provided, revealing a number of common myths regarding fetal monitoring.
- Evidence levels are provided for information regarding various FHR patterns, and several common obstetric myths are laid to rest.
- Appendices now include self-assessment questions as well as fetal monitor tracings for practice in application of the NICHD definitions and principles of standardized interpretation.

ORGANIZATION

Chapter 1 traces the history of fetal monitoring from the use of auscultation in the 17th century to present-day practice and includes a discussion of the resurgence of intermittent auscultation for fetal monitoring in low-risk women.

Chapter 2 provides a review of the physiologic basis for monitoring. The oxygen pathway is discussed, as well as the fetal response to interrupted oxygenation. These core physiologic concepts provide clinicians with the fundamentals of fetal oxygenation that serve as the basis for current practice.

Chapter 3 offers a detailed look at instrumentation for both intermittent auscultation and EFM, including newer approaches such as abdominal electrocardiogram and new display options for dopplers used in intermittent auscultation. Both external and internal monitoring devices and their application are covered in depth, including artifact detection, telemetry, and troubleshooting tips.

Chapter 4, on uterine activity, provides crucial information including a detailed discussion of normal versus excessive uterine activity and the limitations of the summary term *tachysystole*. Consensus guidelines for the diagnosis of active labor are presented, and the link between excessive uterine activity and fetal acidemia is elucidated. Evidence-based tips for managing uterine activity in clinical practice are offered, and oxytocin use is also addressed.

Chapter 5 breaks down clinical practice in fetal monitoring to its three core elements: definitions, interpretation, and management. This chapter includes the NICHD definitions with illustrations to aid in recognition and application. The role of NICHD categories is examined, and evidence- and consensus-based principles of interpretation are explained.

Chapter 6 presents the management of FHR tracings using a systematic approach based on principles of fetal oxygenation. This comprehensive model is based on EFM's value as a screening tool (rather than a diagnostic tool). The management algorithm uses NICHD categories and a structured approach based on the oxygen pathway. Evidence-based corrective measures for hypoxemia are provided in a checklist format. An adapted model specific to the management of Category 2 FHR tracings with significant decelerations is included, with evidence supporting this approach. Chapter 6 elucidates the *primary objective* of intrapartum FHR monitoring: to prevent fetal injury that might result from the progression of hypoxemia during the intrapartum period.

Chapter 7 reviews FHR characteristics in the preterm, late-term, and postterm fetus, including implications for management in both antepartum and intrapartum settings. The chapter includes information on a variety of medications and clinical factors that can affect FHR at various gestational ages.

Chapter 8 explores non-obstetric settings and FHR evaluation, focusing on the importance of collaboration. Settings such as the emergency department, surgical suite, or intensive care unit are discussed with key points for clinical care and FHR assessment. Obstetric triage is reviewed, including the impact of the Emergency Medical Transport and Labor Act (EMTALA).

Chapter 9 focuses on antepartum testing, including the nonstress test, the contraction stress test, vibroacoustic stimulation, ultrasound, and the biophysical profile. Information regarding indication, frequency, and type of antepartum test based on the results of the most recent NICHD panel are provided in a clinically relevant manner.

Chapter 10 focuses on documentation and risk management. Clinical tips for improving documentation are a highlight of this new edition. Intermittent auscultation, EFM, and informed consent are discussed, with suggestions for inter- and intradisciplinary discussion points and patient education. Actual deposition testimony related to documentation reveals the importance of knowing both nomenclature and physiology in detail.

Chapter 11 provides a glimpse of FHR monitoring in select European countries, where paper speed is frequently 1 cm/minute versus the typical 3 cm/minute seen in the United States. Variations in obstetric care models and sample illustrations of a variety of fetal monitor tracings from our European colleagues are provided for review.

Appendix A reflects current practice regarding amnioinfusion, indicated as a potential corrective measure for variable decelerations.

Appendix B has been updated and includes 10 new fetal monitoring tracings, bringing the total number of FHR tracings in the appendix to 40. This appendix provides ample opportunities for education, review, and preparation for certification or credentialing exams. Clinicians can use the tracings to practice application of the NICHD definitions, as well as the principles of standardized interpretation, and an answer key allows clinicians to evaluate their skills.

Appendix C offers a self-assessment consisting of multiple-choice questions related to the content of the textbook. Helpful for reinforcement of information presented herein, it can also be used to study for certification or credentialing examinations or to develop internal competency assessment tools for clinical practice.

Mosby's® Pocket Guide to Fetal Monitoring: A Multidisciplinary Approach continues to be written by clinicians, for clinicians. Nurses, nurse-midwives, medical students, physicians, resident physicians, clinical specialists, educators, and risk management and medical-legal professionals will gain a clear perspective on modalities of fetal monitoring, the role of standardization, as well as the keys to successful collaboration. Meticulously researched and revised, the ninth edition is the most portable and practical reference available for daily clinical practice, education, test prep, and habituation of both knowledge and skills. We are thrilled to be able to offer this valuable tool to all clinicians, in all practice settings.

LISA A. MILLER
DAVID A. MILLER
REBECCA L. CYPHER

CONTENTS

CHAPTER 1

A Brief History of Fetal Monitoring

Shared decision-making, informed choice, and greater public and consumer engagement in obstetrics and obstetric safety has shifted clinical focus in perinatal care. Electronic fetal monitoring (EFM) is only one of the issues being discussed by clinicians and the families they serve. Newer labor curves, intermittent auscultation (IA) of the fetal heart rate (FHR), and continuous labor support are becoming the new normal, especially for healthy, low-risk women [1–3]. The shift to IA for healthy low-risk women relates to a widespread recognition of these facts: research has been unable to definitively show that use of intrapartum FHR monitoring leads to a significant reduction in neonatal neurologic morbidity [4], and both early randomized trials and meta-analyses have shown a trend toward higher cesarean section rates for women who have continuous EFM during labor versus women who do not have continuous EFM [5]. This means that clinicians must be adept at both EFM and IA modalities, and for this reason, a brief overview of the history of FHR assessment is justified.

HISTORICAL OVERVIEW

Jean Alexandre Le Jumeau, Vicomte de Kergaradec, was the first person to speculate in print about the potential clinical uses for FHR auscultation. In 1822 he used a stethoscope hoping to hear the noise of the water in the uterus, and he identified the noise he heard as the FHR [6]. Confirmation of pregnancy, identification of twin gestation, and justification for a postmortem cesarean section were some of the early uses of FHR auscultation. William Kennedy, a British obstetrician, published a description of "fetal distress" in 1833 by describing what would later be classified as a late deceleration. Kennedy correctly associated late decelerations with poor prognoses. He also made the link between fetal head compression and decrease in FHR, now known as *early decelerations* [7]. Other discoveries from early use of FHR assessment via IA included identification of fetal tachycardia in response to maternal fever, FHR decelerations

1

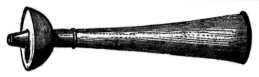

Fig. 1.1 Early obstetric trumpet stethoscope. (Courtesy Wellcome Library, London.)

after excessive uterine activity, and accelerations accompanying fetal movement (Fig. 1.1) [6].

In 1917, the head stethoscope, or DeLee-Hillis fetoscope, was first reported in the literature [8]. Fast forward to the 1950s: physicians throughout the world, including Edward Hon [9–11] in the United States, Caldeyro-Barcia [12,13] in Uruguay, and Hammacher [14] in Germany, developed electronic devices that were able to continuously measure and record the FHR and uterine activity. The simultaneous measurement of FHR and uterine activity came to be called *EFM* or *cardiotocography* (CTG). This new technologic capability permitted systematic study of the relationships between recorded FHR patterns and fetal physiology [10,11,15]. Although investigators worldwide made remarkably similar observations of FHR characteristics, dramatically different terms and definitions were being used and there was no significant standardization (Fig. 1.2).

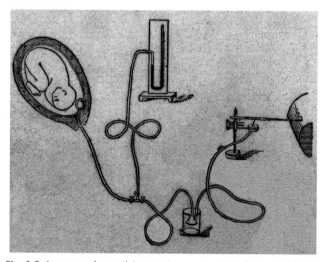

Fig. 1.2 Apparatus for studying uterine contractions during childbirth. (Courtesy Wellcome Library, London.)

RANDOMIZED TRIALS OF ELECTRONIC FETAL MONITORING

Observational studies in the 1960s demonstrated a decrease in intrapartum stillbirth rates in settings that adopted continuous EFM [16–18] and served to drive the widespread adoption of the technology. Although EFM was originally intended for use in high-risk laboring women, it was rapidly incorporated into the management of low-risk laboring women as well and quickly became ubiquitous. Today, observational findings alone would never result in such rapid and widespread practice change.

During the 1970s and 1980s, several randomized clinical [19–27] were conducted comparing continuous EFM with IA using a Pinard stethoscope or a handheld Doppler device. Continuous EFM was not associated with a decrease in low Apgar scores or perinatal mortality. However, there was an increase in the incidence of cesarean section in women who had continuous EFM. Despite these findings, use of continuous EFM did not decrease.

Meta-analyses have reviewed the results of trials comparing continuous intrapartum EFM with IA [5,28,29]. These studies included more than 37,000 women. Compared with IA, continuous EFM showed no significant difference in overall perinatal death but was associated with a significant reduction in neonatal seizures. No significant difference was detected in the incidence of cerebral palsy. However, there was a significant increase in cesarean sections associated with continuous EFM. Interestingly, none of the randomized trials published after 1980 demonstrated a statistically significant increase in the rate of cesarean section in electronically monitored patients. Most important, the majority of newborns in the cohort who later developed cerebral palsy were not in the group of fetuses who had FHR tracings that were considered "ominous" [30].

RESEARCH AT THE END OF THE 20th CENTURY

So what went wrong? Several things. Although the randomized controlled trials (RCTs) followed the usual guidelines for inclusion and exclusion of subjects and used recommended methods for the study protocols, the definitions of FHR patterns reflecting fetal distress varied among the different studies [23–25,31]. In the largest (and most frequently cited) trial, the IA arm and the EFM arm each had fetal scalp blood sampling included as a follow-up test, making the study a comparison of EFM with scalp sampling with IA with scalp sampling rather than a true comparison of EFM versus IA [24]. Many of the studies were conducted before the importance of FHR variability, a critical parameter, was recognized as significant related to fetal acid–base status. Outcome measures evaluated (Apgar scores, perinatal mortality, and cerebral palsy) were nonspecific indicators of the potential for hypoxic injury during the intrapartum period. Finally, the small sample size of published reports is an ongoing issue. It has been noted that more than 50,000 women would need to be randomized to show a difference in mortality [5]; the numbers that would be needed to show a reduction in neonatal encephalopathy related solely to intrapartum events are so high that RCTs for either EFM or IA become implausible [32]. As a result, the conclusions of these studies remain open to alternative interpretations [27,33], and a careful review of the oft-cited Cochrane Database meta-analysis by Alfirevic and colleagues reveals low-quality evidence for all conclusions, save the conclusion regarding neonatal seizures, which was found to be of moderate quality [5]. Clinicians should consider basing decisions regarding the use of continuous EFM on multiple factors, including forthright discussions of risks versus benefits with various patient populations. Informed choice regarding EFM versus IA is challenging with the state of current evidence and is discussed in more detail in Chapter 10.

In 1996, the National Institute of Child Health and Human Development (NICHD) Task Force met and made recommendations [34] for three important aspects of FHR monitoring for both research and clinical practice: (1) the task force developed standard definitions for FHR patterns, (2) they described the FHR pattern (normal baseline rate, moderate variability, presence of accelerations, and absence of decelerations) that consistently reflects an absence of asphyxia, and (3) they described FHR patterns (recurrent late or variable decelerations or substantial bradycardia with absent variability) that are "predictive of current or impending asphyxia" [34].

FETAL MONITORING IN THE 21st CENTURY

The first Task Force on Neonatal Encephalopathy and Cerebral Palsy [35] was convened in 2003 by the American College of Obstetricians and Gynecologists (ACOG) to review the world literature regarding the relationship between FHR patterns in labor and neonatal outcomes. The task force reviewed the literature on Apgar scores, neonatal encephalopathy and cerebral palsy, neonatal seizures, and umbilical cord gases. In 2010 a second task force was convened to update this important work, and in 2014 a second edition was published, which included the review of 1500 references by 17 task force members and 88 consultants [36]. This updated report focuses on neonatal encephalopathy in infants born at 35 weeks' gestation or greater and contains an in-depth review of intrapartum events and their relationship to newborn encephalopathy. Consensus from this work and others forms the basis of the principles of interpretation of EFM that will be elucidated later in this text.

Standardization in research of EFM has been aided by the NICHD definitions that were originally published in 1997 [34]. In 2008 a new NICHD panel on fetal monitoring was convened; the new panel confirmed and provided clarification of the definitions published in 1997 and provided a three-tiered categorization of FHR tracings to replace the traditionally used terms *reassuring* and *nonreassuring*. The panel also reviewed uterine activity and provided guidance for evaluation of uterine activity and definitions for summary terms. Finally, the 2008 NICHD workshop report provided important information regarding consensus on the validity of the negative predictive value of both moderate variability and/or FHR accelerations in relation to fetal metabolic acidemia [37]. Since the report, many healthcare systems have implemented multidisciplinary education and training related to the standardized NICHD definitions.

In an attempt to find a more direct measure of fetal oxygenation to serve as an adjunct to EFM in the assessment of fetal acid–base balance, fetal pulse oximetry made a short-lived appearance on the clinical scene. The first randomized trial of fetal pulse oximetry demonstrated a reduction in the number of cesarean sections performed for nonreassuring FHR patterns but no overall reduction in cesarean sections [38]. At present, fetal pulse oximetry has been a useful tool for research but is no longer available for use in clinical practice. Computer analysis of the fetal electrocardiogram ST segment (STAN Neoventa Medical, Mölndal, Sweden), a technology based on evaluation of the ST segment and the T/QRS ratio of the fetal electrocardiogram complex, continues to be in use, primarily outside the United States. This is further discussed in Chapter 11. The large, multicenter NICHD trial of ST analysis in the United States involving more than 11,000 patients failed to show any decrease in operative deliveries or any differences in perinatal outcomes [39]. It should be noted that this is not the case with ST analysis research outside the United

States, where it has been associated with significant reductions in both hypoxic-ischemic encephalopathy and cesarean birth [40]. This raises the question of whether it is the technology itself or its application in clinical practice that causes the discrepancy.

SUMMARY

The findings of Le Jumeau in 1822 with a stethoscope have evolved significantly, yet fetal monitoring remains fraught with controversy and misinformation. EFM today is a frequently used, much maligned, and often misunderstood technology. Attempts at integration of IA as the preferred mode of monitoring during labor for healthy, low-risk women continues to pose a challenge in many institutions, for a variety of reasons [41]. Clinicians must be able to understand and articulate the appropriate use of EFM and IA to engage in truly informed decision-making with women and their families. Although it is clear that more research is needed on EFM reliability (observer agreement), validity (association with neonatal outcomes), and efficacy (preventive interventions that work), the overall evidence suggests that extreme positions on EFM (either universal use or universal abandonment) are unwarranted. A middle path that encompasses appropriate patient selection, informed choice/shared decision-making, *and a clinical recognition of the limits of both EFM and IA* is perhaps the most reasonable approach to fetal monitoring today. Women want and are entitled to complete information regarding fetal monitoring via auscultation and by electronic means [42]. As the history of fetal monitoring continues to be written, everyone must recognize that technology alone will never be the answer. Standardization of terminology, multidisciplinary education regarding FHR interpretation and underlying physiology, management based on collaboration and teamwork, and the recognition of the role of one-to-one support for laboring women [43] remain the best strategies to ensure safe passage for mother and child.

References

[1] American College of Nurse-Midwives, Intermittent auscultation for intrapartum fetal heart rate surveillance. ACNM Clinical Bulletin Number 13, J. Midwifery Womens Health 60 (2015) 626–632.

[2] American College of Obstetricians and Gynecologists, Approaches to limit intervention during labor and birth, Obstet. Gynecol. 133 (2019) e164–e173, Committee Opinion no. 766. doi: 10.1097/AOG .0000000000003074.

[3] Association of Women's Health, Obstetric and Neonatal Nurses, Fetal heart monitoring, position statement, J. Obstet. Gynecol. Neonatal Nurs 47 (6) (2018) 874–877. https://doi.org/10.1016/j.jogn.2018.09.007.

[4] J.T. Parer, T.L. King, S. Flanders, et al., Fetal acidemia and electronic fetal heart rate patterns: is there evidence of an association? J. Matern. Fetal Neonatal Med. 19 (5) (2006) 289–294.

[5] Z. Alfirevic, D. Devane, G.M.L. Gyte, A. Cuthbert, Continuous car-diotocography (CTG) as a form of electronic fetal monitoring (EFM) for fetal assessment during labour, Cochrane Database of Syst. Rev. (2) (2017). doi:10.1002/14651858.CD006066.pub3.

[6] C. Sureau, Historical perspectives: forgotten past, unpredictable future, Baillieres Clin. Obstet. Gynaecol. 10 (2) (1996) 167–184.

[7] E. Kennedy, Observations of Obstetrical Auscultation, Hodges & Smith, Dublin, 1833, p. 311.

[8] D.S. Hillis, Attachment for the stethoscope, JAMA 68 (1917) 910.

[9] E.H. Hon, Instrumentation of fetal heart rate and electrocardiography II: a vaginal electrode, Am. J. Obstet. Gynecol. 83 (1963) 772.

[10] E.H. Hon, The classification of fetal heart rate. I: a working classifica-tion, Obstet. Gynecol. 22 (1963) 137–146.

[11] E.H. Hon, The electronic evaluation of the fetal heart rate, Am. J. Obstet. Gynecol. 75 (1958) 1215.

[12] R. Caldeyro-Barcia, C. Mendez-Bauer, J. Poseiro, et al., Control of human fetal heart rate during labor, in: D. Cassels (Ed.), The Heart and Circula-tion in the Newborn and Infant, Grune & Stratton, New York, 1966.

[13] R. Caldeyro-Barcia, J.J. Poseiro, C. Negreierosdepaiva, et al., Effects of abnormal uterine contractions on a human fetus, Bibl. Paediatr. 81 (1963) 267–295. http://www.ncbi.nlm.nih.gov/pubmed/14065034 (accessed 05.08.15).

[14] K. Hammacher, New method for the selective registration of the fetal heart beat [German], Geburtshilfe Frauenheilkd. 22 (1962) 1542–1543.

[15] S.T. Lee, E.H. Hon, Fetal hemodynamic response to umbilical cord compression, Obstet. Gynecol. 22 (1963) 553–562.

[16] R. Errkola, M. Gronroos, R. Punnonen, et al., Analysis of intrapartum fetal deaths: their decline with increasing electronic fetal monitoring, Acta Obstet. Gynecol. Scand. 63 (5) (1984) 459–462.

[17] J.T. Parer, Fetal heart rate monitoring, Lancet 2 (8143) (1979) 632–633.

[18] S.Y. Yeh, F. Diaz, R.H. Paul, Ten year experience of intrapartum fetal monitoring in Los Angeles County/University of Southern California Medical Center, Am. J. Obstet. Gynecol. 143 (5) (1982) 496–500.

[19] A.D. Havercamp, M. Orleans, S. Langerdoerfer, et al., A controlled trial of differential effects of intrapartum fetal monitoring, Am. J. Obstet. Gynecol. 134 (4) (1979) 399–408.

[20] A.D. Havercamp, H.E. Thompson, J.G. McFee, et al., The evaluation of continuous fetal heart rate monitoring in high risk pregnancy, Am. J. Obstet. Gynecol. 125 (3) (1976) 310–320.

[21] I.M. Kelso, R.J. Parsons, G.F. Lawrence, et al., An assessment of continuous fetal heart rate monitoring in labor, Am. J. Obstet. Gynecol. 131 (5) (1978) 526–532.

[22] J. Leveno, F.G. Cunningham, S. Nelson, et al., A prospective comparison of selective and universal electronic fetal monitoring in 34,995 pregnancies, N, Engl. J. Med. 315 (10) (1986) 615–641.

[23] D.A. Luthy, K.K. Shy, G. van Belle, et al., A randomized trial of electronic monitoring in labor, Obstet. Gynecol. 69 (5) (1987) 687–695.

[24] D. MacDonald, A. Grant, M. Sheridan-Pereira, et al., The Dublin randomized controlled trial of intrapartum fetal heart rate monitoring, Am. J. Obstet. Gynecol. 152 (5) (1985) 524–539.

[25] S. Neldam, M. Osler, P.K. Hansen, et al., Intrapartum fetal heart rate monitoring in a combined low- and high-risk population: a controlled trial, Eur. J. Obstet. Gynecol. Reprod. Biol. 23 (1–2) (1986) 1–11.

[26] P. Renou, A. Chang, I. Anderson, et al., Controlled trial of fetal intensive care, Am. J. Obstet. Gynecol. 126 (4) (1976) 470–475.

[27] C.L. Winkler, J.C. Hauth, M.J. Tucker, et al., Neonatal complications at term as related to the degree of umbilical artery acidemia, Am. J. Obstet. Gynecol. 164 (2) (1991) 637–641.

[28] S.B. Thacker, D.F. Stroup, H.B. Peterson, Efficacy and safety of intrapartum electronic fetal monitoring: an update, Obstet. Gynecol. 86 (4 Pt 1) (1995) 613–620.

[29] A.M. Vintzileos, D.J. Nochimson, E.R. Guzman, et al., Intrapartum electronic fetal heart rate monitoring versus intermittent auscultation: a meta-analysis, Obstet. Gynecol. 85 (1) (1995) 149–155.

[30] S. Grant, N. O'Brien, M.T. Joy, et al., Cerebral palsy among children born during the Dublin randomized trial of intrapartum monitoring, Lancet 2 (8674) (1989) 1233–1235.

[31] C. Wood, P. Renou, J. Oats, et al., A controlled trial of fetal heart rate monitoring in a low risk obstetric population, Am. J. Obstet. Gynecol. 141 (5) (1981) 527–534.

[32] H.Y. Chen, S.P. Chauhan, C.V. Ananth, et al., Electronic fetal heart rate monitoring and its relationship to neonatal and infant mortality in the United States, Am. J. Obstet. Gynecol. 204 (6) (2011). http://dx.doi.org/10.1016/j.ajog.2011.04.024.

[33] J.T. Parer, T. King, Whither fetal heart rate monitoring? Obstet. Gynecol. Fertil. 22 (5) (1999) 149–192.

[34] National Institute of Child Health and Human Development Research Planning Workshop, Electronic fetal heart rate monitoring; research guidelines for interpretation, Am. J. Obstet. Gynecol. 177 (6) (1997) 1385–1390.

[35] American College of Obstetricians and Gynecologists Task Force on Neonatal Encephalopathy and Cerebral Palsy, Neonatal Encephalopathy and Cerebral Palsy: Defining the Pathogenesis and Pathophysiology, ACOG, AAP, Washington, DC, 2003.

[36] American College of Obstetricians and Gynecologists, Task Force on Neonatal Encephalopathy and Cerebral Palsy, American College of Obstetricians and Gynecologists, American Academy of Pediatrics, Neonatal Encephalopathy and Neurologic Outcome, second ed., American College of Obstetricians and Gynecologists, Washington, DC, 2014, p. 7.

[37] G.A. Macones, G.D. Hankins, C.Y. Spong, et al., The 2008 National Institute of Child Health and Human Development workshop report on electronic fetal monitoring: update on definitions, interpretation, and research guidelines, J. Obstet. Gynecol. Neonatal Nurs. 37 (2008) 510–515.

[38] T.J. Garite, G.A. Dildy, H. McNamara, et al., A multicenter controlled trial of fetal pulse oximetry in the intrapartum management of nonreassuring fetal heart rate patterns, Am. J. Obstet. Gynecol. 183 (5) (2000) 1049–1058.

[39] G. Saade, Fetal ECG analysis of the ST segment as an adjunct to intrapartum fetal heart rate monitoring: a randomized clinical trial, Am. J. Obstet. Gynecol. 212 (1) (2015) S2.

[40] J. Lopez-Pereira, A. Costa, D. Ayres-De-Camps, C. Costa-Santos, J. Amaral, J. Bernardes, Computerized analysis cardiotocograms and ST signals is associated with significant reductions in hypoxic-ischemic encephalopathy and cesarean delivery: an observational study in 38,466 deliveries, Am. J. Obstet. Gynecol. 220 (3) (2019) 269.e1–269.e8. doi:10.1016/j.ajog.2018.12.037.

[41] M. Chuey, R. De Vries, S. Dal Cin, L.K. Low, Maternity providers' perspectives on barriers to utilization of intermittent fetal monitoring: A qualitative study, J. Perinat. Neonatal Nurs. 34 (1) (2020) 46–55. doi:10.1097/JPN.0000000000000453.

[42] S.W.E. Baijens, A.G. Huppelschoten, J. Van Dillen, J.W.M. Aarts, Improving shared decision-making in a clinical obstetric ward by using the three questions intervention, a pilot study, BMC Pregnancy Childbirth 18 (1) (2018) 283. doi:10.1186/s12884-018-1921-z.

[43] M.A. Bohren, G.J. Hofmeyr, C. Sakala, R.K. Fukuzawa, A. Cuthbert, Continuous support for women during childbirth, Cochrane Database Syst. Rev. (7) (2017) CD003766. doi:10.1002/14651858.CD003766.pub6.

CHAPTER 2

Physiologic Basis for Electronic Fetal Heart Rate Monitoring

Intrapartum fetal heart rate (FHR) monitoring is used to assess the adequacy of fetal oxygenation during labor with the dual aims of (1) confirming normal oxygenation so that labor can be continued safely and (2) preventing fetal injury that might result from interruption of normal fetal oxygenation during labor. The underlying assumptions are that (1) certain FHR observations reliably identify normal fetal oxygenation at the time they are observed and (2) interruption of fetal oxygenation leads to characteristic physiologic changes that can be detected by changes in the FHR. The role of intrapartum FHR monitoring in assessing the fetal physiologic changes caused by interrupted oxygenation can be summarized as follows:

1. Fetal oxygenation involves:
   Transfer of oxygen from the environment to the fetus.
   The fetal responses to normal oxygenation and to interruption of oxygen transfer.
2. Certain FHR patterns provide reliable information regarding the basic elements of fetal oxygenation.

This chapter reviews the physiology underlying fetal oxygenation, including transfer of oxygen from the environment to the fetus, and the fetal responses to normal and interrupted oxygenation (Fig. 2.1). Chapters 5 and 6 will review the relationship between fetal oxygenation and FHR patterns.

TRANSFER OF OXYGEN FROM THE ENVIRONMENT TO THE FETUS

Oxygen is transported from the environment to the fetus by maternal and fetal blood along a pathway that includes the maternal lungs, heart, vasculature, uterus, placenta, and umbilical cord (see Fig. 2.1); this is a central concept in FHR monitoring. Interruption of oxygen

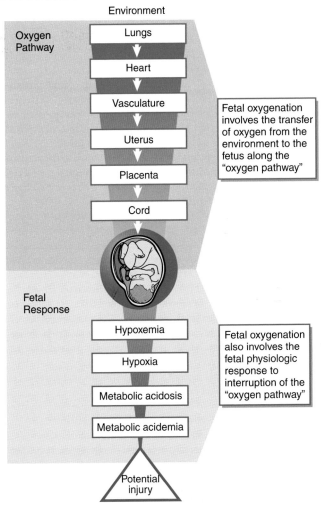

Fig. 2.1 Physiology of fetal oxygenation. (Courtesy David A. Miller, MD.)

transfer can occur at any or all the points along the oxygen pathway. Therefore it is important to understand the physiology and pathophysiology involved in each step.

External Environment

Oxygen comprises approximately 21% of inspired air. In inspired air, the partial pressure exerted by oxygen gas (Po_2) is approximately 21% of total atmospheric pressure (760 mm Hg) minus the pressure exerted by water vapor (47 mm Hg). At sea level, the partial pressure exerted by oxygen gas (Po_2) is approximately 150 mm Hg. As oxygen moves from the environment to the fetus, the partial pressure declines. By the time oxygen reaches fetal umbilical venous blood, the Po_2 is as low as 30 mm Hg. After oxygen is delivered to fetal tissues, the Po_2 of deoxygenated blood in the umbilical arteries returning to the placenta is approximately 15 to 25 mm Hg [1–4]. The sequential transfer of oxygen from the environment to the fetus, along with possible causes of interruption at each step, are described next.

Maternal Lungs

Maternal breathing carries oxygenated air from the external environment to the distal air spaces of the lung, called the *alveoli*. On the way to the alveoli, inspired air mixes with less-oxygenated air leaving the lungs. As a result, the Po_2 of air within the alveoli (PAo_2) is lower than that in inspired air. At sea level, alveolar Po_2 (PAo_2) is approximately 105 mm Hg. From the alveoli, oxygen diffuses across a thin "blood-gas" or "blood-air" barrier into the pulmonary capillary blood. This barrier consists of three layers: a single-cell layer of alveolar epithelium, a layer of extracellular collagen matrix (interstitium), and a single-cell layer of pulmonary capillary endothelium. Interruption of oxygen transfer from the environment to the alveoli can result from airway obstruction or depression of central nervous system control of breathing. Possible examples include conditions such as acute obstruction related to asthma or aspiration, maternal apnea during a convulsion, or medications such as narcotics or magnesium. Interruption of oxygen transfer from the alveoli to the pulmonary capillary blood can be caused by a number of factors, including ventilation-perfusion mismatch and diffusion defects due to conditions such as pulmonary embolus, pneumonia, asthma, atelectasis, or adult respiratory distress syndrome.

Maternal Blood

After diffusing from the pulmonary alveoli into maternal blood, more than 98% of oxygen combines with hemoglobin in maternal red blood cells. Approximately 1% to 2% remains dissolved in the

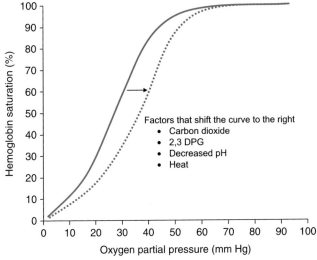

Fig. 2.2 Fetal oxygen dissociation curve. The tendency for hemoglobin to release oxygen is increased by factors that signal an increased requirement for oxygen. Specifically, oxygen release is enhanced by factors that indicate active cellular metabolism. These factors shift the oxyhemoglobin saturation curve to the right and include products of aerobic metabolism (reflected by increased CO_2), productions of anaerobic glycolysis (reflected by increased 2,3-diphosphoglycerate [2,3-DPG] concentration), production of lactic acid (reflected by increased hydrogen ion concentration and decreased pH), and heat. (Courtesy David A. Miller, MD.)

blood, and it is measured by the partial pressure of oxygen in arterial blood (Pao_2). The amount of oxygen bound to hemoglobin depends directly on the Pao_2. Hemoglobin saturations at various Pao_2 levels are illustrated by the oxyhemoglobin dissociation curve (Fig. 2.2). A normal adult Pao_2 value of 95 to 100 mm Hg results in hemoglobin saturation of approximately Pao_2 indicating that hemoglobin is carrying 95% to 98% of the total amount of oxygen it is capable of carrying. A number of factors can affect the affinity of hemoglobin for oxygen and can shift the oxyhemoglobin dissociation curve to the left or right. In general, the tendency for hemoglobin to release oxygen is increased by factors that reflect an increased requirement for oxygen. Specifically, oxygen release is enhanced by factors that indicate active cellular metabolism. These factors shift the oxyhemoglobin saturation curve to the right and include by-products of aerobic metabolism (reflected by increased CO_2 concentration), by-products of anaerobic metabolism (reflected by increased organic phosphate 2,3-diphosphoglycerate [2,3-DPG] concentration), production of lactic acid (reflected by increased hydrogen ion concentration and decreased pH), and heat. Interruption of oxygen transfer from the environment to the fetus due to abnormal maternal oxygen carrying capacity can result from severe anemia or from hereditary or acquired abnormalities affecting oxygen binding, such as hemoglobinopathies, carbon monoxide poisoning, or methemoglobinemia. In an obstetric population, reduced maternal oxygen carrying capacity rarely interferes with fetal oxygenation. Maternal hemoglobin saturation can be estimated noninvasively by transmission pulse oximetry (Spo_2). In recent years, investigators studying the efficacy of fetal oxygen saturation ($FSpo_2$) monitoring have provided valuable insights into fetal physiology (see Chapters 5 and 6).

Maternal Heart

From the lungs, maternal pulmonary veins carry oxygenated blood to the heart. Blood enters the maternal heart from the lungs with a Pao_2 of approximately 95 mm Hg. Oxygenated blood is then pumped out of the maternal heart through the aorta for systemic distribution. Normal transfer of oxygen from the environment to the fetus is dependent on normal cardiac function, reflected by cardiac output. Cardiac output is the product of heart rate and stroke volume. Heart rate is determined by intrinsic cardiac pacemakers (sinoatrial [SA] node, atrioventricular [AV] node), the cardiac conduction system, autonomic regulation (sympathetic, parasympathetic), humoral factors (catecholamines), extrinsic factors (medications), and local factors (calcium, potassium). Stroke volume is determined by preload, contractility, and afterload. Preload is the amount of stretch on myocardial fibers at the end of diastole when the ventricles are full of blood. It is determined in part by the volume of venous blood returning to the heart. Contractility is the force and speed with which myocardial fibers shorten during systole to expel blood from the heart. Afterload is the pressure that opposes the shortening of myocardial fibers during systole and is estimated by the systemic vascular resistance or systemic blood pressure. Interruption of oxygen transfer from the environment to the fetus at the level of the maternal heart can be caused by conditions that reduce cardiac output, including altered heart rate (arrhythmia), reduced preload (hypovolemia, compression of the inferior vena cava), impaired contractility (ischemic heart disease, diabetes, cardiomyopathy, congestive heart failure), and/or increased afterload (hypertension). In addition, structural abnormalities of the heart and/or great vessels may impede the ability to pump blood (valvular stenosis, valvular insufficiency, pulmonary hypertension, coarctation of the aorta). In a healthy obstetric patient, the most common cause of reduced cardiac output is reduced preload resulting from hypovolemia or compression of the inferior vena cava by the gravid uterus.

Maternal Vasculature

Oxygenated blood leaving the heart is carried by the systemic vasculature to the uterus. The path includes the aorta, common and internal iliac arteries, the anterior division of the internal iliac artery, and the uterine artery. From the uterine artery, oxygenated blood travels through the arcuate arteries, the radial arteries, and finally the spiral arteries before exiting the maternal vasculature and entering the intervillous space of the placenta. Acute interruption of oxygen transfer from the environment to the fetus at the level of the maternal vasculature commonly results from hypotension following regional anesthesia, hypovolemia, impaired venous return, impaired cardiac output, or medications. Alternatively, it may result from vasoconstriction of distal arterioles in response to endogenous vasoconstrictors or medications. Conditions associated with chronic vasculopathy, such as chronic hypertension, long-standing diabetes, collagen vascular disease, thyroid disease, and renal disease may result in chronic, rather than acute, suboptimal transfer of oxygen and nutrients to the fetus at the level of the maternal vasculature. Preeclampsia is associated with abnormal vascular remodeling at the level of the spiral arteries and can impede perfusion of the intervillous space. Acute maternal vascular injury (trauma, aortic dissection) is rare. In a healthy obstetric patient, transient hypotension is the most common cause of interrupted oxygen transfer at the level of the maternal vasculature. Chronic vascular conditions can exacerbate this interruption and should be considered under appropriate circumstance in the course of a thorough evaluation.

Uterus

Between the maternal uterine arteries and the intervillous space of the placenta, the arcuate, radial, and spiral arteries traverse the muscular wall of the uterus. Interruption of oxygen transfer from the environment to the fetus at the level of the uterus commonly results from uterine contractions that can compress intramural blood vessels and impede the flow of maternal blood into and out of the intervillous space of the placenta. Uterine injury (rupture, trauma) is uncommon, but must be considered under appropriate clinical circumstances. Uterine activity is discussed in Chapter 4.

Placenta

The placenta facilitates the exchange of gases, nutrients, wastes, and other molecules (for example, antibodies, hormones, medications) between maternal blood in the intervillous space and fetal blood in the villous capillaries. On the maternal side of the placenta, oxygenated blood exits the spiral arteries and enters the intervillous space to surround and bathe the chorionic villi. On the fetal side of the placenta, paired umbilical arteries carry blood from the fetus through the umbilical cord to the placenta (Fig. 2.3). At term, the umbilical arteries receive 40% of fetal cardiac output. On reaching the placental cord insertion site, the umbilical arteries divide into multiple branches and fan out across the surface of the placenta. At each cotyledon, placental arteries dive beneath the surface en route to the chorionic villi (Fig. 2.4). The chorionic villi are microscopic branches of trophoblast that protrude into the intervillous space. Each villus is perfused by a fetal capillary bed that represents the terminal distribution of an umbilical artery. At term, fetal villous capillary blood is separated from maternal blood in the intervillous space by a thin "blood-blood" barrier similar to the blood-gas barrier in the maternal lung. The placental blood-blood barrier is comprised of a layer of placental trophoblast and a layer of fetal capillary endothelium with intervening basement membranes and villous stroma. Substances are exchanged between maternal and fetal blood by a number of mechanisms, including simple diffusion, facilitated diffusion, active transport, bulk flow, pinocytosis, and leakage. These mechanisms are summarized in Table 2.1. Oxygen is transferred from the intervillous space to the fetal blood by a complex process that depends on the Pao_2 of maternal blood perfusing the intervillous space, maternal blood flow within the intervillous space, chorionic villous surface area, and diffusion across the placental blood-blood barrier.

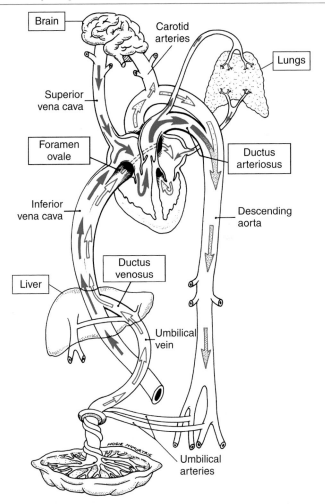

Fig. 2.3 Fetal circulation. Oxygenated and nutrient-rich blood is carried to the fetus by the umbilical vein to the fetal heart. Oxygen-poor and waste product–rich blood circulates back to the placenta via the umbilical arteries. Three anatomic shunts (ductus venosus, foramen ovale, and ductus arteriosus) permit fetal blood to bypass the liver and the lungs. (From R.S. Bloom, Delivery room resuscitation of the newborn, in: R.J. Martin, A.A Fanaroff, M.C. Walsh (Eds.), Fanaroff and Martin's Neonatal-Perinatal Medicine: Diseases of the Fetus and Infant, eighth ed., Mosby, Philadelphia, 2006.)

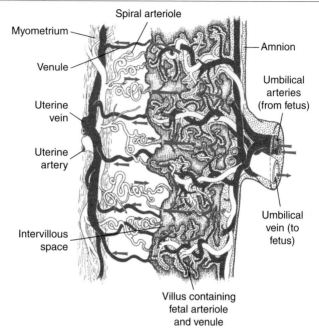

Fig. 2.4 Schema of placenta. As maternal blood enters the intervillous space, it spurts from the uterine spiral arterioles and spreads laterally through the space. *White vessels* carry oxygenated blood. *Gray vessels* carry oxygen-poor blood.

Intervillous Space Pao$_2$

As described previously, oxygenated maternal blood leaves the maternal heart with a Pao$_2$ of approximately 95 mm Hg. Oxygenated maternal blood exiting the spiral arteries and entering the intervillous space has a Pao$_2$ of approximately 95 mm Hg. Oxygen is released from maternal hemoglobin and diffuses across the placental blood-blood barrier into fetal blood where it becomes bound to fetal hemoglobin. As a result, maternal blood in the intervillous space becomes relatively oxygen depleted and exits the intervillous space via uterine veins with a Pao$_2$ of approximately 40 mm Hg (Fig. 2.5). Therefore the average Pao$_2$ of maternal blood in the intervillous space is between the Pao$_2$ of blood entering the intervillous space (95 mm Hg) and the Pao$_2$ of blood exiting the intervillous space (40 mm Hg). The average intervillous space Pao$_2$ is approximately 45 mm Hg. Interruption of fetal oxygenation can result from conditions that reduce the Pao$_2$ of

TABLE 2.1   Mechanisms of Exchange Between Fetal and Maternal Blood

Mechanism	Description	Substances
Simple diffusion	Passage of substances from a region of higher concentration to one of lower concentration along a concentration gradient that is passive and does not require energy	Oxygen Carbon dioxide Small ions (sodium chloride) Lipids Fat-soluble vitamins Many drugs
Facilitated diffusion	Passage of substances along a concentration gradient with the assistance of a carrier molecule involved	Glucose Carbohydrates
Active transport	Passage of substances against a concentration gradient; carrier molecules and energy are required	Amino acids Water-soluble vitamins Large ions
Bulk flow	Transfer of substances by a hydrostatic or osmotic gradient	Water Dissolved electrolytes
Pinocytosis	Transfer of minute, engulfed particles across a cell membrane	Immune globulins Serum proteins
Breaks and leakage	Small breaks in the placental membrane allowing passage of plasma and substances	Maternal or fetal blood cells (potentially resulting in isoimmunization)

maternal blood entering the intervillous space. These conditions have been discussed previously.

Intervillous Space Blood Flow

At term, uterine perfusion accounts for 10% to 15% of maternal cardiac output, or approximately 700 to 800 cc/min. Much of this blood makes its way to the intervillous space of the placenta surrounding the chorionic villi. Conditions that can reduce the volume of the intervillous space include collapse or destruction of the

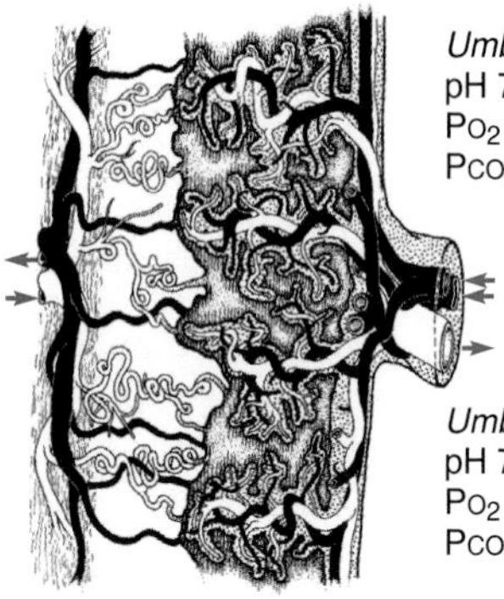

Uterine vein
pH 7.3
Po$_2$ 40 mm Hg
Pco$_2$ 40-50 mm Hg

Uterine artery
pH 7.4-7.45
Po$_2$ 95-100 mm Hg
Pco$_2$ 30-35 mm Hg

Umbilical arteries
pH 7.2-7.3
Po$_2$ 15-25 mm Hg
Pco$_2$ 45-55 mm Hg

Umbilical vein
pH 7.3-7.4
Po$_2$ 25-35 mm Hg
Pco$_2$ 35-45 mm Hg

Fig. 2.5 Approximate maternal and fetal blood gas values.

intervillous space due to placental abruption, infarction, thrombosis, or infection.

Chorionic Villous Surface Area

Optimal oxygen exchange requires normal chorionic villous surface area. Normal transfer of oxygen from the environment to the fetus at the level of the placenta can be interrupted by conditions that limit or reduce the chorionic villous surface area available for gas exchange. These conditions can be acute or chronic and include primary abnormalities in the development of the villous vascular tree or secondary destruction of normal chorionic villi by infarction, thrombosis, hemorrhage, inflammation, or infection.

Diffusion Across the "Blood-Blood" Barrier

Diffusion of a substance across the placental blood-blood barrier is dependent on concentration gradient, molecular weight, lipid solubility, protein binding, and ionization. In addition, diffusion rate is inversely proportional to diffusion distance. At term, the placental blood-blood barrier is very thin, and the diffusion distance is short. Under normal circumstances, oxygen and carbon dioxide diffuse readily across this thin barrier. However, normal diffusion can be impeded by conditions that increase the distance between maternal and fetal blood. These conditions can be acute, subacute, or chronic and include villous hemorrhage, inflammation, thrombosis, infarction, edema, fibrosis, and excessive cellular proliferation (syncytial knots).

Interruption of Placental Blood Vessels

Rarely, fetal blood loss can be caused by injury to blood vessels at the level of the placenta. Damaged chorionic vessels can allow fetal blood to leak into the intervillous space, leading to fetal-maternal hemorrhage. This may be a consequence of abdominal trauma, but can occur in association with abnormal placental development, placental abruption, or invasive procedures. A specific cause is not always identified. Ruptured vasa previa is a rare cause of fetal hemorrhage. Vasa previa is a placental vessel that traverses the chorioamniotic membrane in close proximity to the cervical os. Such a vessel may be damaged by normal cervical change during labor or injured inadvertently during membrane rupture or digital examination.

Summary of Placental Causes of Disrupted Oxygenation

Many conditions can interfere with the transfer of oxygen across the placenta. Those involving the microvasculature frequently are diagnosed by histopathologic examination after delivery. Clinically detectable causes, such as placental abruption, bleeding placenta previa, or vasa previa, should be considered but may not be amenable to conservative corrective measures.

Fetal Blood

After oxygen has diffused from the intervillous space across the placental blood-blood barrier and into fetal blood, the Pao_2 is in the range of 30 mm Hg and fetal hemoglobin saturation is between 50% and 70%. Although fetal Pao_2 and hemoglobin saturation are low compared with adult values, adequate delivery of oxygen to the fetal tissues is maintained by a number of compensatory mechanisms. For example, fetal cardiac output per unit weight is greater than that of the adult. Hemoglobin concentration and affinity for oxygen are greater in the fetus as well, resulting in increased oxygen carrying capacity. Finally, oxygenated blood is directed preferentially toward vital organs by way of anatomic shunts at the level of the ductus venosus, foramen ovale, and ductus arteriosus. Conditions that can interrupt the transfer of oxygen from the environment to the fetus at the level of the fetal blood are uncommon but may include fetal anemia (alloimmunization, infections, fetomaternal hemorrhage, vasa previa, hemolysis) and conditions that reduce oxygen carrying capacity (Bart's hemoglobinopathy, methemoglobinemia).

Umbilical Cord

After oxygen combines with fetal hemoglobin in the villous capillaries, oxygenated blood returns to the fetus by way of villous veins that coalesce to form placental veins on the surface of the placenta. Placental surface veins unite to form a single umbilical vein within the umbilical cord. Interruption of the transfer of oxygen from the environment to the fetus at the level of the umbilical cord can result from simple mechanical compression. Other uncommon causes may include vasospasm, thrombosis, atherosis, hypertrophy, hemorrhage, inflammation, or a "true knot."

From the environment to the fetus, maternal and fetal blood carry oxygen along the "oxygen pathway" illustrated in Fig. 2.1. Common causes of interrupted oxygen transfer at each step along the pathway are summarized in Table 2.2. In the interest of simplicity, the foregoing discussion was limited to one gas, oxygen. It is critical to note that gas exchange also involves the transfer of carbon dioxide in the opposite direction—from the fetus to the environment. Any condition that interrupts the transfer of oxygen from the environment to the fetus has the potential to interrupt the transfer of carbon dioxide from the fetus to the environment. However, carbon dioxide diffuses across the placental blood-blood barrier more rapidly than does oxygen. Therefore interruption of the pathway is likely to affect oxygen transfer to a greater extent than carbon dioxide transfer. As summarized previously, oxygen transfer from the environment to the fetus represents the first basic component of fetal oxygenation. The second basic component of fetal oxygenation involves the fetal physiologic responses to normal oxygenation and to interrupted oxygen transfer.

FETAL RESPONSE TO INTERRUPTED OXYGEN TRANSFER

If recurrent or sustained, interruption of oxygen transfer at any point along the oxygen pathway can result in progressive deterioration of fetal oxygenation. The cascade begins with hypoxemia, defined as decreased oxygen content in the blood. At term, hypoxemia is characterized by an umbilical artery Pao_2 below the expected range of 15 to 25 mm Hg. Recurrent or sustained hypoxemia can lead to decreased delivery of oxygen to the tissues and reduced tissue oxygen content, termed *hypoxia*. Normal homeostasis requires an adequate supply of oxygen and fuel to generate the energy required for cellular

TABLE 2.2 Some Causes of Interrupted Transfer of Oxygen from the Environment to the Fetus

Oxygen Pathway	Causes of Interrupted Oxygen Transfer
Lungs	Respiratory depression (narcotics, magnesium)
	Seizure (eclampsia)
	Pulmonary embolus
	Pulmonary edema
	Pneumonia/ARDS
	Asthma
	Atelectasis
	Rarely pulmonary hypertension
	Rarely chronic lung disease
Heart	Reduced cardiac output
	Hypovolemia
	Compression of the inferior vena cava
	Regional anesthesia (sympathetic blockade)
	Cardiac arrhythmia
	Rarely congestive heart failure
	Rarely structural cardiac disease
Vasculature	Hypotension
	Hypovolemia
	Compression of the inferior vena cava
	Regional anesthesia (sympathetic blockade)
	Medications (hydralazine, labetalol, nifedipine)
	Vasculopathy (chronic hypertension, SLE, preeclampsia)
	Vasoconstriction (cocaine, methylergonovine)
Uterus	Excessive uterine activity
	Uterine stimulants (prostaglandins, oxytocin)
	Uterine rupture
Placenta	Placental abruption
	Rarely vasa previa
	Rarely fetomaternal hemorrhage
	Placental infarction, infection (usually confirmed retrospectively)
Umbilical cord	Cord compression
	Cord prolapse
	"True knot"

ARDS, adult respiratory distress syndrome; *SLE,* systemic lupus erythematosus.

function. When oxygen is readily available, aerobic metabolism efficiently generates energy in the form of adenosine triphosphate (ATP). By-products of aerobic metabolism include carbon dioxide and water. When oxygen is in short supply, tissues may be forced to convert from aerobic to anaerobic metabolism, generating energy less efficiently and resulting in the production of lactic acid. Accumulation of lactic acid in the tissues results in metabolic acidosis. Lactic acid accumulation can lead to utilization of buffer bases (primarily bicarbonate) to help stabilize tissue pH. If the buffering capacity is exceeded, the blood pH may begin to fall, leading to metabolic acidemia. Eventually, recurrent or sustained tissue hypoxia and acidosis can lead to loss of peripheral vascular smooth muscle contraction, reduced peripheral vascular resistance, and hypotension, in turn leading to potential hypoxic-ischemic injury to many tissues, including the brain and heart.

Acidemia is defined as increased hydrogen ion content (decreased pH) in the blood. With respect to fetal physiology, it is critical to distinguish between respiratory acidemia, caused by accumulation of CO_2, and metabolic acidemia, caused by accumulation of fixed (lactic) acid. These distinct categories of acidemia have entirely different clinical implications and are discussed later in this chapter.

Mechanisms of Injury

If interrupted oxygen transfer progresses to the stage of metabolic acidemia and hypotension, as described earlier, multiple organs and systems (including the brain and heart) can face hypoperfusion, reduced oxygenation, lowered pH, and reduced delivery of fuel for metabolism. These changes can trigger a cascade of cellular events, including altered enzyme function, protease activation, ion shifts, altered water regulation, disrupted neurotransmitter metabolism, free radical production, and phospholipid degradation. Disruption of normal cellular metabolism can to lead to cellular dysfunction, tissue dysfunction, and even death.

Injury Threshold

The relationship between fetal oxygen deprivation and neurologic injury is complex. Electronic FHR monitoring was introduced with the expectation that it would reduce the incidence of neurologic injury (specifically cerebral palsy) caused by intrapartum interruption of fetal oxygenation. In recent years, it has become apparent that most cases of cerebral palsy are unrelated to intrapartum events and therefore cannot be prevented by intrapartum FHR monitoring. Nevertheless, some cases of cerebral palsy may be related to intrapartum events and continue to generate controversy.

In 1999, the International Cerebral Palsy Task Force published a consensus statement identifying specific criteria that must be met to establish intrapartum interruption of fetal oxygenation as a possible cause of cerebral palsy [5]. In January 2003, the American College of Obstetricians and Gynecologists (ACOG) and the American Academy of Pediatrics Cerebral Palsy Task Force published a monograph titled *Neonatal Encephalopathy and Cerebral Palsy: Defining the Pathogenesis and Pathophysiology,* summarizing the world literature regarding the relationship between intrapartum events and neurologic injury [6].

In 2014, another publication from the ACOG Task Force on Neonatal Encephalopathy reevaluated and clarified the scientific evidence underlying the relationship among intrapartum events, neonatal encephalopathy, and neurologic outcome [7]. This publication, titled *Neonatal Encephalopathy and Neurologic Outcome* (second edition), was supported by the Royal College of Obstetricians and Gynecologists and endorsed by the American College of Nurse-Midwives, the American Gynecologic and Obstetrical Society, the American Society for Reproductive Medicine, the Association of Women's Health, Obstetric and Neonatal Nurses, the Australian Collaborative Cerebral Palsy Research Group, the Child Neurology Society, the Japan Society of Obstetrics and Gynecology, the March of Dimes Foundation, the Royal Australian and New Zealand College of Obstetricians and Gynaecologists, the Society for Maternal-Fetal Medicine, and the Society of Obstetricians and Gynaecologists of Canada. Broad international consensus supports the conclusion that "in a fetus exhibiting either moderate variability or accelerations of the FHR, damaging degrees of hypoxia-induced metabolic acidemia can reliably be excluded" [7].

Subsequent research has challenged the assumption that moderate variability excludes all cases of fetal metabolic acidemia [8]. This study found that 18% of cases of neonatal metabolic acidemia (pH <7.0 and base deficit ≥12 mmol/L) were associated with the presence of moderate variability in the last hour before birth. However, the authors found that only 11% of cases of neonatal metabolic acidemia were associated with low 5-minute Apgar scores, and only 29% were associated with admission to the neonatal intensive care unit (NICU), suggesting that most cases of neonatal metabolic acidemia were not clinically significant and did not reflect "damaging degrees of hypoxia-induced metabolic acidemia." In fact, potentially significant neonatal metabolic acidemia accompanied by a low 5-minute Apgar score was encountered in the presence of moderate variability in only 0.3/1000 deliveries. Potentially significant metabolic acidemia associated with NICU admission was encountered in the presence of moderate variability in only 0.9/1000 deliveries. In other words, the likelihood of "missing" clinically significant neonatal metabolic acidemia because moderate variability was present shortly before birth was in the range of 0.3 to 0.9 per 1000, a false-negative rate similar

TABLE 2.3   Key Concepts of the Physiologic Basis of Intrapartum Fetal Heart Rate Monitoring

1. The objective of intrapartum FHR monitoring is to assess fetal oxygenation during labor.
2. Fetal oxygenation involves the transfer of oxygen from the environment to the fetus along the oxygen pathway and the fetal physiologic response to interruption of the oxygen pathway.
3. Oxygen is transferred from the environment to the fetus by maternal and fetal blood along a pathway that includes the maternal lungs, heart, vasculature, uterus, placenta, and umbilical cord.
4. The fetal response to interrupted oxygen transfer involves the sequential progression from hypoxemia to hypoxia, metabolic acidosis, and metabolic acidemia.
5. Damaging degrees of hypoxia-induced metabolic acidemia can reliably be excluded in the fetus exhibiting either moderate variability or accelerations of the FHR [7,8].

FHR, fetal heart rate monitoring.

to the false-negative rates of common forms of antepartum testing, such as the biophysical profile (~0.7 per 1000) and nonstress test with amniotic fluid volume assessment (~0.8 per 1000). This analysis is consistent with the conclusion of the ACOG Task Force that "in a fetus exhibiting either moderate variability or accelerations of the FHR, damaging degrees of hypoxia-induced metabolic acidemia can reliably be excluded" [7].

SUMMARY

The physiology of fetal oxygenation involves the sequential transfer of oxygen from the environment to the fetus and the subsequent fetal response to interruption of this pathway (see Fig. 2.1). Interruption of oxygen transfer can occur at any point along the oxygen pathway. Examples of causes that might be encountered in a typical obstetric population are summarized in Table 2.2. Recurrent or sustained interruption of oxygen transfer can lead to progressive deterioration of fetal oxygenation and potential fetal injury. There is broad consensus in the literature that the presence of moderate variability or accelerations of the FHR reliably exclude hypoxic injury at the time they are observed. The physiologic basis of FHR monitoring can be summarized in a few key concepts (Table 2.3). Later chapters expand on these concepts and apply them to standardized interpretation and management of FHR patterns.

References

[1] J.T. Helwig, J.T. Parer, S.J. Kilpatrick, R.K. Laros, Umbilical cord blood acid–base state: what is normal? Am. J. Obstet. Gynecol. 174 (1996) 1807–1812.

[2] A. Nodwell, L. Carmichael, M. Ross, B. Richardson, Placental compared with umbilical cord blood to assess fetal blood gas and acid–base status, Obstet. Gynecol. 105 (2005) 129–138.

[3] B. Richardson, A. Nodwell, K. Webster, M. Alshimmiri, R. Gagnon, R. Natale, Fetal oxygen saturation and fractional extraction at birth and the relationship to measures of acidosis, Am. J. Obstet. Gynecol. 178 (1998) 572–579.

[4] R. Victory, D. Penava, O. Da Silva, R. Natale, B. Richardson, Umbilical cord pH and base excess values in relation to adverse outcome events for infants delivering at term, Am. J. Obstet. Gynecol. 191 (6) (2004) 2021–2028.

[5] A. MacLennan, A template for defining a causal relation between acute intrapartum events and cerebral palsy: international consensus statement, BMJ 319 (7216) (1999) 1054–1059.

[6] American College of Obstetricians and Gynecologists' Task Force on Neonatal Encephalopathy and Cerebral Palsy, American College of Obstetricians and Gynecologists, American Academy of Pediatrics, Neonatal Encephalopathy and Cerebral Palsy: Defining the Pathogenesis and Pathophysiology, American College of Obstetricians and Gynecologists, Washington, DC, 2003.

[7] American College of Obstetricians and Gynecologists' Task Force on Neonatal Encephalopathy and Cerebral Palsy, American College of Obstetricians and Gynecologists, American Academy of Pediatrics, Neonatal Encephalopathy and Neurologic Outcome, second ed., American College of Obstetricians and Gynecologists, Washington, DC, 2014.

[8] S.L. Clark, E.F. Hamilton, T.J. Garite, A. Timmins, P.A. Warrick, S. Smith, The limits of electronic fetal heart rate monitoring in the prevention of neonatal metabolic acidemia, Am. J. Obstet. Gynecol. 216 (2017) 163 e1–6.

CHAPTER 3

Methods and Instrumentation

During the labor process, information about the fetal heart rate (FHR) and uterine activity (UA) is collected so that a collaborative management plan can be created. To correctly interpret the FHR and UA, clinicians should have a basic understanding of the instrumentation that is used to collect these data. Two primary methods gather this information: traditional FHR auscultation usually accompanied by uterine palpation or electronic fetal monitoring (EFM). The latter of these two monitoring options can either be external, internal, or a combination of both methods. This chapter describes the two principal approaches to fetal monitoring and reviews the application and instrumentation of the various techniques.

INTERMITTENT AUSCULTATION OF THE FETAL HEART RATE

Description

Whereas EFM is based on visual assessment, auscultation is an *auditory* assessment in which an instrument or device collects specific FHR characteristics that occur in a prescribed amount of time at predefined intervals and in relation to uterine contractions. In some situations, intermittent auscultation (IA) can assist clinicians with differentiation of maternal heart rate (MHR) from FHR. Auscultation can be performed nonelectronically with a regular stethoscope, such as a *DeLee-Hillis fetoscope* or a *Pinard stethoscope.* From an electronic perspective, a *Doppler ultrasound* device also may be used (Fig. 3.1). There are significant differences between nonelectronic and electronic equipment in relationship to FHR characteristics, and these are summarized in Table 3.1. Fetal ventricular heart valves are heard opening and closing with the stethoscope and fetoscope versus sound waves from Doppler technology [1,2]. In particular, the DeLee-Hillis and Pinard devices are worn on the clinician's head so that bone conduction can amplify the fetal heart sounds for counting. The *Doppler ultrasound* device transmits ultra high-frequency sound waves to the moving interface

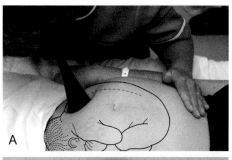

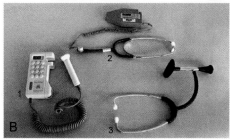

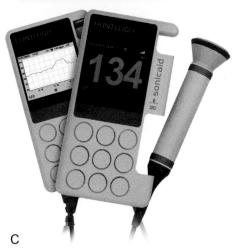

Fig. 3.1 (A) Auscultation of the fetal heart rate (FHR) with a Pinard stethoscope. Vertex left occipitoanterior. (B) *1,* Ultrasound fetoscope; *2,* ultrasound stethoscope; *3,* DeLee-Hillis fetoscope. (C) Ultrasound Doppler with FHR display. (A, From D.M. Fraser, M.A. Cooper (Eds.), Myles Textbook for Midwives, fourteenth ed., Churchill Livingstone, London, 2003. B, Courtesy Michael S. Clement, MD, Mesa, Arizona. C, Courtesy Huntleigh Healthcare.)

TABLE 3.1   Fetal Heart Rate Characteristics Determined Via Auscultation Versus Electronic Fetal Monitoring Characteristics

FHR Characteristic[a]	Fetoscope	Doppler Without Paper Printout	Electronic Fetal Monitor
Variability	No	No	Yes
Baseline rate	Yes	Yes	Yes
Accelerations	Detects increases[b]	Detects increases[b]	Yes
Decelerations	Detects decreases	Detects decreases	Differentiates types of decelerations
Rhythm	Yes	Yes	Yes
Double-counting or half-counting FHR	Can clarify	May double-count or half-count	May double-count or half-count
Differentiation of maternal heart rate and FHR	Yes	May detect maternal heart rate	May detect and record maternal heart rate

[a] Definitions of each FHR characteristic per the National Institute of Child Health and Human Development 2008 criteria.
[b] Per method described by L.L. Paine, R.G. Payton, T. Johnson, Auscultated fetal heart rate accelerations, part I: accuracy and documentation, J. Nurse Midwifery 31 (1986) 68–72.
FHR, fetal heart rate.
From American College of Nurse-Midwives, Intermittent auscultation for intrapartum fetal heart rate surveillance. ACNM Clinical Bulletin Number 13, J. Midwifery Womens Health 60 (2015) 626–632; K. Wisner, C. Holschuh, Fetal heart rate auscultation, Nurs Womens Health 22 (6) (2018) e1–e32.

of the fetal heart valves and deflects these back to the device, converting them into an electronic signal that can be counted [3,4]. Newer devices have interchangeable probes, a digital FHR display, and with the proper equipment an ability to print out a hard copy of the tracing. The practice of using the fetal monitor's ultrasound transducer is not recommended as machines have autocorrelation that averages an FHR that is different from counting an FHR for a prespecified time such as 60 seconds [2]. Although auscultation with Doppler technology is most frequently performed transabdominally in the first trimester, a transvaginal ultrasound (TVUS) probe may also be used to detect and measure fetal cardiac activity by two-dimensional video or M-mode imaging [5]. TVUS provides closer proximity to the uterus, enabling the detection of fetal cardiac activity in the first trimester and in clinically difficult examinations such as a patient who is obese.

Leopold's Maneuver

Leopold's maneuver is a systematic abdominal assessment technique that includes four separate actions to determine the lie, presentation, and position of the fetus [6,7]. Fetal lie is the relationship between the long axis or the spine of the fetus in relationship to the maternal spine and is described as *longitudinal, transverse,* or *oblique.* Fetal presentation is the fetal part that overlies the pelvic inlet and is closest to the cervical os; these are described as *cephalic, breech,* or *shoulder* presentations. Position is the relationship of the presenting part to a quadrant of the maternal pelvis, such as left occiput anterior. This organized approach facilitates the optimal placement location of the auscultation or Doppler device. Performing Leopold's maneuver also can assist in correctly placing the external Doppler transducer used in EFM [8].

Ensure the woman's bladder is empty.

Position the woman supine with one pillow under her head and with her knees slightly flexed.

Place a small rolled towel under her right hip to displace the uterus (prevents supine hypotensive syndrome).

If right-handed, stand on the woman's right, facing her:

1. Identify the fetal part that occupies the fundus to assist with identifying the fetal position. The head feels round, firm, freely movable, and palpable by ballottement; the breech feels less regular and softer (Fig. 3.2A).
2. Using the palmar surface of one hand, locate and palpate the smooth convex contour of the fetal back and the irregularities that identify the small parts (feet, hands, elbows). This assists in identifying fetal lie and position (see Fig. 3.2B).
3. With the right hand, determine which fetal part is presenting over the inlet to the true pelvis. Gently grasp the lower pole of the uterus between the thumb and fingers, pressing in slightly (see Fig. 3.2C). If the head is presenting and not engaged, determine the attitude of the head (flexed or extended). This maneuver defines the fetal lie and position according to the presenting part. It is referred to as *Pawlak's maneuver.*
4. Turn to face the woman's feet. Using both hands, outline the fetal head (see Fig. 3.2D) with the palmar surface of the fingertips.

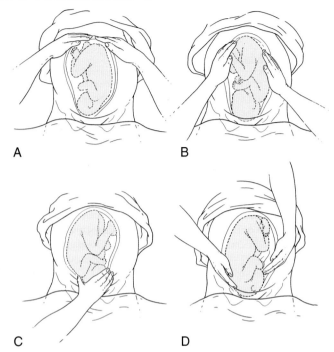

A   B

C   D

Fig. 3.2 Leopold's maneuvers. (From D. Kachlik, I. Kästner, V. Baca, Christian Gerhard Leopold: fascinating history of a productive obstetrician gynecologist. Obstet. Gynecol. Surv. 67 (1) (2012) 1–5.)

When the presenting part has descended deeply, only a small portion of it may be outlined. The fourth maneuver assists in defining the approximate distance between the presenting part and the maternal pelvis.

Palpation of cephalic prominence assists in identifying the attitude of head.

If the cephalic prominence is found on the same side as the small parts, the head must be flexed, and the vertex is presenting. If the cephalic prominence is on the same side as the back, the presenting head is extended, and the face is presenting.

Utilization, Procedure, and Frequency of Intermittent Auscultation

IA instead of continuous EFM in low-risk obstetric patients is the preferred method of fetal surveillance by healthcare professionals in many countries. Benefits include mobility in labor, less distraction, ease of use with hydrotherapy, and providing a more natural birthing experience for women who desire less interventions. In an attempt to limit interventions during labor and birth, the American College of Obstetricians and Gynecologists (ACOG) suggested that obstetric care teams be familiar with low interventional approaches to intrapartum management in low-risk women with spontaneous labor [9]. One recommendation is adopting protocols and facilitating training for use of IA in low-risk women instead of continuous monitoring. In the United States reliance on the electronic monitor is more prevalent, most likely because of staffing patterns, staffing mix, and liability concerns [8,10,11].

Suggested IA counting methods in the literature are typically based on protocols evaluated in randomized trials [3,8]. At this time, there is insufficient evidence on the best counting method for auscultating FHR characteristics. The technique used for IA and suggested methods to identify rate, rhythm, and increases and decreases are outlined in Table 3.2. In general, the first element of IA is to auscultate the FHR for 30 to 60 seconds when the fetus is not moving and between uterine contractions. The rhythm (regular or irregular) is typically identified during this time. A multicount strategy is typically used as the second component of auscultation in which the FHR is counted during several 5- to 15-second increments. Increases indicate an acceleration and decreases indicate a deceleration [3,8,12]. Regardless of the counting method used to assess the FHR, the standard practice is to evaluate and document the FHR at specific time intervals to provide factual and accurate information [3,8].

There is a lack of clear evidence and clinical trials to guide the optimal frequency intervals for FHR auscultation during latent and active phase labor [2,8]. Some sources recommend using a more conservative approach of assessing more frequently based on certain risk factors, although it should be noted that there are inconsistent definitions of what qualifies as low risk and high risk. Consequently, professional organizations have provided general guidelines for assessment frequency of low- and high-risk patients during labor.

TABLE 3.2   Procedure for Intermittent Auscultation

1. Determine fetal position, lie, and presentation by performing Leopold's maneuvers (see Fig. 3.2).
2. Place the listening device over the fetal back or shoulder where maximum intensity of the FHR sounds is the loudest. If using a regular *stethoscope,* the dome or bell end of the device is used.
3. Palpate and count the maternal radial pulse to differentiate FHR from maternal heart rate. Simultaneous palpation of the maternal pulse while listening assists in distinguishing between both fetal and maternal heart rates.
4. Palpate the abdomen for the presence or absence of uterine activity. If present, frequency, duration, intensity, and resting tone are assessed.
5. Auscultate the FHR for 30–60 seconds to establish a baseline. If UA is present, auscultate between contractions. Suggested counting techniques include:
   Count for one full minute.
   Count for two intervals of 30 seconds and add together.
   Count for four intervals of 15 seconds and add together.
6. Determine whether FHR rhythm is regular or irregular. If an irregular rhythm is detected, further assessment by other methods (e.g., ultrasound, echocardiography) may be necessary to diagnose the type of arrhythmia present or to rule out artifact.
7. Time auscultation in relationship to UA to confirm whether an FHR is consistent with the established baseline and to detect audible increases or decreases from the baseline. Suggested auscultation techniques include:
   - Throughout and after a contractions
   - In the latter portion of a contraction and after a contraction
   - Immediately after a contraction
8. Determine the presence of FHR increases and decreases. Suggested strategies include:
   - Count the FHR during several 5- to 15-second increments.
   - Count the FHR in consecutive 6-second intervals and multiply the number of beats for each interval by 10.
9. When there are distinct discrepancies in FHR during listening periods, auscultate for a longer period of time during, after, and between contractions. EFM also may be initiated.

FHR, fetal heart rate; *UA,* uterine activity.

From K. Wisner, C. Holschuh, Fetal heart rate auscultation, Nurs Womens Health 22 (6) (2018) e1–e32; S. Dore, W. Ehman, Fetal health surveillance: intrapartum consensus guideline, No. 396, J Obstet Gynaecol Can. 42 (3) (2020) 316–348; American College of Nurse-Midwives, Intermittent auscultation for intrapartum fetal heart rate surveillance, J Midwifery Womens Health. 60 (5) (2015) 626–632.

However, the American College of Nurse-Midwives (ACNM) suggests that low risk be defined as the absence of obstetric or medical conditions, such as hypertension, that are associated with utero-placental insufficiency or conditions that are associated with an increased incidence of an umbilical artery pH less than 7.1 at birth [3]. Furthermore, the latent and active phases of labor were redefined in a consensus statement regarding the safe prevention of primary cesarean delivery, with active labor defined as ≥6 cm as opposed to ≥4 cm [13]. Frequency of fetal assessment was not addressed in the statement. These definitions are not reflected in several auscultation position statements or guidelines distributed by international professional organizations, except for the Association of Women's Health, Obstetric and Neonatal Nurses (AWHONN; [Table 3.3]). Regardless of which definition of latent and active phase is used, assessment frequency must take into account the maternal–fetal status and may need to occur more often on the basis of individual patient characteristics. Because of the scarcity of high-quality evidence regarding the optimal frequency of IA, clinicians may be best served by a multidisciplinary review of the limited evidence and formulation of consensus-based institutional protocols. Chapter 10 addresses assessment frequency versus documentation frequency in greater detail.

TABLE 3.3   Suggested Frequency of Intermittent Auscultation

Professional Organization	Latent Phase	Active Stage Labor	Second Stage Labor
ACOG/AAP (2017)	Insufficient evidence to make recommendations	Defined as ≥ 6 cm Low risk: every 30 minutes High risk: every 15 minutes	Low risk: every 15 minutes High risk: every 5 minutes Does not differentiate passive and active pushing
ACOG (2009)	Insufficient evidence to make recommendations	Does not differentiate between low and high risk every 15 minutes	Every 5 minutes Does not differentiate between low and high risk Does not differentiate between passive and active pushing

Continued

TABLE 3.3   Suggested Frequency of Intermittent Auscultation—cont'd

Professional Organization	Latent Phase	Active Stage Labor	Second Stage Labor
ACNM (2015)	Insufficient evidence to make recommenda-tions	Low risk: every 15-30 minutes High risk: EFM	*Active second stage pushing* Low risk: every 5 minutes High risk: EFM
AWHONN (2018)	*< 4 cm and low risk without oxytocin* Insufficient evidence to make recom-mendations; frequency determined by midwife or physi-cian *4–5 cm every 15–30 minutes*	*≥ 6 cm and low risk without oxytocin* Low risk: every 15–30 minutes	*Passive second stage and low risk without oxytocin* Every 15 minutes *Active pushing and low risk without oxytocin* Low risk: every 5–15 minutes

Note: At this time, professional organizations including AWHONN, ACNM, ACOG, or the AAP have not published detailed definitions differentiating "low risk" and "high risk." ACNM has suggested criteria for low-risk women only. Generally, continuous EFM is recommended for women who have obstetric or medical conditions (e.g., intrauterine growth restriction or chronic hyperten-sion requiring antihypertensive medication) that place the maternal–fetal dyad at risk for adverse perinatal/neonatal outcomes or metabolic acidemia.

AAP, American Academy of Pediatrics; *ACNM,* American College of Nurse-Midwives; *ACOG,* American College of Obstetricians and Gynecologists; *AWHONN,* Association of Women's Health, Obstetric and Neonatal Nurses.

Adapted from American Academy of Pediatrics (AAP), American College of Obstetricians and Gynecologists (ACOG), Guidelines for Perinatal Care, seventh ed., AAP, ACOG, Washington, DC, 2012; American College of Nurse-Midwives (ACNM), Intermittent auscultation for intrapartum fetal heart rate surveillance. ACNM Clinical Bulletin Number 13, J. Midwifery Womens Health 60 (2015) 626–632; N.F. Feinstein, A. Sprague, M.J. Trepanier, Fetal Heart Rate Auscultation, second ed., Association of Women's Health, Obstetric and Neonatal Nurses (AWHONN), Washington, DC, 2008; American College of Obstetricians and Gynecologists (ACOG), Intrapartum fetal heart rate monitoring: nomenclature, interpretation, and general management principles. ACOG Practice Bulletin No. 106, Obstet. Gynecol. 114 (2009) 192–202; Association of Women's Health, Obstetric and Neonatal Nurses (AWHONN), Fetal heart monitoring. AWHONN Position Statement, J. Obstet. Gynecol. Neonatal Nurs. 44 (5) (2015) 683–686.

Documentation of Auscultated Fetal Heart Rate

Similar to EFM, clinical information about the FHR and UA is documented on a regular basis during the intrapartum period. This includes the counted FHR, the rhythm, the presence of increases and decreases, and whether these changes are abrupt or gradual.

NOTE: It is *not* appropriate to record the descriptive terms *early, late,* and *variable decelerations* or *absent, minimal, moderate,* or *marked variability* when documenting the auscultated FHR because these patterns can only be interpreted with a visual assessment of a monitor tracing. However, terms that are numerically defined, such as *bradycardia* and *tachycardia,* can be used [3,8]. The UA findings assessed during palpation also are included in the documented entry. Documentation of an auscultated FHR is accompanied by other routine parameters that are assessed and documented during labor including but not limited to maternal observations and assessment, interventions, maternal–fetal responses to these interventions, and communication with other healthcare professionals [8]. These entries are to be documented concurrently at the time of assessment [8,14].

Interpretation of Auscultated Fetal Heart Rate

The three-tiered category system introduced by the National Institute of Child Health and Human Development [15] has been adapted by AWHONN and ACNM to a two-tier category system that reflects FHR characteristics acquired via IA [3,8]. Other international professional organizations have not adopted a category system for IA. Category I auscultated FHR characteristics include a FHR baseline (BL) range of 110 to 160 bpm, regular rhythm, presence or absence of FHR increases from the FHR BL range, and absence of decreases from the FHR BL range. Category I characteristics are strongly predictive of normal fetal acid–base status at the time of observation and do not require specific interventions other than routine management [15]. Category II auscultated FHR characteristics include everything that is not classified as Category I [3,8]. Management options for a Category II include increasing IA frequency, implementation of corrective measures such as lateral positioning, application of the EFM to clarify the FHR pattern visually, and notification of the midwife or physician [3,8].

Benefits and Limitations of Auscultation

Benefits

- Widely available and easy to use
- Less invasive
- Outcomes comparable to EFM with 1:1 nursing care
- Inexpensive
- Comfortable for the woman
- Provides freedom of movement for the woman

- 1:1 nursing care promotes "doula effect" benefits
- Allows easy FHR assessment during use of hydrotherapy

Limitations

- May be difficult to obtain the FHR in some situations, such as hydramnios and maternal obesity
- Does not provide a permanent, documented visual record of the FHR
- Counting of the FHR is intermittent
- Cannot assess visual patterns of the FHR variability or periodic changes
- Significant events may occur during periods when the FHR is not auscultated
- May not allow early detection of the FHR changes that reflect hypoxemia
- Not recommended for high-risk pregnancies

   In summary, IA is an effective method of fetal surveillance if performed in a consistent manner by a clinician caring for a woman according to a prescribed frequency. Internationally, IA is frequently and successfully employed as the first line of fetal surveillance in the obstetric population. Continued research regarding auscultation, especially studies related to nurse/patient ratios, counting methods and frequency of assessments during labor, and inter- and intraobserver reliability could prove beneficial in incorporating IA into daily clinical practice.

Palpation of the Uterus

There are several approaches to uterine contraction assessment during the intrapartum period to include manual palpation, tocodynamometry, measurement of intrauterine pressure, and uterine electrohysterography (EHG). Uterine palpation is the primary method that is used in conjunction with auscultation but is also recommended in combination with other electronic modes of monitoring UA. Refer to Chapter 4 for further information.

ELECTRONIC FETAL MONITORING

Overview

EFM equipment is designed to recognize and process FHR data and UA information [16]. Several entities manufacture EFM equipment. Each have various computer programming capabilities, buttons, cable port entrances, keyboards, displays, and names for various parts and pieces. Fetal monitoring and UA data can be obtained via an external, internal, or a combined approach using either method. The external mode of monitoring employs the use of transducers placed on the maternal abdomen to assess the FHR and UA. The internal mode uses a fetal spiral electrode (FSE) to assess the FHR and an intrauterine pressure catheter (IUPC) to assess UA and intrauterine pressure. In some countries, EFM is called *cardiotocography* (CTG). Further information about CTG can be found in Chapter 11. The following table compares the external and internal modes of monitoring and gives a brief description of the equipment used for each.

External Mode	Internal Mode
FHR	
Ultrasound (Doppler) transducer: High-frequency sound waves reflect mechanical action of the fetal heart.	**Fetal spiral electrode:** Electrode converts FECG (as obtained from presenting part) to FHR via cardiotachometer by measuring consecutive fetal R wave intervals. The cervix must be sufficiently dilated to allow placement. The electrode penetrates the fetal presenting part 1.5 mm, and it must be securely attached to ensure an adequate signal.
UA	
Tocodynamometer (tocotransducer): This instrument monitors the approximate frequency and duration of contractions by means of a pressure-sensing device applied to the abdomen.	**Intrauterine pressure catheter:** This instrument quantitatively monitors frequency, duration, and intensity of contractions and resting tone. The catheter is compressed during contractions, placing pressure on a transducer tip and then converting the pressure into millimeters of mercury (mm Hg) on the UA panel of the monitor tracing. The membranes must be ruptured and the cervix sufficiently dilated for placement. Catheters are available with a second lumen that can be used for amnioinfusion.

FECG, fetal electrocardiogram; *FHR,* fetal heart rate; *UA,* uterine activity.

Converting Raw Data Into a Visual Display of Fetal Heart Rate

The FHR data collected, whether by external or internal means, is converted into a visual display (Figs. 3.3 and 3.4). This display may be on paper, on a computer screen, or both. Interpretation is based on a visual assessment of data presented on a Cartesian graph. The gridlines on the horizontal (x) axis of the graph represent time in increments of 10 seconds. The gridlines on the vertical (y) axis represent the FHR in increments of 10 bpm. As illustrated in Fig. 3.5, the FHR appears on

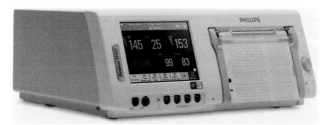

Fig. 3.3 Philips Avalon FM50 fetal monitor provides measurement of the fetal heart rate (FHR) including noninvasive triplet monitoring, FHR high/low audible and visual alarms, and fetal electrocardiogram (FECG). Maternal parameters include toco and intrauterine pressure, blood pressure, pulse rate, pulse oximetry, and ECG. It has cross-channel verification of maternal and fetal heart rate, displays FECG and maternal ECG on the color display touch screen, and has a LAN interface for compatibility with hospital IT networks. (Courtesy Philips Medizin Systemes, Böblingen, Germany.)

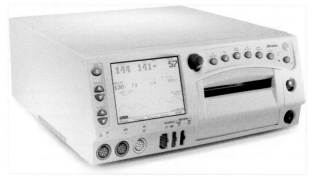

Fig. 3.4 Corometrics 250CX fetal monitor. (Courtesy GE Healthcare, Milwaukee, WI.)

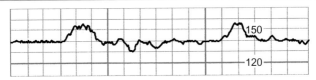

Fig. 3.5 A fetal heart rate tracing has the appearance of an irregular horizontal line. (Courtesy David A. Miller, MD.)

the graph as an irregular horizontal line representing the FHR over a period of time. However, as demonstrated in Fig. 3.6, closer inspection reveals that the "irregular horizontal line" is not a line at all. Instead, a series of individual, closely spaced points are observed. Each point represents an individual heart rate that is calculated from the time between two successive heartbeats. This is a fundamental principle of EFM and merits a brief review.

Fetal monitoring equipment used in clinical practice detects the fetal heartbeat in one of two ways. An FSE detects the actual electrical impulses that originate in the fetal heart and make up the fetal electrocardiogram (FECG). An external transducer uses Doppler ultrasound to detect cardiac motion. Regardless of the method of detecting the fetal heartbeat, the monitor uses the same basic principles to process the raw data for visual display. If the FHR is derived from a direct fetal electrode detecting the FECG, as illustrated in Fig. 3.6, the monitor measures the distance between two successive R waves and calculates a heart rate

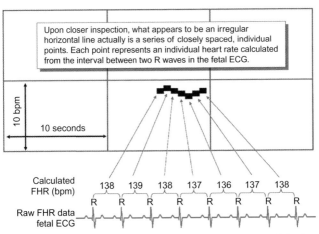

Fig. 3.6 Converting raw fetal heart rate (FHR) data for visual display. ECG, electrocardiogram. (Courtesy David A. Miller, MD.)

based on that single R-R interval. The individual heart rate is plotted as a single point on the FHR graph. The monitor then measures the next R-R interval, calculates a new heart rate, and plots it as a new point on the graph. This process is repeated with every subsequent R wave. If the FHR is derived from an external Doppler ultrasound transducer, the monitor uses the peak of the Doppler waveform in place of the R wave and performs the same basic calculations. A normal FHR BL rate of 120 bpm will yield approximately 120 individual graph points every minute, each representing an individual heart rate. To the eye, these individual points are spaced so closely together that they appear as a line. Variations in the FHR cause the line to appear irregular. The physiologic significance of these variations is discussed in Chapter 5.

EXTERNAL MODE OF MONITORING

Ultrasound Transducer

Description

The ultrasound transducer device is placed on the maternal abdomen and transmits high-frequency ultrasound waves of approximately 2.5 MHz into the fetal tissues [16] (Fig. 3.7). Once ultrasound waves

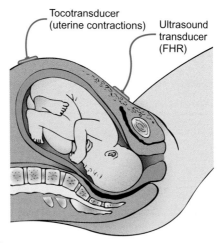

Fig. 3.7 Placement of external transducers. The tocotransducer transmits uterine activity. The ultrasound transducer transmits fetal heart rate (FHR). (From D.L. Lowdermilk, S.E. Perry, K. Cashion, et al., Maternity & Women's Health Care, twelfth ed., Mosby, St. Louis, 2020.)

reach the fetal heart interface, waves are reflected back toward the transducer device in different sound frequencies and converted into electric signals. This phenomenon is known as the *Doppler effect.* This change in frequencies is used to calculate the motion of the fetal heart. As described previously, Doppler-detected fetal heart motion is converted to a continuous graphic display of the FHR printed on the upper portion of the monitor tracing. Simultaneously, the Doppler-detected FHR is converted electronically to an audible sound and flashing light on a monitor screen.

The Doppler signal can be affected by changes in the position of the transducer, the woman, or the fetus. Changes in the direction of the sound beam with UA may cause a loss of signal and make the resulting tracing uninterpretable. Therefore the ultrasound transducer may need frequent repositioning to attain an FHR tracing that can be interpreted correctly. Furthermore, certain equipment errors and clinical conditions may produce artifacts or data that make interpretation confusing and difficult.

Placement of Ultrasound Transducer

A sequential procedure with rationales is provided for the application of the ultrasound transducer.

Procedure	Rationale
1. Position the woman in a comfortable sitting or side-lying position.	Maximizes uteroplacental blood flow to avoid supine hypotension.
2. Perform Leopold's maneuvers (see Fig. 3.2).	Determines fetal position, lie, and presentation.
3. Align and insert the ultrasound transducer plug into the appropriate monitor port (labeled Cardio or US [for ultrasound]).	Provides connection without damaging connector pins that result in a faulty signal.
4. Apply a small amount of ultrasound gel to the ultrasound transducer surface placed on the maternal abdomen.	Aids in the transmission of ultrasound waves.
5. Place the ultrasound transducer on the abdomen, preferably over the fetal back, which is usually the point of maximum intensity. Adjust the monitor's volume control to aid in correct placement.	Assists in achieving a clear signal.

Continued

Procedure	Rationale
6. Palpate the maternal radial pulse and compare with the FHR.	Differentiates between maternal and fetal heart rates.
7. Secure the ultrasound transducer with the abdominal straps or other fixation device.	Prevents ultrasound transducer from being displaced.
8. Observe the signal-quality indicator.	Verifies clarity of input based on correct placement of the transducer.
9. Confirm paper speed is set at 3 cm/min. NOTE: A speed of 1 or 2 cm/min is used in some countries.	Confirms that the paper feeds correctly and that a recording is clear.
10. Reposition the ultrasound transducer whenever the fetal signal becomes uninterpretable (e.g., when the woman moves or when the fetus descends in the pelvis).	Ensures a clear, contiguous tracing during fetal surveillance.
11. Carefully remove the ultrasound transducer at the completion of monitoring and cleanse the abdomen of gel.	Removal of accumulated substances from the abdomen assists in preventing or decreasing skin irritation.
12. Box 3.1 provides guidelines for care, cleaning, and storage of external transducers.	Prevents damage and ensures cleanliness of equipment.

FHR, fetal heart rate.

BOX 3.1   General Guidelines for Care, Cleaning, and Storage of External Ultrasound and Tocotransducers and Internal Monitoring Cables

- Exercise caution when removing and handling the ultrasound and tocotransducers so that they are not dropped or allowed to swing against any equipment to protect from damage.
- Clean transducers and cables according to the manufacturer's operating manual, usually with a soft cloth using mild soap and water. Avoid submerging transducers or placing them beneath running water. Do not use alcohol or other cleaning solutions that may damage equipment.
- Gently and loosely coil transducers and cables for storage. Avoid tight coiling and sharp bending of the cables, which will result in damage to the wires or casing.
- Cables between monitor models and manufacturers are usually not interchangeable. Forced insertion into an incompatible monitor port is likely to result in damage.
- Dispose of disposable abdominal belts and leg straps.

Tocotransducer

Description

The tocotransducer, often referred to as a *toco,* monitors UA transabdominally by means of a pressure-sensing button that is depressed by uterine contractions or fetal movement. The UA panel of the monitor paper or computer screen displays the frequency and duration of contractions and relaxation time between contractions. Intensity and resting tone can be assessed only with palpation or the use of an IUPC. Thus palpation of UA to assess intensity and resting tone is mandatory when using the tocotransducer.

Placement of Tocotransducer

A sequential procedure with rationales is provided for the placement of the tocotransducer.

Procedure	Rationale
1. Position the woman in a comfortable sitting or side-lying position.	Maximizes uteroplacental blood flow by avoiding supine hypotension.
2. Perform Leopold's maneuvers (see Fig. 3.2).	Determines fetal position, lie, and presentation.
3. Align and insert the tocotransducer plug into the appropriate monitor port labeled Toco or UA (for uterine activity).	Provides connection without damaging connector pins that result in a faulty signal.
4. Place the tocotransducer on the maternal abdomen over the upper uterine segment, which is the more active portion of the uterus. No gel is required for this task.	Confirms that the upper uterine segment is as close as possible to the pressure-sensing button. Gel accumulation impedes tocotransducer functioning.
5. Secure the tocotransducer with the abdominal straps or other fixation device.	Prevents tocotransducer from being displaced.
6. Confirm paper speed is set at 3 cm/min. NOTE: A speed of 1 or 2 cm/min is used in some countries.	Confirms that the paper feeds correctly and that a recording is clear.
7. Between contractions, press the UA or Toco reference button for the resting baseline to print at the 10- to 20-mm Hg line on the monitor strip.	Establishes baseline parameter to be used when determining the start and end of a uterine contraction.

Continued

Procedure	Rationale
8. Monitor frequency and duration of uterine contractions and palpate resting tone and intensity.	Tocotransducer *cannot* measure resting tone and intensity of uterine contractions because depression of the pressure-sensing button varies with amount of maternal adipose tissue.
9. When monitoring is in progress, readjust abdominal belt periodically, and massage any reddened skin areas.	Promotes maternal comfort and maintains proper positioning of the tocotransducer.
10. Reposition the tocotransducer periodically after palpation and secure the abdominal belt snugly.	Ensures a clear, contiguous tracing during fetal surveillance.
11. Carefully remove the tocotransducer at the completion of monitoring and cleanse the abdomen of any accumulation of perspiration or other solutions.	Removal of accumulated substances from the abdomen assists in preventing or decreasing skin irritation.
12. See Box 3.1 for guidelines for care, cleaning, and storage of external transducers.	Prevents damage and ensures cleanliness of equipment.

Advantages and Limitations of External Transducers

Advantages

- Noninvasive
- Easy to apply
- May be used during the antepartum period
- May be used with telemetry
- Does not require ruptured membranes or cervical dilation
- No known risks to woman or fetus
- Provides continuous recording of the FHR and UA

Limitations

- May limit maternal movement.
- Frequent repositioning of transducers is often needed to maintain an accurate tracing.
- Ultrasound transducer may double-count a slow FHR of less than 60 bpm, resulting in an apparently normal FHR during a bradycardia,

or it may half-count an elevated FHR of more than 180 bpm, resulting in an apparently normal FHR during a tachycardia.

- MHR may be counted if the ultrasound transducer is placed over the maternal arterial vessels, such as the aorta.
- Tocotransducer provides information limited to frequency and duration of uterine contractions; it cannot accurately assess strength or intensity of uterine contractions.
- Obese women and preterm or multifetal gestations may be difficult to monitor.

Integrated Abdominal Fetal Heart Rate and Uterine Activity Monitoring

Noninvasive monitoring for FHR and UA using transabdominal detection continues to evolve in obstetric practice. As previously discussed, Doppler technology has two main issues that affect reliability of the data presented: separation of the FHR from the MHR and loss of signal during maternal position changes or fetal movement. Signal loss using Doppler technology occurs approximately 10% to 40% of the time a monitor is in place and is related to but not limited to maternal and fetal position changes, maternal body habitus, and the stage of labor [17]. Integrated systems are alternatives to traditional external monitoring because this technology incorporates FECG and EHG into a singular piece of technology and has been found to be beneficial in the obese population [17–20]. Integrated monitoring systems do not replace traditional internal FHR or UA monitoring when clinically indicated, such as when Montevideo units need to be calculated for oxytocin management.

Wireless, adhesive patches, similar to adult ECG pads, are placed on the maternal abdomen in several locations (Fig. 3.8). These patches collect the electrical activity emitted from the MHR, fetal R-R interval, and uterine contraction activity [17]. Once the monitor filters and converts the abdominal signals to electrophysiologic data, the MHR, FHR, and UA are transmitted wirelessly in a digital format, via Bluetooth technology, to a monitor interface [21]. Data are then displayed on the fetal monitor and central display. More precisely, these devices simultaneously monitor the electrophysiologic signals on separate channels using a sophisticated technology to uniquely identify the maternal ECG and subtract it from the signal leaving only the FECG complex [22,23]. This complex process eliminates some of the difficulty that is often found with Doppler technology, such as signal interruption with fetal movement and signal coincidence. Additionally, adipose tissue has less of an effect on the electrical signals monitored on the abdomen than it does on the

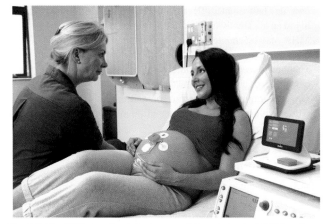

Fig. 3.8 Novii Wireless Patch System providing abdominal fECG and contraction monitoring via EMG. (Courtesy GE Healthcare, Milwaukee, WI.)

transmission of ultrasound, so there is less signal loss in women with elevated body mass indices [17,18,24].

UA is created from a small amount of electrical activity at the level of the myometrial smooth muscle cell [20]. In turn this results in an increase in intrauterine pressure, which is reflected as UA frequency, occurrence of the peak, and duration. Actual intrauterine pressure reflected in millimeters of mercury is not measured. Palpation is used to assess contraction strength and uterine resting tone. Studies have reported higher sensitivity and accuracy in laboring women, regardless of the body mass index, when this monitoring mode was compared with a tocotransducer [20]. Contraction consistency index and sensitivity were also reported to be better versus traditional monitoring with a toco.

Benefits of the abdominal FECG and EHG approach include improved signal quality, elimination of maternal–fetal signal coincidence, and maternal mobility and comfort. This device is now waterproof and can be used for hydrotherapy. These devices eliminate the need for belts and frequent tocotransducer readjustments common in traditional monitoring, and now there are models available for home use that may aid in telehealth initiatives. Although availability of the noninvasive FECG is a clear benefit, there are some fetuses that generate a poor FECG as measured on the abdomen and cannot be monitored with this technology. Clinicians should refer to the manufacturer's guidelines for further guidance.

INTERNAL MODE OF MONITORING

Fetal Spiral Electrode

Description

The FSE monitors the FECG from the presenting part. Application of this device occurs once the amniotic membranes have been ruptured, although it may be applied through intact membranes if clinically indicated. Additionally, the cervix must be sufficiently dilated to allow placement, and the presenting part must be accessible and identifiable (Fig. 3.9). Care is taken to avoid skull suture lines and fontanels or the gluteal area of the fetal buttocks. Therefore the FSE is used only during the intrapartum period. A licensed registered nurse (RN) may place the FSE if approved by the institution policies and there is documentation of successful completion of the skills competency. The state nursing licensing board regulations for FSE placement by an RN also should be reviewed with special attention on placement in the setting of intact membranes if applicable.

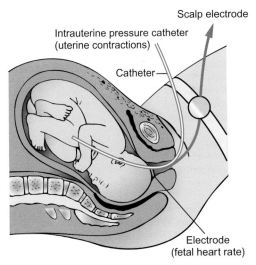

Scalp electrode

Intrauterine pressure catheter
(uterine contractions)

Catheter

Electrode
(fetal heart rate)

Fig. 3.9 Internal mode of monitoring with intrauterine pressure catheter and spiral electrode attached to the fetal scalp. (From D.L. Lowdermilk, S.E. Perry, K. Cashion, et al., Maternity & Women's Health Care, twelfth ed., Mosby, St. Louis, 2020.)

Contraindications

- Planned application to the fetal face, fontanels, or genitalia
- Inability to identify the portion of the fetus where application is contemplated
- Presence or suspicion of placenta previa
- Presence of active herpes lesions or human immunodeficiency virus
- Maternal infection with hepatitis B or C

Situations Requiring Caution

- Woman is positive for group B *Streptococcus*, syphilis, or gonorrhea
- The fetus is premature

It is important to refer to the manufacturer's directions and guidelines, current professional guidelines, and institutional policies related to use of the FSE.

Placement of Fetal Spiral Electrode

Procedure	Rationale
1. Perform a sterile vaginal examination to determine presenting fetal part and cervical dilation.	Assists in avoiding placement on fetal face, fontanels, and genitalia.
2. Retract FSE until tip is approximately 1 inch into drive handle and introduce the guide tube into the vagina with nonexamining hand, keeping examining fingers on target area.	Prevents injury to the vaginal wall and clinician's fingers after glove puncture. Also ensures proper placement.
3. Rotate the drive and guide tubes clockwise approximately 1½ rotations until resistance is met. Do not continue to rotate the device.	Ensures proper depth of placement and to avoid tissue injury from excessive placement depth.
4. Release the electrode wires from the locking device or handle notch and slide the drive and guide tubes off the electrode wires and out of the vagina. Discard the outer drive tube when the application procedure is completed.	Maintains proper placement and safe removal of device.

Procedure	Rationale
5. Connect to the leg plate cable and secure on the woman's thigh. Avoid tension, pulling, or dislodging the spiral electrode.	Promotes an adequate signal from the electrode.
6. During monitoring, check the attachment plate periodically, and reposition for comfort as needed.	Ensures transmission of the signal.
7. When removing the spiral electrode, prior to an operative vaginal birth or cesarean birth, turn 1½ rotations counterclockwise or until it is free from the fetal presenting part. Do not pull the electrode from the fetal skin. Do not cut wires and pull apart to remove electrode from the fetus. Disconnect the electrode from the leg plate, remove the attachment pad, and dispose of the electrode and the attachment pad according to facility policy.	Pulling the electrode straight out results in unnecessary trauma to the fetal skin, produces an observable wound, and predisposes the site to infection. In cesarean delivery if the FSE does not attach, cut the wires at the perineum and notify the physician.
8. See Box 3.1 for guidelines for care, cleaning, and storage of cables.	Prevents damage and ensures cleanliness of equipment.

FSE, fetal spiral electrode.

Intrauterine Pressure Catheter

Description

In certain clinical scenarios, an internal assessment of the uterine environment is warranted, such as an inability to effectively monitor UA in an obese woman. The IUPC monitors uterine contraction frequency, duration, intensity, resting tone, and relaxation time (Fig. 3.10). A small catheter is introduced transcervically into the uterus after the amniotic membranes have been ruptured and the cervix is sufficiently dilated to identify the presenting part. The catheter is compressed during uterine contractions, placing pressure on a transducer. The pressure is then reflected on the monitor tracing in units of millimeters of mercury.

Similar to FSE placement, a licensed RN may insert the IUPC as long as state licensing board regulations have been verified and the nurse is competency-verified according to the institution's policies. There are two types of IUPCs available for labor management: transducer tipped and sensor tipped. Each one has specific benefits, limitations, troubleshooting procedures, and capabilities including

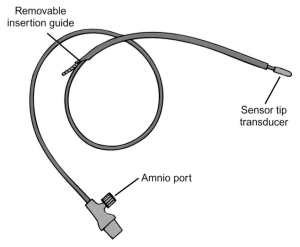

Removable insertion guide

Sensor tip transducer

Amnio port

Fig. 3.10 Intrauterine catheter with the sensor transducer located in the tip of the catheter provides uninterrupted uterine activity monitoring. Note that this catheter has an amnioport that may be used for amnioinfusion. The procedure of amnioinfusion is used to treat variable decelerations in the presence of oligohydramnios. See Appendix A for more information.

ease of use, placement technique, ability to allow amnioinfusion, and rezeroing capability. Clinicians are advised to refer to the manufacturer's directions and guidelines, along with the facility's policies and procedures, for information on use and insertion.

Placement of Intrauterine Pressure Catheter

Procedure	Rationale
1. Turn the power on and insert the reusable cable into the appropriate monitor connector labeled UA, Toco, or Utero.	Activates the pressure transducer.
2. Refer to manufacturer's directions for zeroing instructions as each IUPC has specific instructions.	Establish a zero baseline for the catheter system based on normal atmospheric pressure.
3. Perform a sterile vaginal examination to determine presenting fetal part and cervical dilation.	Identifies an optimal location for catheter insertion.

Procedure	Rationale
4. Insert the sterile catheter and introducer guide inside the cervix between the examining fingers; do not extend introducer guide beyond fingertips.	Prevents injury to the vaginal wall.
5. Advance only the catheter according to the insertion depth indicator or until the blue/black or stop mark on it reaches the vaginal introitus.[a]	Confirms that sufficient catheter is inside the uterus (approximately 30–45 cm) to maintain a quality tracing.
6. Separate and remove or slide the catheter introducer guide away from the introitus and remove; dispose of the guide appropriately.	Prevent the guide from sliding toward the introitus causing injury or retraction of the catheter device.
7. Secure the catheter to the woman's leg or abdomen; it avoids tension, pulling, or dislodging the IUPC.	Promotes an adequate signal from the IUPC.
8. Encourage the woman to cough or briefly perform Valsalva's maneuver. Observe the graph during this time; a sharp spike should appear when the IUPC is properly positioned.	Confirms placement and functioning.
9. Rezero monitor if indicated during labor, according to manufacturer's directions.	Ensure that uterine activity information is correct.
10. Gently remove catheter after use and disconnect from the cable.	
11. See Box 3.1 for guidelines for care, cleaning, and storage of cables.	

[a] Remove catheter immediately in the event of *extraovular* placement outside of the amniotic fluid space (between the chorionic membrane and endometrial lining), as evidenced by blood in the catheter.
IUPC, intrauterine pressure catheter; *UA,* uterine activity.

Advantages and Limitations of Internal Monitoring

Advantages

- Capability of accurately displaying some fetal cardiac arrhythmias when linked to ECG recorder.
- Accurately displays an FHR between 30 and 240 bpm.
- Only truly accurate measure of all UA (e.g., frequency, duration, intensity, and resting tone).

- Allows for use of amnioinfusion.
- Positional changes do not usually affect quality of FHR tracing (may affect IUPC accuracy).
- May be more comfortable than external transducer belt.

Limitations

- Presenting part must be accessible and identifiable to place the FSE.
- Internal electrode may record MHR in presence of fetal demise.
- May not achieve adequate ECG conduction when excessive fetal hair is present.
- Requires (or will result in) rupture of membranes.
- Cervix must be dilated sufficiently to allow placement.
- Improper insertion can cause maternal or placental trauma.
- May increase risk for infection.

DISPLAY OF FETAL HEART RATE, UTERINE ACTIVITY, AND OTHER INFORMATION

The front of the EFM will display the FHR and the intrauterine pressure, while identifying each signal source, including when there is a change in the mode of monitoring. Additional data that are collected depending on the model of the EFM and whether these monitoring options are enabled include maternal noninvasive blood pressure, MHR, maternal pulse oximetry, maternal ECG in real time, and gross fetal body movements. Several of these parameters are displayed on the front or face of the monitor and may be viewed on the tracing or the paper printout (Fig. 3.11). The MHR and maternal ECG can be trended on the upper (or heart rate) section of the monitor strip. Maternal noninvasive blood pressure is printed as whole numbers. Additional recorded information includes the time of day, date, and paper speed. The manufacturer's operating manual should be readily available and be referred to for more information, especially troubleshooting equipment or when further assistance is needed when women require concurrent monitoring of multiple parameters.

Monitor Tracing Scale

The FHR and UA are printed on scaled paper with the FHR printed on the upper section and the UA on the lower section of the paper or computer display (Fig. 3.12). Monitors are preset by the manufacturers for the countries in which they are used. Note the differences in the range and scale of the FHR and UA sections, and in the paper/recorder

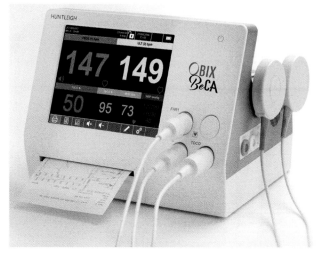

Fig. 3.11 OBIX BeCA fetal monitor displaying vital signs. (Courtesy Clinical Computer Systems, Inc., Hoffman Estates, IL and Huntleigh Healthcare LTD. Cardiff, UK.)

speed, in Fig. 3.13. In North America, the paper speed is 3 cm/min and is depicted in Fig. 3.13A. One minute is represented by 10-second boxes with dark lines printed every 60 seconds. Other countries may set the paper speed to either 1 cm/min or 2 cm/min as further discussed in Chapter 11. The monitor strip in Fig. 3.13B represents a tracing that has been set at 1 cm/min. Tracings that are set at a lower speed will show a compressed pattern in which variability will appear increased. Accelerations and decelerations will give the impression that each is shorter in duration. Therefore clinicians should confirm that the correct scale is being used for fetal monitoring and the equipment's capabilities.

Vertical Axis: 3 cm/min	
Fetal heart rate range	30–240 bpm
Fetal heart rate scale	Increments of 10 bpm
Uterine activity range	0–100 mm Hg
Uterine activity scale	Increments of 10 mm Hg
Horizontal Axis: 3 cm/min	
Paper/recorder speed	3 cm/min = 6 10-second subsections within 1 minute
Fetal heart rate range	30–210 bpm
Fetal heart rate scale	Increments of 5 bpm
Uterine activity range	0–100 mm Hg pressure
Uterine activity scale	Increments of 10 mm Hg

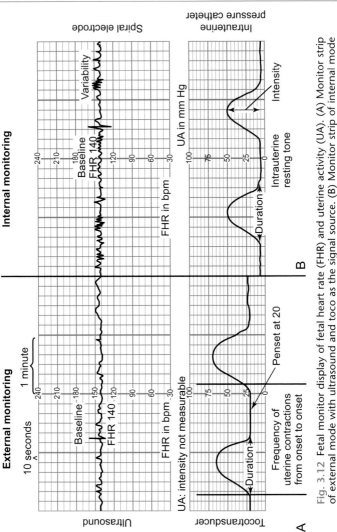

Fig. 3.12 Fetal monitor display of fetal heart rate (FHR) and uterine activity (UA). (A) Monitor strip of external mode with ultrasound and toco as the signal source. (B) Monitor strip of internal mode with spiral electrode and intrauterine catheter as the signal source.

Monitoring Multiple Gestations

Today's fetal monitors have the capability of monitoring multiple gestations simultaneously. This is accomplished with two or three separate ultrasound transducers, or one fetus may be monitored via an FSE during labor, with the remaining FHRs monitored with ultrasound transducers (Fig. 3.14). An alert may occur if both fetuses have coincidental heart rates in which case the ultrasound transducer is repositioned. Newer generation monitors offer the unique capability of distinguishing between two or three FHRs by displaying a distinguishing thick or dark line for one FHR and a thin or light line for another (Fig. 3.15). The computer display may show two or three

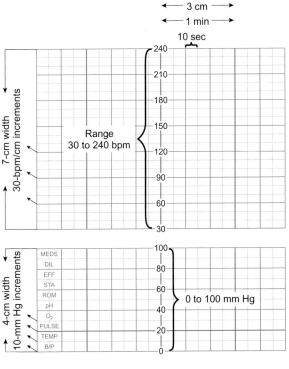

A

Fig. 3.13 (A) Fetal monitor paper scale: 3-cm/min speed used in North America.

Continued

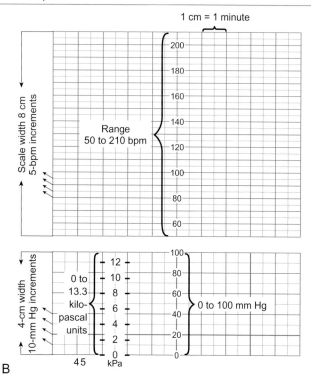

Fig. 3.13—cont'd (B) Fetal monitor paper scale: 1-cm/min speed used in countries outside North America, with key points identified.

separate colors for twin or triplet gestations. Another option to distinguish the tracings in multiple gestations is a "twin offset" mechanism, which separates the two FHRs on the tracing by a distance of about 20 bpm. Thus one fetus appears to have an FHR that is higher than the actual heart rate. The manufacturer's instruction manual should be consulted to have a clear understanding of this capability.

Prior to placement of the ultrasound transducers, twin and triplet FHRs must be clearly differentiated. In some situations, a bedside ultrasound may be performed by an appropriately trained physician or midwife. RNs also may perform this task if appropriate didactic education and competency training has been accomplished in accordance with the AWHONN recommendations for performance of limited ultrasound [25]. Fetal positions in the uterus are documented and ultrasound transducers identified accordingly. Fetuses are often labeled as "presenting" or "A" versus "nonpresenting" or "B" based on the location

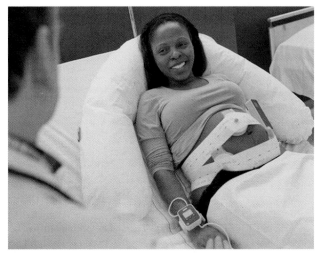

Fig. 3.14 Monitoring of multiple gestations with separate ultrasound transducers. (Courtesy Philips Medizin Systemes, Böblingen, Germany.)

and proximity to the internal cervical os during the antepartum period [26,27]. In many cases the first fetus and second fetus that are birthed are in the same order as in utero. On occasion, a nonpresenting fetus may birth first, which results in a reversal of the preestablished intrauterine designation. This is a serious patient safety concern and may result in unnecessary procedures or interventions in the neonatal period [26,27]. One potential solution that will not affect the antepartum identification in the outpatient clinic setting is to assign each neonate as "1" or "2" at the time of birth. Shortly after birth, each would be identified as A-1 and B-2 if A was born first and B was second. If the nonpresenting fetus is birthed first, the labeling would reflect A-2 and B-1 [27].

Artifact Detection and Signal Ambiguity (Coincidence) With Maternal Heart Rate

Several sources of artifact are recognized in EFM interpretation. These include electrical or signal discrepancies and monitor limitations [16]. Signal error is often related to incorrect transducer placement or maternal–fetal signal interference, such as UA or fetal movement, which results in a weak or undetectable FHR signal. Errors may be

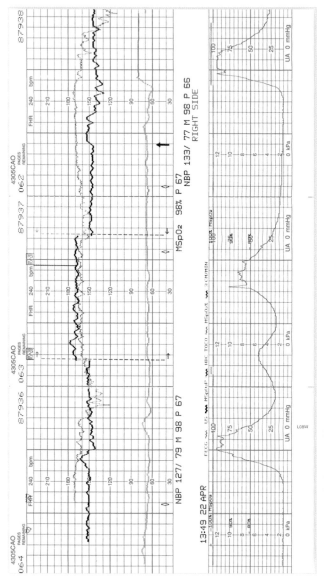

Fig. 3.15 Dual ultrasound heart rate monitoring strip demonstrates the simultaneous external monitoring of twins. (Courtesy GE Medical Systems Information Technologies, Milwaukee, WI.)

assessed as gaps or noncontiguous segments on an FHR tracing. Device limitations may originate from an audible FHR bradycardia or tachycardia resulting in a tracing that appears to be doubled or halved. Finally, incorrect interpretation may be caused by fetal arrhythmias, recording of the MHR, or the wrong paper speed [16,28,29].

Modern fetal monitors have built-in artifact rejection software, referred to as *logic function* or *circuitry*, that is in operation with the external mode of EFM. Older equipment may have a switch located in the back of the monitor. This feature can reject data or "extraneous noise" when there is a greater variation than expected between successive fetal heartbeats. Essentially logic circuitry filters and eliminates FHR data that are recognized as invalid. When logic is enabled on an EFM, an accurate FHR is not recorded because repetitive R-R interval rates are either too rapid or too slow based on the manufacturer's recommended guidelines. If the logic function is off, the computer software will automatically record all FHR signals without filtering, including regular and extraneous rates. If a fetal cardiac arrythmia is present, such as premature atrial contractions or atrial flutter, these extra beats will be recorded by the EFM.

During internal monitoring, artifact is rare, and the logic system will miss only those changes that exceed the predetermined limits of the system. If there is an accessible switch to select a logic or no-logic mode, it is preferable to have the monitor in the off position when using the FSE to detect fetal arrhythmias.

Signal ambiguity or *signal coincidence* refers to a circumstance in which the signal source transitions from the FHR to the MHR, which is recorded on the tracing by the external ultrasound transducer. Despite current technology in which the external transducer detects high-frequency ultrasound waves from the fetal heart, the device may mistakenly capture MHR. This is concerning as this rate may lie in the range of a normal FHR BL rate. This can lead to a failure to diagnose an intrauterine fetal demise or a deteriorating fetal status because of the inability to recognize a shift from the FHR to the MHR on the tracing printout or computer display [28–30] (Fig. 3.16). Clinical conditions that are related to this include second-stage active pushing when the MHR may become elevated and appears as FHR accelerations, obesity, twin gestations, active fetal movement, and patient positioning during epidural placement [28–31]. Certain manufacturers offer a tocotransducer device that allows for automatic maternal pulse detection and automatic coincidence detection using cross-channel verification, allowing confirmation of both maternal and fetal signals without use of maternal pulse oximetry or manual confirmation.

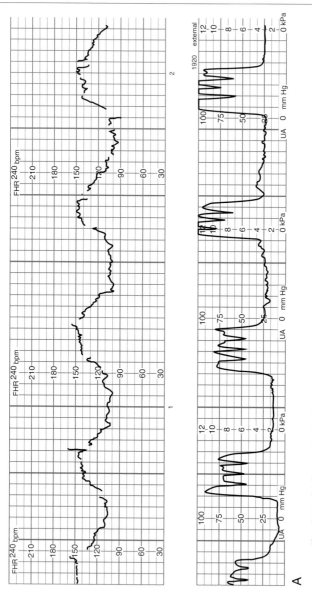

Fig. 3.16 (A) Example of a fetal heart rate (FHR) tracing showing maternal heart rate of 90 to 100 bpm being recorded as fetal. Note appearance of "accelerations" with maternal pushing efforts.

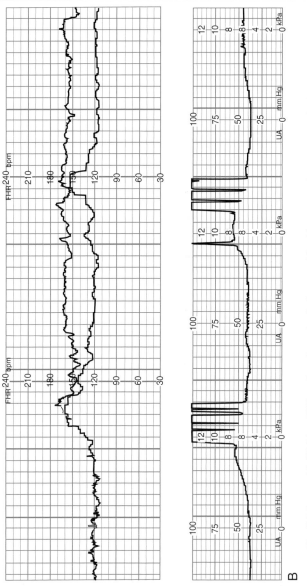

Fig. 3.16—cont'd (B) Now FHR tracing shows both the actual fetal heart rate (upper tracing line) concomitantly with the maternal heart rate (lower tracing line). Maternal heart rate accelerations are seen with pushing efforts. *UA*, uterine activity.

B

Telemetry

Remote internal or external FHR monitoring via radio wave telemetry (Fig. 3.17) allows women to ambulate without the loss of continuous

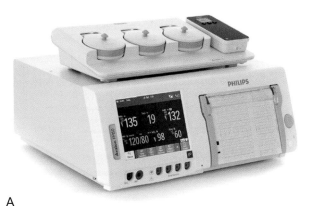

A

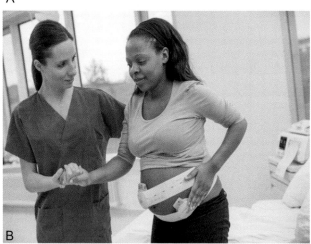

B

Fig. 3.17 (A) The Avalon cableless solution (Avalon CL) offers a complete wireless obstetric area while providing all traditional fetal monitoring measurements without cables, including monitoring of twins, triplets, maternal Spo$_2$ and noninvasive blood pressure. The measurement device transmits information to a base station that is connected to a fetal monitor. The waterproof transducers may be used for the patient who is in bed, ambulating, or in the bath. (B) Cordless ultrasound and tocotransducer are applied to the maternal abdomen for external monitoring. (Courtesy Philips Medizin Systemes, Böblingen, Germany.)

monitoring data. A woman may feel less confined, more relaxed, and more content if she is mobile. The transducer is worn by means of an abdominal belt or other device. FHR and UA signals are continuously transmitted to a receiver that is connected to the fetal monitor. The monitor then processes and displays the data via a central display feature facilitating clinician surveillance of the telemetry-monitored patient. In addition, external watertight transducers are available for fetal surveillance via telemetry during hydrotherapy or water birth.

Electronic Fetal Monitoring Troubleshooting

With advancing technology, electronic devices have become more sophisticated leading to potential problems that may require actions to resolve. The following chart suggests troubleshooting measures to identify electromechanical problems.

Troubleshooting Actions

Problem	Action
Power	Verify location of power cord in back of monitor and in wall location.
Ultrasound 1. Half or double rate 2. Erratic trace or display	■ Assess FHR with fetoscope, stethoscope, or bedside ultrasound. ■ Check maternal pulse to rule out maternal signal, and document maternal pulse. ■ Reapply ultrasound gel and recheck. ■ Move transducer to search for a better signal. ■ Consider applying spiral electrode. ■ Reposition transducer or patient. ■ Tighten ultrasound belt if too loose. ■ Check gel on transducer to ensure an adequate amount is present to conduct sound waves. Reapply gel if needed. Move transducer if fetus is out of range.
Spiral Electrode 1. Erratic trace or display 2. Inadequate signal quality; indicator light red	■ Check attachment pad on leg for adherence to skin. ■ Ensure that connection of FSE is secure on the attachment pad and that the connector is securely inserted into the leg-plate cable. ■ Ensure that logic switch is off to assess for fetal arrhythmia. ■ Apply a new FSE.

Continued

Problem	Action
Tocotransducer 1. UA not recording 2. Numbers in high range 3. Toco not picking up contractions	■ Check that cable is plugged into the monitor and power is on. ■ Readjust toco on abdomen; ensure that cable is fully attached to monitor. ■ Zero monitor with toco/UA button between contractions or replace with another toco. ■ Palpate abdomen for best location to sense contractions, and reapply toco. ■ Test toco by *lightly* depressing pressure transducer and observing readout on monitor. ■ Tighten belt or use another device to hold toco firmly against abdomen. ■ Consider placement of an IUPC.
IUPC 1. Not recording 2. Resting tone (>25 mm Hg) 3. Not recording contractions 4. Elevated resting tone (*hypertonus*)	■ Recheck cable insertion. ■ Palpate abdomen to identify uterine tonus before making equipment adjustments. ■ Zero or recalibrate non–fluid-filled catheter. ■ Verify IUPC markings are correct at the introitus (catheter may have slipped out). ■ Replace IUPC. ■ Higher resting tone may be noted with multiple gestations, uterine malformation or myoma, use of oxytocin, amnioinfusion, or extraovular placement. ■ Rezero monitor. ■ Replace IUPC.
Potential Problems 1. Suspected fetal arrhythmia 2. Errors caused by incorrect paper speed or paper with different scale 3. Cross-channel verification alert	■ Auscultate FHR with fetoscope or stethoscope. ■ Consider bedside ultrasound by qualified physician. ■ Check annotation with paper speed: it should be 3 cm/min in North America. ■ Check scale: it should be 30–240 bpm for FHR if paper speed is 3 cm/min or 50–210 bpm if paper speed is 1 or 2 cm/min. ■ Alert occurs with two coincidental heart rates. Verify maternal heart rate. Reposition ultrasound transducer(s) to detect second fetal heart rate.

FHR, fetal heart rate; *FSE,* fetal spiral electrode; *IUPC,* intrauterine pressure catheter; *UA,* uterine activity.

Computerized Perinatal Data Systems

The ability to have multiple points of data entry, information retrieval, and reproduction of a woman's record and fetal monitor tracing is a significant advancement in patient care. Coupled with the appropriate interface to the hospital admission, discharge, and other hospital-based information systems, computer technology in the 21st century is revolutionizing how patients are cared for on a daily basis. Many state-of-the-art perinatal centers have computerized obstetric data systems that offer central surveillance, visual and sounds alerts, documentation, and electronic archiving capabilities. Archiving allows for a reproducible copy of the record, including the fetal tracing, to be retrieved. Additionally, clinical decision support systems have been integrated into selected fetal surveillance technology.

Clinical decision support systems are software technologies that improve evaluation, assessment, and treatment of patients [32]. The focus of decision support is to change a clinician's behavior at the point of care, improving patient safety [32–34]. These customized hospital-driven tools and checklists assist clinicians in improving evaluation, assessment, and treatment of patients resulting in an opportunity to improve patient safety [32]. For example, an electronic message or visual notification may be sent when an oxytocin management protocol is deviated from during clinical care. Benefits of this technology include the following list [32,35]:

1. *Patient safety:* reduces incidence of medication errors and adverse events
2. *Clinical management:* adherence to clinical guidelines, follow-up and treatment reminders, and other tasks
3. *Cost savings:* reduction in test and order duplication, alternative medication, and treatment options, automating tedious steps to reduce clinician workload
4. *Enhanced administrative function:* diagnostic code selection, automated documentation in some data fields, and auto-fill notes
5. *Diagnostic support:* provide diagnostic suggestions based on inputted patient data, automated output of test results
6. *Diagnostics support for imaging, laboratory, and pathology:* augments the removal, visualization, and interpretation of medical images and laboratory test results
7. *Patient decision support:* given to patients through personal health records and other processes

8. *Improved documentation*
9. *Improvement in workflow in the clinical setting:* accelerations of existing clinical workflow throughout an electronic health record (EHR) with better data retrieval and presentation

A central monitor display provides an opportunity to view tracings from multiple rooms concurrently when located in a key workflow location such as the unit's main workstation (Fig. 3.18). Single-screen displays of one or more patient rooms can be accessed from remote locations such as the patient's bedside, an outpatient clinic, or a home office setting. Perinatal data systems include the capability of contemporaneous data entry in the form of checkboxes or more detailed notes related to FHR and UA patterns, vaginal examination results, medication administration, and vital signs. These contemporary systems also offer universal EHRs that incorporate the entire perinatal and neonatal spectrum, from prenatal care through delivery, and postpartum and neonatal care. Reports and paper charts can be generated with a printer linked to the display or shared electronically through the healthcare institution's intranet.

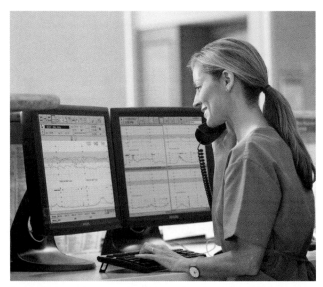

Fig. 3.18 Central monitoring system for electronic fetal monitoring allowing access to multiple records in a variety of formats. (Courtesy Philips Medizin Systemes, Böblingen, Germany.)

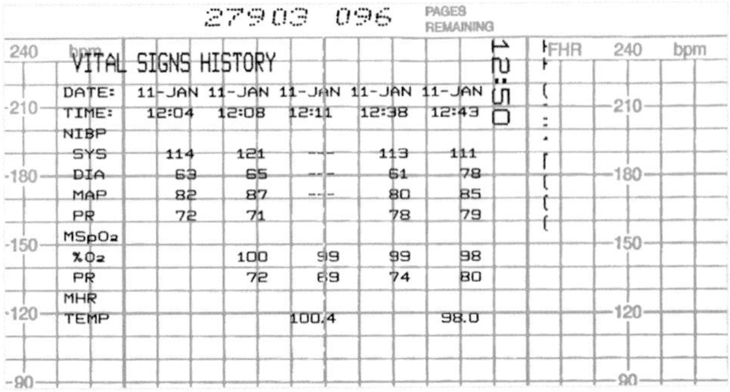

Fig. 3.19 Clinicians can review and print trending data, such as the history of maternal blood pressure readings, and quickly determine status changes. (Courtesy GE Healthcare, Milwaukee, WI.)

Central display systems provide multiple options for accessing and viewing information (Fig. 3.19), including the following:

- A *system status* screen offers an immediate overview of multiple patient beds on the system and indicates alerts by room number. The system can identify the signal source of any woman on the system.
- A *trend screen* provides several minutes of the latest FHR and UA data with immediate warning of critical conditions relating to any patient currently being followed in the system.
- *Scrolling* capabilities allow clinicians to review hours and days of FHR data in a short amount of time helping to identify trends and changes over time, which is an important component of FHR tracing evaluation.
- An *alert screen* delivers an immediate summary of the trend analysis on any woman. These data can be made available to the staff before, during, and after an alert.

The surveillance component of a perinatal data system can be set to alert for any FHR or maternal data that falls outside a predefined alarm limit including those that are greater or less than a hospital-specific setting. This includes fetal bradycardia or tachycardia, signal loss, coincidental fetal and maternal heart rates, and other maternal vital sign parameters such as blood pressure, pulse rate, and pulse oximeter reading. Alert ranges can be set at different levels for each patient depending on the clinical situation.

Computerized perinatal data systems also provide database access for statistical reporting for quality, research, and administration reasons, especially when integrated with other hospital or outpatient information systems. This advance allows multiple data entry points across the continuum of care and serves to link care and services provided at different sites within the healthcare/hospital network [36,37]. For example, if a preterm patient presents to triage on a weekend with labor symptoms, clinicians can readily access the outpatient prenatal record and the operative report from the cerclage procedure performed in the early second trimester.

Additionally, some systems allow clinicians to access information and review FHR using cellular phone displays (Fig. 3.20).

A complete and detailed EHR contains electronic documentation on forms, flow sheets, and checklists, along with annotated FHR tracings and automated data acquisition of information such as maternal blood pressure or the time and date. The *archiving* and *retrieval* of paper FHR tracings have proven to be difficult for medical record departments in hospitals that retain this format type because the process is labor intensive. Storage of paper tracings can be space-consuming, especially if there are several days or weeks of data. Paper strips are also

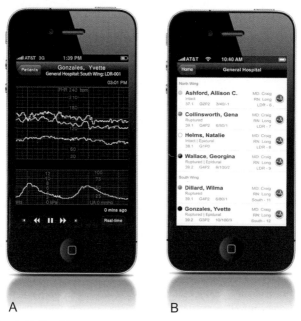

Fig. 3.20 Providers can access near real-time FHR tracings (A) and review patient data using their mobile phones (B). (Courtesy AirStrip Technologies, Inc., San Antonio, TX.)

subject to deterioration. A majority of hospitals have changed the method of record storage from microfiche to computer-based electronic storage systems as the former has become mostly obsolete in the healthcare setting. Computer-based electronic storage systems provide secure archival and retrieval options and can help prevent loss or destruction of fetal monitoring data.

Computer Decision Analysis of the Fetal Heart Rate

One of the major shortcomings of EFM is the considerable inter- and intraobserver variability with visual interpretation of FHR characteristics and patterns [38,39]. This variation in FHR assessment can lead to an FHR tracing being misinterpreted, which in turn can lead to inadequate communication between clinicians and decisions. Ultimately, these differences in FHR interpretation can result in unnecessary interventions or delays in treatment, including an expedited birth [16,39]. Computer decision analysis of an FHR pattern applies artificial intelligence (AI) to a concerning tracing, supporting the clinician when a complex decision-making intervention becomes necessary [40,41]. Multiple international studies have investigated computer analysis and AI against the human component of visual interpretation [41]. There has been supportive literature demonstrating that this technology can facilitate earlier recognition of tracings that are associated with metabolic acidemia [42]. Conversely, other experts have found that FHR decision analysis does not improve neonatal outcome or lead to a significant reduction in the rate of metabolic acidosis or obstetric interventions [40,43]. Further development of this technology may improve with further refinement of the algorithm used in decision support and more research including but not limited to a focus on generalizability in perinatal centers.

Data-Input Devices

Electronic perinatal data systems may use a variety of data-input devices, including barcode readers, keypads for data entry, touch screens, remote event markers, and standard computer keyboards. Information that is input into the system is recorded in the EHR. Data that reflect FHR characteristics, UA, and maternal vital signs are subsequently printed on the tracing (Figs. 3.21 and 3.22). The use of these options promotes accurate documentation if used correctly and can eliminate the need for handwritten annotations, which are

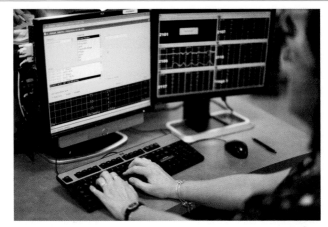

Fig. 3.21 Current systems offer a variety of data entry options as well as display choices. (Courtesy Clinical Computer Systems. Hoffman Estates, IL.)

sometimes illegible. Additionally, ongoing information important to documentation such as the time, date, paper speed, and signal source is routinely entered on the monitor strip automatically. Refer to Chapter 10 for further information on documentation.

SUMMARY

Obstetrics as a specialty has changed over the years, primarily because of advancements in technology. Several methods of fetal surveillance exist ranging from auscultation to electronic modes of monitoring, including the use of other technologies such as decision support analysis.

The care given to the electronically monitored woman is the same as that given to any woman during labor, with the additional consideration of those factors that relate directly to the monitor.

Regardless of the mode of fetal surveillance, clinicians are obliged to have a discussion about the monitoring methods that may be implemented during the intrapartum period because patient education regarding the selection of methodology is an important part of collaborative care. This includes an explanation of equipment operations, the chance of a transition from auscultation and palpation to a higher level of monitoring, and the need for frequent adjustments during labor.

Regardless of the technique chosen, clinicians must understand the proper application, care, and use of related equipment and the benefits, limitations, and specific patient selection criteria.

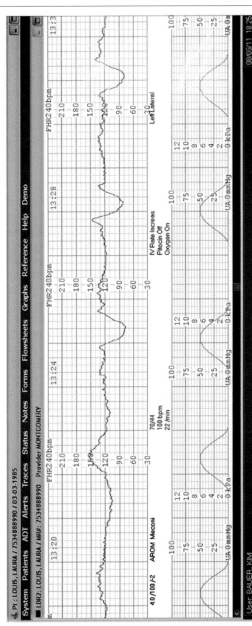

Fig. 3.22 Documentation data are printed on monitor tracing. (Courtesy OBIX Perinatal Data System, Clinical Computer Systems, Inc., Elgin, IL.)

References

[1] L. Goodwin, Intermittent auscultation of the fetal heart rate: a review of general principles, J. Perinat. Neonatal Nurs. 14 (3) (2000) 53–61.

[2] E. Blix, R. Maude, E. Hals, et al., Intermittent auscultation fetal monitoring during labour: A systematic scoping review to identify methods, effects, and accuracy, PLoS One 14 (7) (2019) 1–21.

[3] American College of Nurse-Midwives, Intermittent auscultation for intrapartum fetal heart rate surveillance, J. Midwifery Womens Health 60 (5) (2015) 626–632.

[4] R. Martis, O. Emilia, D.S. Nurdiati, J. Brown, Intermittent auscultation (IA) of fetal heart rate in labour for fetal well-being, Cochrane Database of Syst. Rev. (2017) CD008680.

[5] J. Pellerito, B. Bromley, S. Allison, et al., Practice parameter for the performance of standard diagnostic obstetric ultrasound examinations, J. Ultrasound Med. 37 (11) 2471–2476.

[6] G. Posner, A. Black, G. Jones, J. Dy, Oxorn foote human labor and birth, 6th ed. McGraw Hill, New York, 2013.

[7] D. Kachlik, I. Kästner, V. Baca, Christian Gerhard Leopold, Fascinating history of a productive obstetrician gynecologist, Obstet. Gynecol. Surv. 67 (1) (2012) 1–5.

[8] K. Wisner, C. Holschuh, Fetal heart rate auscultation, Nurs. Womens Health 22 (6) (2018) e1–e32.

[9] American College of Obstetricians and Gynecologists, Approaches to limit intervention during labor and birth. Committee Opinion no. 766, Obstet. Gynecol. 133 (2) (2019) e164–e173.

[10] L.A. Miller, Litigation in perinatal care: The deposition process, J. Perinat. Neonatal Nurs. 32 (1) (2018) 53–58.

[11] L.M. Glaser, F.A. Alvi, M.P. Magdy, Trends in Malpractice Claims for Obstetric and Gynecologic Procedures, 2005–2014, Am. J. Obstet. Gynecol. 217 (3) (2017) 340e1–340e6.

[12] S. Dore, W. Ehman, Fetal health surveillance: Intrapartum consensus guideline, No. 396, J. Obstet. Gynaecol. Can. 42 (3) (2020) 316–348.

[13] American College of Obstetricians and Gynecologists, Society for Maternal-Fetal Medicine, Safe prevention of the primary cesarean delivery: obstetric care consensus, Am. J. Obstet. Gynecol. 210 (3) (2014) 179–193.

[14] American Academy of Pediatrics, American College of Obstetricians and Gynecologists, Guidelines for Perinatal Care, eighth ed., AAP, ACOG, Washington, DC, 2017.

[15] G.A. Macones, G.D. Hankins, C.Y. Spong, et al., The 2008 National Institute of Child Health and Human Development workshop report on electronic fetal monitoring: update on definitions, interpretation, and research guidelines, Obstet. Gynecol. 112 (3) (2008) 661–666.

[16] J.T. Parer, T.L. King, T. Ikeda, Electronic fetal heart rate monitoring: A 5-tier system, third ed., Jones & Bartlett Learning, Burlington, MA, 2018.

[17] M. Monson, C. Heuser, B.D. Einerson, et al., Evaluation of an external fetal electrocardiogram monitoring system: A randomized controlled trial, Am. J. Obstet. Gynecol. 223 (2) (2020) 244.e1–244.e12.

[18] W.R. Cohen, B. Hayes-Gill, Influence of maternal body mass index on accuracy and reliability of external fetal monitoring techniques, Acta Obstet. Gynecol. Scand. 93 (6) (2014) 590–595.

[19] W.R. Cohen, S. Ommani, S. Hassan, et al., Accuracy and reliability of fetal heart rate monitoring using maternal abdominal surface electrodes, Acta Obstet. Gynecol. Scand. 91 (11) (2012) 1306–1313.

[20] M.W. Vlemminx, C. Rabotti, M.B. van der Hout- van derJagt, S.G. Oei, Clinical use of electrohysterography during term labor: A systematic review on diagnostic value, advantages, and limitations, Obstet. Gynecol. Surv. 73 (5) (2018) 303–324.

[21] Monica Novii Wireless Patch System Operation and Maintenance Manual. Available from: http://www.monicahealthcare.com/Monica _Healthcare/media/Monica/Novii%20Support%20Material/107-PT-005 -US-rev2_Novii-Operation-and-Maintenance-Manual-(DOC2111914). pdf 2018 (accessed 9.05.20).

[22] B.C. Jacod, E.M. Graatsma, E. Van Hagen, G.H. Visser, A validation of electrohysterography for uterine activity monitoring during labour, J. Matern. Fetal Neonatal Med. 23 (1) (2010) 17–22.

[23] E.M. Graatsma, B. Jacod, L. van Egmond, et al., Fetal electrocardiography: feasibility of long-term fetal heart rate recordings, BJOG 116 (2009) 334–338.

[24] E.M. Graatsma, J. Miller, E.J. Mulder, C. Harman, A.A. Baschat, G.H. Visser, Maternal body mass index does not affect performance of fetal electrocardiography, Am. J. Perinatol. 27 (7) (2010) 573–577.

[25] Association of Women's Health, Obstetric, and Neonatal Nurses, Ultrasound examinations performed by registered nurses in obstetric, gynecologic, and reproductive medicine settings: Clinical competencies and education guide, 4th ed., 2016.

[26] E. Weiner, J. Barrett, M. Ram, et al., Delivery of the nonpresenting twin first: Rates and associated factors, Obstet. Gynecol. 131 (6) (2018) 1049–1056.

[27] E. Kontopoulos, R. Quintero, J. Barrett, R. Chmait, Which twin is which? A proposed solution for the labeling of twins at birth, Am. J. Obstet. Gynecol. 213 (2) (2015) 245–246.

[28] D.J. Kiely, L.W. Oppenheimer, J.C. Dornan, Unrecognized maternal heart rate artefact in cases of perinatal mortality reported to the United States Food and Drug Administration from 2009 to 2019: A critical patient safety issue, BMC Pregnancy Childbirth 19 (1) (2019) 1–10.

[29] R.L Cypher, When signals become crossed: Maternal-fetal signal ambiguity, J. Perinat. Neonatal Nurs. 33 (2) (2019) 105–107.

[30] D.R. Neilson, R.K. Freeman, S. Mangan, Signal ambiguity resulting in unexpected outcome with external fetal heart rate monitoring, Am. J. Obstet. Gynecol. 198 (6) (2008) 717–724.

[31] D.J. Sherman, E. Frenkel, Y. Kurzweil, A. Padua, S. Arieli, M. Bahar, Characteristics of maternal heart rate patterns during labor and delivery, Obstet. Gynecol. 99 (4) (2002) 542–547.

[32] S.K. Hasley, Decision support and patient safety: the time has come, Am. J. Obstet. Gynecol. 204 (6) (2011) 461–465.

[33] P.R. McCartney, Computer fetal heart rate pattern analysis, MCN, Am. J. Matern. Child Nurs. 36 (6) (2011) 397.

[34] Nunes, D. Ayres-de-Campos, C. Figueiredo, J. Bernardes, An overview of central fetal monitoring systems in labour, J. Perinat. Med. 41 (1) (2013) 93–99.

[35] R.T. Sutton, D. Pincock, D.C. Baumgart, et al., An overview of clinical decision support systems: Benefits, risks, and strategies for success, NPJ Digit. Med. 3 (1) (2020) 1–10.

[36] C. Kelly, Perinatal computerized patient record and archiving systems: pitfalls and enhancements for implementing a successful computerized medical record, J. Perinat. Neonatal Nurs. 12 (4) (1999) 1–14.

[37] P.R. McCartney, E.E. Drake, Perinatal and Neonatal Health Information Technology, J. Perinat. Neonatal Nurs. 30 (3) (2016) 209–213.

[38] L.D. Devoe, Future perspectives in intrapartum fetal surveillance, Best Pract. Res. Clin. Obstet. Gynaecol. 30 (2016) 98–106.

[39] J. Balayla, G. Shrem, Use of artificial intelligence (AI) in the interpretation of intrapartum fetal heart rate (FHR) tracings: A systematic review and meta-analysis, Arch. Gynecol. Obstet. 300 (1) (2019) 1–8.

[40] Nunes, D. Ayres-de-Campos, A. Ugwumadu, et al., Central fetal monitoring with and without computer analysis, Obstet. Gynecol. 129 (1) (2017) 83–90.

[41] J.E. Lutomski, S. Meaney, R.A. Greene, A.C. Ryan, D. Devane, Expert systems for fetal assessment in labour, Cochrane Database Syst. Rev. (4) (2015) CD010708.

[42] P. Brocklehurst, D. Field, K. Greene, et al., Computerised interpretation of fetal heart rate during labour (INFANT): A randomised controlled trial, Lancet. 389 (10080) (2017) 1719–1729.

[43] S.L. Clark, E.F. Hamilton, T.J. Garite, et al., The limits of electronic fetal heart rate monitoring in the prevention of neonatal metabolic acidemia, Am. J. Obstet. Gynecol. 216 (2) (2017) 163e1–163e6.

CHAPTER 4

Uterine Activity Evaluation and Management

Uterine contractions during labor result in a decrease in perfusion at the level of the intervillous space, making labor a period of oxidative stress for the fetus. This stress does not pose a challenge for most healthy term fetuses for a variety of reasons, including the increased affinity for oxygen in fetal hemoglobin, the vascular shunts in fetal circulation, fetal cardiac output, and high glycogen store in fetal myocardium [1]. However, even in healthy term fetuses, excessive uterine activity can have an adverse effect on fetal oxygenation and acid–base status [2–8], making the understanding and assessment of uterine activity during labor a crucial patient safety issue. Prompt response and intervention for excessive uterine activity and *physiologic support of normal uterine activity* in the different phases and stages of labor must be common skills for nurses, physicians, and midwives. The primary focus of this chapter is the evaluation of uterine activity in labor, including defining clinical parameters for both normal and excessive uterine activity. Additionally, a brief review of current parameters for the diagnosis and management of abnormal labor patterns are reviewed, along with specific issues regarding the use of oxytocin for both induction and augmentation of labor.

ASSESSMENT METHODS: PALPATION AND ELECTRONIC MONITORING

Uterine activity may be assessed by manual palpation or by electronic monitoring with an external tocotransducer, an abdominal "patch" using electromyogram (EMG), or an internal intrauterine pressure catheter (IUPC). A complete assessment of uterine activity includes the identification of contraction frequency, duration, strength or intensity, and resting tone. The relative sensitivities of various methods of contraction monitoring are illustrated in Fig. 4.1.

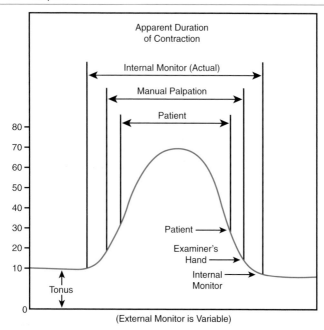

Fig. 4.1 Comparison of relative sensitivities of assessing uterine contractions by internal monitoring (intrauterine pressure catheter), manual palpation, and patient perception. The tocodynamometer and abdominal electromyogram methods are not included as they are variable in sensitivity. (Reprinted from Fetal Heart Rate Monitoring by R.K Freeman, T.J Garite, M.P. Nageotte, and L.A. Miller, 2012, Lippincott Williams & Wilkins, Philadelphia, p.79.)

Manual Palpation

Manual palpation is the traditional method of monitoring contractions. This method can measure contraction frequency, duration, and relative strength. Palpation is a learned skill that is best performed with the fingertips to feel the uterus rise upward as the contraction develops. *Mild, moderate,* and *strong* are the terms used to describe the strength of uterine contractions as determined by the examiner's hands during palpation and based on the degree of indentation of the abdomen [9,10]. For learning and for the purpose of comparison, the degree of indentation corresponds to the palpation sensation when feeling the parts of the adult face, as described in the following chart:

Contraction Strength	Palpation Sensation
Mild	Tense fundus but easy to indent (feels like touching finger to tip of nose)
Moderate	Firm fundus, difficult to indent with fingertips (feels like touching finger to chin)
Strong	Rigid, board-like fundus, almost impossible to indent (feels like touching finger to forehead)

Palpation of uterine activity is an important clinical skill that is used concomitantly with all modes of contraction monitoring. When using the tocodynamometer (Toco) or abdominal EMG, palpation is the only method to gauge the strength of contractions. When an IUPC is in use, manual palpation is used to confirm the findings both at the time of initial insertion and on an ongoing basis throughout labor.

Electronic Monitoring of Uterine Activity

External uterine activity monitoring is typically achieved using a tocotransducer (to provide information about uterine contraction frequency and duration) combined with manual palpation (to evaluate relative strength). Abdominal fetal electrocardiogram (FECG) and EMG are other methods of external electronic fetal monitoring. Both methods provide continuous data and a permanent record of uterine activity. The electronic display of a contraction, when using a tocodynamometer, depends on the depression of a pressure-sensing device placed on the maternal abdomen. Issues such as placement of the transducer, belt tightness, and maternal adipose tissue result in variations of depression and will affect the graphic representation on the fetal heart rate (FHR) tracing (Fig. 4.2). These factors may result in contractions appearing stronger (or less strong) than they truly are, making it imperative to assess strength of the uterine contraction by manual palpation when uterine activity is externally monitored.

Internal uterine activity monitoring uses an IUPC that measures actual intrauterine pressure in millimeters of mercury during both contractile and acontractile (resting) periods. As demonstrated in Fig. 4.1, the IUPC allows clinicians to evaluate the frequency, duration, and strength of contractions in millimeters of mercury with improved accuracy. The following chart contrasts the data obtained with these external versus internal modes of monitoring:

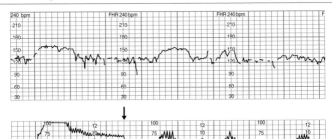

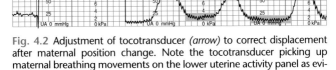

Fig. 4.2 Adjustment of tocotransducer *(arrow)* to correct displacement after maternal position change. Note the tocotransducer picking up maternal breathing movements on the lower uterine activity panel as evidenced by jagged lines (highlighted). *BPM,* beats per minute; *FHR,* fetal heart rate, *UA,* uterine activity. (Courtesy Lisa A. Miller, CNM, JD.)

External Mode: Tocotransducer or Abdominal EMG	Internal Mode: IUPC
Frequency of Contractions	
Measured from the onset of one contraction to the onset of the next contraction.	Measured from the onset of one contraction to the onset of the next contraction.
Duration of Contractions	
Measured from contraction onset to offset.	Measured from contraction onset to offset.
Strength/Intensity of Contractions	
The abdomen must be palpated to assess the strength of the contraction based on the degree of indentation of the fundus. The more difficult it is to indent the fundus during palpation, the stronger the contraction. *Strength* of contractions using a toco is usually documented as *mild, moderate,* or *strong* to palpation. The tracing produced using external methods will reflect contraction strength *relative* to other contractions, i.e., stronger contractions will generally produce higher waveforms.	Intrauterine pressure is measured directly and recorded on the tracing in millimeters of mercury. *Strength* is usually documented as the numerical value at the peak of the contraction, e.g., 50 mm Hg, 70 mm Hg, etc. *Intensity* of contractions is technically a term used to identify the peak of the contraction less the resting tone, expressed in millimeters of mercury. In clinical practice, the terms *strength* and *intensity* are often used interchangeably; it is important that whichever term is used, it is defined and used consistently.

External Mode: Tocotransducer or Abdominal EMG	Internal Mode: IUPC
Resting Tone	
The abdomen must be palpated to assess resting tone based on whether the fundus palpates as soft or firm (rigid). During periods of palpated resting tone, the external monitor is generally set/reset to a level of 10 on the uterine activity portion of the fetal monitoring tracing.	Resting tone is measured directly and reflected on the tracing based on the intrauterine pressure in millimeters of mercury. Resting tone is recorded as the numerical value when the uterus is completely relaxed (acontractile), e.g., 10 mm Hg, 15 mm Hg, etc.

EMG, electromyogram; *IUPC,* intrauterine pressure catheter.

Electronic Display of Uterine Activity

Uterine activity is monitored and recorded on the lower section of the monitor strip (Fig. 4.3). The range of the scale is from 0 to 100 mm Hg. There are five major vertical divisions of 20 mm Hg each, divided again into minor vertical representations of 10 mm Hg each. Some tracing paper manufactured in North America has four major vertical sections of 25 mm Hg each, with the smaller divisions representing 5 mm Hg of pressure in the uterine activity section. For further information on instrumentation, please refer to Chapter 3.

PARAMETERS FOR NORMAL LABOR

The assessment of normal labor progress has changed, and updated labor curves and consensus guidelines are having an effect on labor support and management [9–13]. Research indicates that current labor patterns are different from those reported by Friedman in the 1950s [14,15]. This has led to the development of partograms (labor progress graphs) that reveal significantly slower curves, and a later onset of active labor, with a median closer to 6 cm of dilation [12,13] (Fig. 4.4). Regardless of these updated parameters, basic definitions for *the stages of labor* are unchanged. The first stage of labor begins with the onset of contractions and ends with complete dilation of the cervix. It is divided into two phases: *latent* and *active*. During the latent phase, irregular and infrequent uterine contractions are associated with gradual cervical softening, dilation, and effacement (thinning). During the active phase of labor, the rate of cervical dilation increases and the fetal presenting part descends. The second stage of labor begins with complete dilation of the cervix and ends with

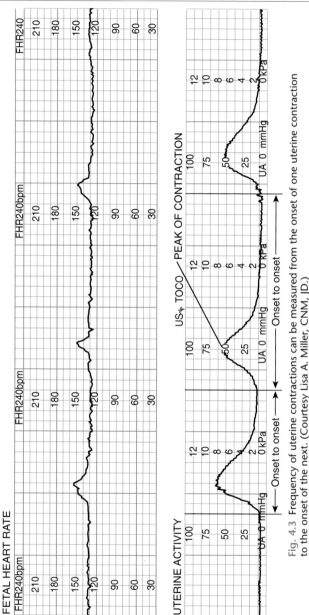

Fig. 4.3 Frequency of uterine contractions can be measured from the onset of one uterine contraction to the onset of the next. (Courtesy Lisa A. Miller, CNM, JD.)

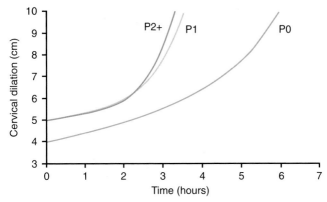

Fig. 4.4 Average labor curves by parity in singleton term pregnancies with spontaneous onset of labor, vaginal delivery, and normal neonatal outcomes. *P0,* nulliparous women; *P1,* women of parity 1; *P2+,* women of parity 2 or higher. (From J. Zhang, H.J. Landy, D. Ware Branch, et al., Contemporary patterns of spontaneous labor with normal neonatal outcomes, Obstet. Gynecol. 116 (2010) 1281–1287, used with permission.)

delivery of the fetus. Although some clinicians may continue to differentiate the second stage into two phases, a passive phase of rest and an active phase of maternal pushing efforts, current research (including a meta-analysis) regarding delayed pushing indicates it has significant disadvantages, including increases in maternal blood loss, chorioamnionitis, and decreased umbilical cord pH [16–18]. Although the practice of delayed pushing may be acceptable in certain select situations, its routine use is no longer recommended. A detailed review of labor management is outside the scope of this textbook, but a discussion of the evaluation of uterine activity and labor abnormalities and oxytocin use is warranted.

DEFINING ADEQUATE UTERINE ACTIVITY

Uterine contractions during labor result in the progressive dilation and effacement of the cervix and descent of the fetal presenting part, culminating in spontaneous vaginal delivery. Much of the data defining the "normal" range of uterine activity was derived from the research of Caldeyro-Barcia and colleagues in the late 1950s and 1960s [19–23]. Using intraamniotic pressure catheters,

Caldeyro-Barcia and Poseiro [20] evaluated uterine activity and coined the term *Montevideo units (MVUs)* as a method of measuring uterine activity. The original formula was calculated by multiplying the average *intensity* in millimeters of mercury (peak of contraction less resting tone) times the frequency of uterine contractions in a 10-minute period. Thus, if there are four contractions in 10 minutes with an average intensity of 40 mm Hg, the MVUs for that period would be 4×40, or 160 MVUs. Over time, it became obvious that the simple *addition* of the individual contraction *intensities* over 10 minutes resulted in essentially similar numbers to the multiplication method; since then the addition method has become common practice [9].

Early research showed that spontaneous labor began clinically when MVUs rose to between 80 and 120, with contraction strength needing to reach at least 40 mm Hg [20,21]. This would equate to two to three contractions with intensities of 40 mm Hg or more every 10 minutes for the initiation of labor. In normal labor, contractions increase in intensity and frequency as labor progresses through the first stage and into the second stage. Caldeyro-Barcia and colleagues [20–22] found that uterine activity in the first stage of normal labors generally ranged between 100 and 250 MVUs, with contractions increasing in intensity from 25 to 50 mm Hg and in frequency from three to five over 10 minutes. In the second stage, MVUs can rise to 300 to 400 [3,19–23] as contraction intensities may increase to 80 mm Hg or more and five or six contractions may be seen every 10 minutes.

Baseline uterine tone, also known as *resting tone,* averages 10 mm Hg during labor, rising from 8 to 12 mm Hg from the beginning of the first stage to the onset of the second stage. Resting tone is assessed during the time between contractions, known as *relaxation time.* Relaxation times are generally longer (60 seconds or more) in first-stage labor and tend to shorten (45–60 seconds) during the second stage. Contraction duration of 60 to 80 seconds remains relatively stable from active phase labor through the second stage [24]. These findings provide a basis for logical definitions of "adequate" uterine activity when using internal pressure catheters for assessment of uterine contractions.

Caldeyro-Barcia and Poseiro also provided crucial information related to contraction assessment when using palpation, or palpation and a tocotransducer. They found that until the intensity (peak less baseline tonus) reaches 40 mm Hg, the wall of the uterus is easily indented by palpation [21]. This correlates well with the premise that uterine contractions that palpate as moderate or stronger are likely to have peaks of 50 mm Hg or greater if they are measured by internal means, whereas palpated contractions identified as mild are likely

---

BOX 4.1   Components of Uterine Activity During Labor

Frequency	Contraction frequency overall generally ranges from 2 to 5 per 10 minutes during labor, with lower frequencies seen in the first stage of labor and higher frequencies seen during the second stage of labor.
Duration	Contraction duration remains fairly stable throughout the first and second stages, ranging from 45 to 80 seconds, not generally exceeding 90 seconds.
Strength	Uterine contractions generally range from peaking at 40–70 mm Hg in the first stage of labor and may rise to over 80 mm Hg in the second stage. Contractions palpated as "mild" would likely peak at <50 mm Hg if measured internally, and contractions palpated as "moderate" or greater would likely peak at 50 mm Hg or greater if measured internally.
Resting tone	Average resting tone during labor is 10 mm Hg; if using palpation, should palpate as "soft," i.e., easily indented, no palpable resistance.
Relaxation time	Relaxation time is usually 60 seconds or more in the first stage and 45 seconds or more in the second stage.
Montevideo units (MVUs)	Usually range from 100 to 250 MVUs in the first stage, may rise to 300–400 in the second stage. Contraction intensities of ≥40 mm Hg and MVUs of 80–120 are generally sufficient to initiate spontaneous labor.

to have peaks of less than 50 mm Hg if measured internally. These findings offer guidance for clinicians in identifying reasonable definitions of "adequate" uterine activity when using palpation (with or without a tocotransducer) for assessment of uterine contractions. Box 4.1 provides a summary of normal parameters of uterine activity in labor, and Fig. 4.5 illustrates a variety of common uterine contraction patterns in normal labor.

In summary, applying what is known about parameters of uterine activity during normal labor:

1. Allows clinicians to promote and support adequate and effective uterine activity during the different phases and stages of labor, influencing management decisions when abnormal labor progress or dystocia is diagnosed;
2. Forms a basis for the safe and proper use of labor stimulants; and
3. Provides a foundation on which to define excessive uterine activity by professional consensus.

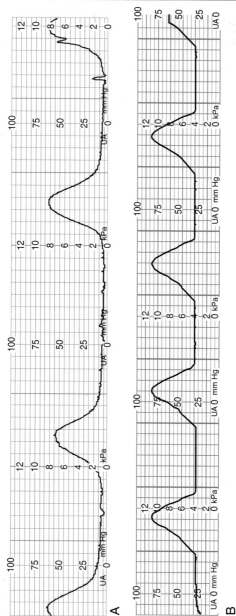

Fig. 4.5 Examples of normal uterine activity (UA) during labor. (A) Normal contraction pattern in latent phase labor. (B) Normal contraction pattern in active phase labor; note that contractions are more frequent, but there is still adequate relaxation time.

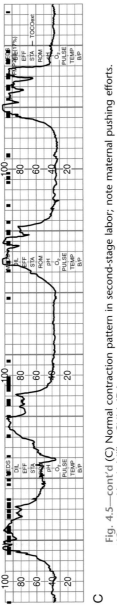

Fig. 4.5—cont'd (C) Normal contraction pattern in second-stage labor; note maternal pushing efforts. (Courtesy Lisa A. Miller, CNM, JD.)

DEFINING EXCESSIVE UTERINE ACTIVITY

Summary terms related to uterine activity were first published in 2008, when the National Institute of Child Health and Human Development (NICHD) issued a workshop report on fetal monitoring [25]. Prior to this report, the lack of sound, standardized definitions for uterine activity hindered both effective communication and the development of consensus-based multidisciplinary guidelines. The summary terms suggested by the NICHD are for the classification of uterine activity using *frequency of contractions averaged over a 30-minute period* [25,26]:

Normal: less than or equal to five contractions in 10 minutes

Tachysystole: greater than five contractions in 10 minutes

Tachysystole is to be further qualified by the presence or absence of FHR decelerations and applies to spontaneous and stimulated labors. The workshop report stressed the *importance of other parameters* such as *duration, intensity,* and *relaxation time* in the evaluation of uterine activity, specifically stating that "frequency alone is a partial assessment of uterine activity" [25]. The report also suggested abandonment of previously used summary terms *hyperstimulation* and *hypercontractility.* Although the NICHD workshop report is clearly important progress toward the standardization of terminology, standardized terminology alone does not provide clinicians with sufficient guidance for the safe and effective management of uterine activity in labor. Tachysystole is a fairly common event and has been linked to an increase in composite neonatal morbidity [5]. Clinicians must be familiar with the normal physiology of uterine activity (described previously) and the relationship between excessive uterine activity and fetal acid–base status.

The link between excessive uterine activity and untoward effects on FHR is well established [4,27]. Peebles and colleagues [6] noted decreased fetal cerebral oxygen saturation with shorter contraction intervals. Bakker and colleagues [3] found that fetal acidemia (umbilical artery pH ≤7.11) of all types (respiratory, metabolic, and mixed) was more prevalent in patients with excessive uterine activity during labor, both first and second stages. Specifically, a first-stage average MVU value of 261 and relaxation time of 51 seconds was noted in the acidemic group, versus average MVU value of 236 and relaxation time of 63 seconds in the nonacidemic group. In the second stage, an average MVU value of 442 and relaxation time of 36 seconds were noted in the acidemic group versus average MVU value of 402 and relaxation time of 47 seconds in the nonacidemic group [3]. Logic would therefore dictate that *avoiding* MVUs exceeding the previously discussed norm of 250 in the first stage of labor and 300 to 400 in the second stage could *decrease* the incidence of significant fetal acidemia at birth. Furthermore, in cases of external monitoring or any situation in which MVU evaluation is not feasible, *ensuring* adequate relaxation times of 60 seconds or more in the first stage and 45 seconds or more in the second stage also could prevent fetal acidemia at birth. Clinicians using frequency of contractions alone ("counting bumps"), without ensuring adequate relaxation time, may be unwittingly creating a negative effect on fetal acid–base status (Fig. 4.6).

In addition to evaluating frequency, strength, and relaxation time, it is important to understand that for the fetus to be able to maintain oxygenation, *resting tone* also must be normal. *Hypertonus,* or elevated resting tone, is most commonly defined as *uterine resting tone greater than 20 to 25 mm Hg,* or *a uterus that does not return to soft if using palpation.* The information in Box 4.2 can be used by clinicians and multidisciplinary committees to reach consensus on definitions for terms related to uterine activity and evidence-based guidelines for management of all types of excessive uterine activity. This information should serve as the starting point for the development of clear, physiologically sound, and clinically useful approaches to excessive uterine activity that include *all parameters* of uterine activity versus focusing on frequency (tachysystole) alone.

Some clinicians erroneously contend that the management of excessive uterine activity should be based on the presence or absence of FHR changes. This approach is directly in conflict with what limited evidence exists regarding uterine activity and fetal oxygenation. Bakker and colleagues [3] found no difference in the occurrence of late decelerations between the acidemic and nonacidemic fetuses, suggesting that the key to avoiding acidemia is not dependent on the appearance of FHR changes but on the presence of excessive uterine activity itself. Simpson and James [7] found that in the first stage of labor, even five uterine contractions in 10 minutes ("normal" uterine activity by definition) over a 30-minute period resulted in a 20% decrease in fetal oxygen saturation as measured by fetal pulse oximetry. Both of these studies make it clear that premising the management of uterine activity on frequency alone or basing the management of excessive uterine activity on FHR changes may lead to less than optimal fetal oxygenation and potentially the deterioration of fetal acid–base. *Waiting to respond to excessive uterine activity until there are significant changes in FHR is not appropriate.* Rather, to

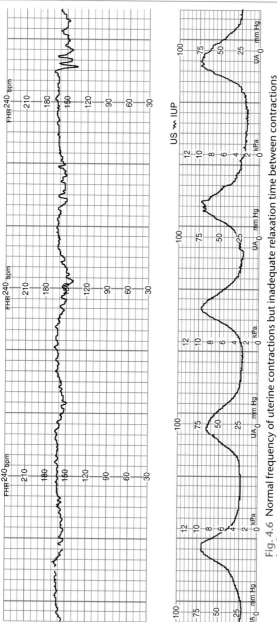

Fig. 4.6 Normal frequency of uterine contractions but inadequate relaxation time between contractions for first-stage labor. Recommended relaxation time in first stage is 60 seconds; note possible fetal heart rate (FHR) decelerations. *IUP*, intrauterine pressure; *UA*, uterine activity; *US*, ultrasound. (Courtesy Lisa A. Miller, CNM, JD.)

BOX 4.2   Evaluation of Uterine Activity During Labor

Preliminary Assumptions

- Normal uterine activity in first-stage labor generally does not exceed 250 MVUs.
- Normal uterine activity in second-stage labor should not exceed 400 MVUs.
- Normal contraction duration generally ranges from 45 to 90 seconds.
- Normal contraction intensity (peak less resting tone) generally ranges from 25 to 80 mm Hg, with higher intensities common as labor progresses.
- Normal uterine resting tone ranges from 8 to 12 mm Hg and is generally not greater than 20 to 25 mm Hg.
- Fetal acid–base status can be affected by excessive uterine activity *before* as evidenced by fetal heart rate changes.

Excessive Uterine Activity

All definitions for excessive uterine activity apply to both spontaneous and/or stimulated labor; management of excessive uterine activity should be based on clinical context.

- Tachysystole

Contraction frequency of greater than 5 in 10 minutes, averaged over 30 minutes; applies to spontaneous or stimulated labor.

- Hypertonus

Uterine resting tone exceeding 20 to 25 mm Hg with an intrauterine pressure catheter or a uterus that does not return to soft by palpation during relaxation time.

- Inadequate relaxation time

Less than 60 seconds' uterine relaxation between contractions during the first stage of labor; less than 45 to 50 seconds' uterine relaxation between contractions in second stage.

- Excessive contraction duration (also known as tetanic *contractions* or *uterine tetany*)

A series of single contractions lasting 2 minutes or more.

Data from references 3, 4, 6, 8, 9, 19–24, and 28–32.

---

prevent fetal acidemia at birth, clinicians should focus on *identifying and promoting normal (adequate) uterine activity* and correcting underlying causes of any type of excessive uterine activity.

Common Underlying Causes of Excessive Uterine Activity

- Use of pharmacologic cervical ripening agents
- Use of synthetic oxytocin for augmentation or induction (more common with high-dose, high-frequency administration protocols)

- Abruptio placentae
- Uterine overdistention, whether iatrogenic from amnioinfusion or as a result of multiple gestation, hydramnios, or macrosomia

Corrective Measures to Decrease Excessive Uterine Activity

1. Change maternal position to lateral side-lying.
2. Administer a bolus of intravenous (IV) fluids and/or increase the maintenance IV rate.
3. Remove cervical ripening agents or, in the case of oxytocin usage, decrease or discontinue the infusion.
4. If excessive uterine activity related to the use of cervical ripening agents or oxytocin administration is noted in association with FHR changes indicative of interrupted oxygenation, clinicians may consider the use of a tocolytic [33].

These interventions are *specific to excessive uterine activity.* Note that the management of FHR patterns is addressed in detail in Chapter 6. It is imperative that clinicians respond appropriately to FHR changes regardless of the nature of uterine activity because uterine activity is only one of several causes of interrupted fetal oxygenation. However, FHR changes are not a prerequisite for clinical response to excessive uterine activity. It cannot be overemphasized: Excessive uterine activity should trigger clinician response **whether or not FHR changes are observed**.

CURRENT TRENDS IN LABOR SUPPORT AND MANAGEMENT

Recognizing the differences in contemporary patterns of labor progression, professional organizations are working collaboratively to enhance the clinician's knowledge regarding normal labor and to provide new parameters for the approach to labor management, including emphasizing the importance of individualization and shared decision-making [11]. Labor abnormalities have been described historically using a variety of expressions, such as *slow progress in labor, failure to progress, dystocia, dysfunctional labor,* or *cephalopelvic disproportion* [34]. Up to 68% of unanticipated cesarean deliveries in patients with vertex presentation are reported to be caused by dystocia, and given the number of repeat cesarean deliveries that follow a primary cesarean for dystocia, the diagnosis of dystocia may account for as many as 60% of all cesarean births [34].

Because fetal monitoring includes the evaluation of the adequacy of uterine activity and the progress of labor, a brief overview of different labor abnormalities and possible management strategies is warranted. A clear understanding of labor progress can be helpful when interdisciplinary discussions arise regarding management of uterine activity, especially discussions regarding the utilization of oxytocin, the most common treatment for dystocia.

Latent Phase Abnormalities

Labor onset is defined as effacement and dilation of the cervix caused by regular uterine contractions. The latent phase of labor begins with the onset of labor (regular contractions, cervical change) and ends at the beginning of the active phase of first stage. Latent phase is considered prolonged if it is >20 hours in nulliparous patients and >14 hours in multiparous patients [34]. Contrary to what may be seen in clinical practice, both the American College of Obstetricians and Gynecologists (ACOG) and the Society for Maternal-Fetal Medicine (SMFM) do not recommend cesarean delivery for either slow progress in latent phase or a prolonged latent phase, noting that most women will enter active phase with expectant management [11]. Research now also provides specific management strategies for management of the latent phase in nulliparous women being induced at term [35]. Considerations for the management of prolonged latent phase labor are listed next.

*Management Strategies for Latent Phase Disorders**

1. For women in spontaneous labor, avoid admission to the labor unit in early latent phase labor. Unless otherwise indicated, admit only if the cervix is >3 cm dilated or 100% effaced. Educate patients antenatally about the benefits of this approach, and provide instructions for comfort measures while laboring at home.
2. Assess the woman's level of fatigue, and provide appropriate labor support.
3. Encourage adequate fluid intake and small, frequent meals while the mother is at home.
4. Set specific intervals to reevaluate status, even if symptoms remain unchanged.
5. Encourage ambulation to provide comfort and increase tolerance to latent phase labor.

---

*Adapted from references 11, and 34–38.

6. Provide adequate time for latent phase labor to progress during induction of labor. This may mean up to 18 to 20 hours of adequate uterine activity in nulliparous women.

7. Diagnose prolonged latent phase only after the presence of adequate uterine activity for >20 hours in nulliparas and >14 hours in multiparas. Use of oxytocin and/or amniotomy should be considered as opposed to cesarean delivery.

8. For nulliparous women at term undergoing induction, do not consider cesarean delivery for failed induction until at least 15 hours after both rupture of membranes and oxytocin initiation.

9. Evaluate patients for appropriate methods of cervical ripening for induction of labor in the presence of an unripe cervix.

Active Phase Abnormalities

There are three main categories of active phase labor abnormalities:

1. *Protraction disorders:* a slow rate of cervical dilation, defined as less than the fifth percentile statistically

2. *Arrest disorders:* where labor progresses normally initially in active phase, then stops, for a period of at least 2 hours

3. *Combined disorders:* where slow progress precedes arrest [34]

ACOG recommends that oxytocin augmentation be considered for these disorders [11]. Although traditionally the diagnosis of an arrest disorder required 2 hours without cervical change in the presence of a uterine contraction pattern that exceeded 200 MVUs, studies [39–41] now suggest that 4 hours of uterine activity exceeding 200 MVUs (or 6 hours if the average uterine activity pattern was <200 MVUs) will result in up to a 92% vaginal delivery rate with no increased risk to the newborn. The suggested management approaches for active phase disorders are listed next.

*Management Strategies for Active Phase Disorders**

1. Ensure that cervix is dilated at least to 6 cm before diagnosing the active phase of labor.

2. Use standardized oxytocin titration to achieve adequate uterine activity while avoiding tachysystole.

3. Consider an increase in the amount of hourly IV fluids to improve uterine muscle performance.

4. Consider use of an IUPC to document adequacy of contractions; a minimum of 200 MVUs is required.

*Adapted from references 11, 12, 27, 28, 32, 38–45, and 53.

5. Consider amniotomy if membranes are intact.
6. Limit active management of labor to nulliparous patients with singleton, cephalic presentations.
7. Require a diagnosis of active phase arrest as follows: no cervical change after at least 4 hours of adequate uterine activity or 6 hours of oxytocin administration with inadequate uterine activity.
8. Provide continuous labor support.

Second-Stage Abnormalities

Failure of the fetus to rotate and descend is called *arrest of descent,* and it is the labor abnormality associated with the second stage. ACOG and SMFM now state that before confirming an arrest diagnosis in the second stage, there should be at least 2 hours of active pushing in multiparous women and at least 3 hours of active pushing in the nullipara [11]. They also note that longer durations may be appropriate based on individual clinical factors. Contrary to some clinicians' practices, these are not mandates for cesarean delivery but rather parameters for guiding assessment and intervention. Prolonged second stage should trigger clinical reevaluation of the three Ps: *powers, passenger,* and *passage.* Evaluation of adequacy of uterine contractions, fetal position, and pelvic diameters may provide direction regarding interventions to facilitate rotation and descent. Although it may be considered appropriate in certain cases, delaying active pushing once complete dilation has been reached should no longer be a routine practice because of the increased risks [16,17].

UTERINE ACTIVITY AND OXYTOCIN USE

Disagreements related to oxytocin management are a frequent source of conflict between nurses, midwives, and physicians, and allegations regarding oxytocin management are common in obstetric litigation. Designated as a high-alert medication [46], oxytocin remains the most common treatment choice for labor abnormalities, making its use a daily issue in most labor and delivery suites in the United States. There are many sound, evidence-based protocols for the administration of oxytocin, ranging from high-dose, high-frequency to low-dose, low-frequency and hybrids that combine aspects of both regimens. Closely and accurately monitoring uterine activity is important during the care of all laboring women, but especially in labors being either induced or augmented with oxytocin, because oxytocin usage can result in excessive uterine activity even at low dosages.

Studies [43–45,47] regarding the pharmacologic characteristics of oxytocin use in relation to dysfunctional labor and dystocia show that 40 minutes are needed to achieve the maximum dose level. Regarding oxytocin pharmacokinetics, reviews by Arias [48] and Sanchez-Ramos [42] concluded that lower doses and less frequent increases of oxytocin are preferable as they allow time for a more physiologic approach and decrease the risk of tachysystole that is associated with higher doses and shorter dosing intervals. Simpson and Creehan [31,32] suggested starting doses of 0.5 to 2 mU/min with increases every 30 to 60 minutes of 1 to 2 mU/min. This approach is in keeping with one of the primary tenets of pharmacology, which is *use the lowest amount of drug needed to achieve the desired effect.* A systematic review of high-dose versus low-dose oxytocin for labor *induction* at term [49] found no benefit and noted an increase in tachysystole in the high-dose group. A randomized controlled trial comparing high-dose to low-dose for labor *augmentation* in nulliparous women at term [50] showed no difference in cesarean section between the two groups, and although the high-dose group did have slightly shorter labors, they had more tachysystole and more instrumental vaginal births for fetal indications. Couple this information with the liability aspects related to uterine activity and oxytocin, a low-dose approach is the preferred approach from both an evidence-based viewpoint and for risk management considerations. Clinicians should carefully consider all the data, and the differences in use of oxytocin for induction versus augmentation, when deciding on oxytocin management schemes. Suggestions for the safe and effective use of oxytocin in labor are summarized in Box 4.3.

Oxytocin dosage should be titrated to uterine activity, with a goal of attaining adequate or normal uterine activity. *Coupling or tripling* of uterine contractions (Fig. 4.7) is a phenomenon that may be seen during oxytocin administration. Suggested treatment for this pattern is temporary discontinuation of oxytocin, lateral positioning of the mother, initiation of a fluid bolus, and a restart of oxytocin after 30 minutes or more [32]. Oxytocin rest has also been shown to be a safe and effective way to decrease the cesarean rate in term nulliparas experiencing a prolonged latent phase; rest periods of 8 hours or longer reduced cesarean delivery without any increase in maternal or neonatal morbidity [52].

When administering oxytocin and using internal monitoring during labor induction or augmentation, the titration of oxytocin to establish uterine activity patterns reaching MVUs of 200 to 240 is an appropriate goal. When external monitoring and palpation are

BOX 4.3   Suggestions for Safe and Effective Oxytocin Usage

1. Use isotonic intravenous fluids during oxytocin administration to avoid dilutional hyponatremia.
2. Administer oxytocin for both induction and augmentation of labor using a low-dose, low-frequency protocol to maximize pharmacologic dose response and avoid tachysystole.
3. Use standardized definitions for adequate and excessive uterine activity; ensure that all team members are in accord.
4. Resolve any episodes of excessive uterine activity, regardless of whether fetal heart rate changes are present. Note that the goal of oxytocin use is *adequate* but not *excessive* uterine activity.
5. To promote optimal fetal oxygenation in first-stage labor, train team members to decrease oxytocin *before* tachysystole occurs by responding to contraction frequencies less than every 2 minutes before 30 minutes have elapsed.
6. Attempt to maintain average relaxation times of 60 seconds between contractions in first stage and 45 seconds during second stage.
7. Once an adequate pattern of uterine activity has been established, wean the oxytocin to the lowest amount necessary to maintain adequate contractions.
8. If coupling and tripling of uterine contractions occur, discontinue oxytocin for 30–60 minutes, administer an intravenous fluid bolus (isotonic), and encourage the woman to a side-lying position.

Data from references 3, 6–8, 24, 27, 28, 31, 32, 34, 36, 37, 40–45, and 49–51.

used, palpable contractions of normal duration every 2.5 to 3 minutes should correlate well with adequate MVUs (Fig. 4.8). If labor progress is not occurring with what seems to be adequate uterine activity by palpation, the proper clinical response is not to increase the oxytocin, but rather *to consider internal monitoring to assess uterine activity more accurately.* Once accurate evaluation of uterine activity is achieved via IUPC, then oxytocin can be safely increased.

Even using a low-dose, low-frequency approach with oxytocin, contraction frequency of less than every 2 minutes during the course of labor is a common occurrence; if it persists over a 30-minute period, it is considered tachysystole. Management must be based on clinical context and institutional protocol but should be geared toward returning uterine activity to adequate and appropriate for the stage of labor. In other words, clinicians should not try to achieve second-stage labor patterns in the latent or active phase of first-stage labor because this may interfere with fetal gas exchange. Continuous and ongoing evaluation of fetal status using a systematic approach can prevent fetal acidemia, improve outcomes, and reduce medicolegal

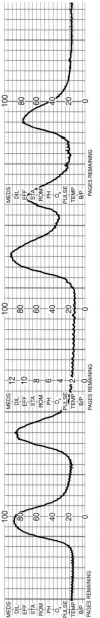

Fig. 4.7 Oxytocin administration may result in coupling and tripling of uterine contractions. Treatment consists of discontinuation of oxytocin, maternal position change, and intravenous hydration. (Courtesy Lisa A. Miller, CNM, JD.)

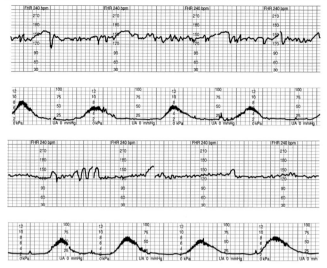

Fig. 4.8 Example of adequate uterine activity (UA) during oxytocin augmentation using external monitoring. Note adequate relaxation time between contractions. According to nursing documentation, the contractions palpated were of moderate strength. *FHR,* fetal heart rate. (Courtesy Lisa A. Miller, CNM, JD.)

risk. Safety related to oxytocin use is achieved by avoidance of the injudicious use of oxytocin, adherence to evidence-based multidisciplinary guidelines regarding oxytocin administration, and appropriate and consistent team management of excessive uterine activity.

SUMMARY

Uterine activity during labor results in normal oxidative stress for the fetus, and fetal gas exchange and acid–base status are directly affected by uterine activity during labor. Excessive uterine activity is related to fetal acidemia at birth and should be avoided by careful monitoring and cautious use of labor stimulants. Parameters for normal, or adequate, uterine activity are easily defined on the basis of normal labor physiology. Clinicians must reach consensus on definitions related to excessive uterine activity and recognize that the term *tachysystole* addresses only one aspect of uterine activity, that of frequency. Recognition of the importance of other parameters of uterine activity, such as strength, duration, resting tone, and relaxation time are equally important components of the evaluation of uterine activity during labor.

Crucial to the promotion of improved outcomes for mother and fetus is clinician understanding of both the normal progress of labor and labor abnormalities. The availability of continuous labor support, patient education regarding appropriate admission criteria, and adequate hydration play key roles in minimizing labor abnormalities. Familiarity with various labor curves, individualization of labor management, and incorporation of shared decision-making regarding induction or augmentation are crucial to ensuring safe passage. An understanding of the pharmacologic characteristics of oxytocin, combined with a goal to attain adequate uterine activity, will lead to safe and effective use of this high-alert medication.

As Bakker [3] so aptly states, "contraction monitoring deserves full attention." The evaluation of uterine activity and FHR patterns is inextricably intertwined in the care and support of the laboring mother. Historically, focus on uterine activity assessment and management has been inconsistent in clinical practice. Nurses, midwives, and physicians must have the requisite knowledge and skills to give uterine activity evaluation and management the same attention and care given to FHR pattern assessment.

References

[1] J.M. Turner, M.D. Mitchell, S.S. Kumar, The physiology of intrapartum fetal compromise at term, Am. J. Obstet. Gynecol. 222 (1) (2020) 17–26.

[2] A.I. Ahmed, L. Zhu, S. Aldhaheri, et al., Uterine tachysystole in spontaneous labor at term, J. Matern. Fetal Neonatal Med. 29 (20) (2016) 3335–3339.

[3] P.C.A.M. Bakker, P.H.J. Kurver, D.J. Kuik, et al., Elevated uterine activity increases the risk of fetal acidosis at birth, Am. J. Obstet. Gynecol. 196 (4) (2007) 313e1–313e6.

[4] R. Caldeyro-Barcia, Intrauterine fetal reanimation in acute intrapartum fetal distress, Early Hum. Dev. 29 (1992) 27–33.

[5] C.C. Heuser, S. Knight, M.S. Esplin, et al., Tachysystole in term labor: incidence, risk factors, outcomes, and effect on fetal heart tracings, Am. J. Obstet. Gynecol. 209 (1) (2013) 32e1–32e6.

[6] D. Peebles, J. Spencer, A. Edwards, et al., Relation between frequency of uterine contractions and human fetal cerebral oxygenation saturation studied during labour by near infrared spectroscopy, Br. J. Obstet. Gynaecol. 101 (1) (1994) 44–48.

[7] K.R. Simpson, D.C. James, Effects of oxytocin-induced uterine hyperstimulation on fetal oxygen status and fetal heart rate patterns during labor, Am. J. Obstet. Gynecol. 199 (2008) 34e1–34e5.

[8] K.R. Simpson, L.A. Miller, Assessment and optimization of uterine activity during labor, Clin. Obstet. Gynecol. 54 (1) (2011) 40–49.

[9] Association of Women's Health, Obstetric and Neonatal Nurses, Fetal Heart Monitoring: Principles and Practices, fifth ed., Kendal Hunt, Dubuque, IA, 2015.

[10] D.L. Lowdermilk, S.E. Perry, Maternity & Women's Health Care, twelfth ed., Mosby, St. Louis, MO, 2020.

[11] American College of Obstetricians and Gynecologists, Safe prevention of the primary cesarean delivery. Obstetric Care Consensus No. 1, Obstet. Gynecol. 123 (2014) 693–711.

[12] J. Zhang, H.J. Landy, D. Ware Branch, et al., Contemporary patterns of spontaneous labor with normal neonatal outcomes, Obstet. Gynecol. 116 (6) (2010) 1281–1287.

[13] S.M. Norman, M.G. Tuuli, A.O. Odibo, et al., The effects of obesity on the first stage of labor, Obstet. Gynecol. 120 (1) (2012) 130–135.

[14] E.A. Friedman, Labor in multiparas: a graphicostatistical analysis, Obstet. Gynecol. 8 (1956) 691–703.

[15] E.A. Friedman, Primigravid labor: a graphicostatistical analysis, Obstet. Gynecol. 6 (1955) 567–589.

[16] A.G. Cahill, S.K. Srinivas, A.T.N. Tita, et al., Effect of immediate vs delayed pushing on rates of spontaneous vaginal delivery among nulliparous women receiving neuraxial analgesia: A randomized clinical trial, JAMA 320 (14) (2018) 1444–1454.

[17] A. Fiedler, R. Brun, D. Randegger, et al., Adverse effect of delayed pushing on postpartum blood loss in nulliparous women with epidural analgesia, Int. J. Gynaecol. Obstet. 150 (1) (2020) 92–97.

[18] D. Di Mascio, G. Saccone, F. Bellussi, et al., Delayed versus immediate pushing in the second stage of labor in women with neuraxial analgesia: a systematic review and meta-analysis of randomized controlled trials, Am. J. Obstet. Gynecol. (2020 Feb 15) pii: S0002-9378(20)30140-X. doi:10.1016/j.ajog.2020.02.002.

[19] R. Caldeyro-Barcia, Oxytocin in pregnancy and labour, Acta Endocrinol 34 (Suppl 50) (1960) 41–49 Suppl. (Copenhagen).

[20] R. Caldeyro-Barcia, J.J. Poseiro, Physiology of uterine contractions, Clin. Obstet. Gynecol. 3 (1960) 386–408.

[21] R. Caldeyro-Barcia, J.J. Poseiro, Oxytocin and contractility of the pregnant human uterus, Ann. N.Y. Acad. Sci. 75 (1959) 813–830.

[22] R. Caldeyro-Barcia, Y. Sica-Blanco, J.J. Poseiro, et al., A quantitative study of the action of synthetic oxytocin on the pregnant human uterus, J. Pharmacol. Exp. Ther. 121 (1) (1957) 18–31.

[23] R. Caldeyro-Barcia, G. Theobald, Sensitivity of the pregnant human myometrium to oxytocin, Am. J. Obstet. Gynecol. 102 (8) (1968) 1181.

[24] G. Pontonnier, F. Puech, H. Grandjean, et al., Some physical and biochemical parameters during normal labour, Biol. Neonate 26 (3–4) (1975) 159–173.

[25] G.A. Macones, G.D. Hankins, C.Y. Spong, et al., The 2008 National Institute of Child Health and Human Development workshop report on electronic fetal monitoring: update on definitions, interpretation, and research guidelines, J. Obstet. Gynecol. Neonatal Nurs. 37 (2008) 510–515.

[26] American College of Obstetricians and Gynecologists, Intrapartum fetal heart rate monitoring: nomenclature, interpretation, and general management principles Practice Bulletin no. 106, Obstet. Gynecol. 114 (2009) 192–202.

[27] K.R. Simpson, Intrauterine resuscitation during labor: review of current methods and supportive evidence, J. Midwifery Womens Health 52 (3) (2007) 229–237.

[28] American College of Obstetricians and Gynecologists, Induction of labor, Practice Bulletin no. 107, ACOG, Washington, DC, 2009.

[29] S.B. Effer, R.P. Bértola, A. Vrettos, et al., Quantitative study of the regularity of uterine contractile rhythm in labor, Am. J. Obstet. Gynecol. 105 (6) (1969) 909–915.

[30] A.J. Krapohl, G.G. Myers, R. Caldeyro-Barcia, Uterine contractions in spontaneous labor: a quantitative study, Am. J. Obstet. Gynecol. 106 (3) (1970) 378–387.

[31] K.R. Simpson, Cervical Ripening and Induction and Augmentation of Labor, fourth ed., AWHONN, Washington, DC, 2013.

[32] K.R. Simpson, P.A. Creehan, Perinatal Nursing, fifth ed., Lippincott Williams & Wilkins, Philadelphia, PA, 2020.

[33] American College of Obstetricians and Gynecologists, Clinical management guidelines for obstetricians-gynecologists: management of intrapartum fetal heart rate tracings. Practice Bulletin no. 116, Obstet. Gynecol. 116 (2010) 1232–1240.

[34] A. Ness, J. Goldberg, V. Berghella, Abnormalities of the first and second stages of labor, Obstet. Gynecol. Clin. North Am. 32 (2) (2005) 201–220.

[35] W.A Grobman, J. Bailit, Y. Lai, et al., Defining failed induction of labor, Am. J Obstet. Gynecol. 218 (1) (2018) 122e1–122e8.

[36] B.M. Mercer, Induction of labor in the nulliparous gravida with an unfavorable cervix, Obstet. Gynecol. 105 (4) (2005) 688–689.

[37] D.W. Dowding, H.L. Cheyne, V. Hundley, Complex interventions in midwifery care: reflections on the design and evaluation of an algorithm for the diagnosis of labor, Midwifery 27 (5) (2010) 654–659. http://dx.doi.org/10.1016/j.midw.2009.11.01.

[38] M.A. Bohren, G. Hofmeyr, C. Sakala, et al., Continuous support for women during childbirth, Cochrane Database of Systematic Reviews (Issue 7) (2017). Art. No.: CD003766. doi: 10.1002/14651858.CD003766.pub6E.

[39] S. Shields, S. Ratcliffe, P. Fontaine, et al., Dystocia in nulliparous women, Am. Fam. Physician 75 (11) (2007) 1671–1678.

[40] D.J. Rouse, J. Owen, J.C. Hauth, Criteria for failed labor induction: prospective evaluation of a standardized protocol, Obstet. Gynecol. 96 (5 Pt 1) (2000) 671–677.

[41] D. Rouse, J. Owen, K. Savage, et al., Active phase labor arrest: revisiting the 2-hour minimum, Obstet. Gynecol. 98 (4) (2001) 550–554.

[42] L. Sanchez-Ramos, Induction of labor, Obstet. Gynecol. Clin. North Am. 32 (2) (2005) 181–200.

[43] J. Seitchik, The management of functional dystocia in the first stage of labor, Clin. Obstet. Gynecol. 30 (1) (1987) 42–49.

[44] J. Seitchik, J.A. Amico, M. Castillo, Oxytocin augmentation of dysfunctional labor. V. An alternative oxytocin regimen, Am. J. Obstet. Gynecol. 151 (6) (1985) 757–761.

[45] J. Seitchik, J. Amico, A.G. Robinson, et al., Oxytocin augmentation of dysfunctional labor. IV. Oxytocin pharmacokinetics, Am. J. Obstet. Gynecol. 150 (3) (1984) 225–228.

[46] Institute for Safe Medical Practices, High alert medications. Available from: https://www.ismp.org/sites/default/files/attachments/2018-08/highAlert2018-Acute-Final.pdf. Accessed May 1, 2020.

[47] H.D. Crall, D.R. Mattison, Oxytocin pharmacodynamics: effect of long infusions on uterine activity, Gynecol. Obstet. Invest. 31 (1) (1991) 17–22.

[48] F. Arias, Pharmacology of oxytocin and prostaglandins, Clin. Obstet. Gynecol. 43 (3) (2000) 455–468.

[49] A. Budden, L.J.Y. Chen, A. Henry, High-dose versus low-dose oxytocin infusion regimens for induction of labour at term, Cochrane Database of Systematic Reviews, (Issue 10) (2014). Art. No.: CD009701. doi: 10.1002/14651858.CD009701.pub2.

[50] L. Selin, U.B. Wennerholm, M. Jonsson, et al., High-dose versus low-dose of oxytocin for labour augmentation: a randomised controlled trial, Women Birth 32 (4) (2019) 356–363.

[51] L.A. Miller, Oxytocin, excessive uterine activity, and patient safety: time for a collaborative approach, J. Perinat. Neonatal Nurs. 23 (1) (2009) 52–58.

[52] M. McAdow, X. Xu, H. Lipkind, et al., Association of oxytocin rest during labor induction of nulliparous women with mode of delivery, Obstet. Gynecol. 135 (3) (2020) 569–575.

[53] R.M.D. Smyth, C. Markham, T. Dowswell, Amniotomy for shortening spontaneous labour, Cochrane Database Syst. Rev. (6) (2013) CD006167.

CHAPTER 5

Pattern Recognition and Interpretation

The clinical application of electronic fetal heart rate (FHR) monitoring consists of three distinct, interdependent elements:

1. Definition
2. Interpretation
3. Management

This chapter focuses on standardized definitions of FHR patterns and standard, evidence-based interpretation of FHR patterns with respect to underlying physiology. The principles developed in this chapter are used during the discussion of FHR management in Chapter 6.

THE EVOLUTION OF STANDARDIZED FETAL HEART RATE DEFINITIONS

Electronic FHR monitoring was introduced into clinical practice almost 50 years ago before consensus was achieved regarding standardized definitions and interpretation of FHR patterns. In 1995 and 1996, the National Institute of Child Health and Human Development (NICHD) convened a workshop to develop "standardized and unambiguous definitions for fetal heart rate tracings" [1]. These definitions have been endorsed by the American College of Obstetricians and Gynecologists (ACOG), the Association of Women's Health, Obstetric and Neonatal Nurses (AWHONN), and the American College of Nurse-Midwives (ACNM). In 2008 a second NICHD consensus panel was convened to review and update the standardized definitions published in 1997 [2]. Standardized NICHD FHR definitions are summarized in Table 5.1. Detailed discussion of individual pattern definitions, along with evidence-based review of the underlying fetal physiology, will be presented later in this chapter.

The 2008 National Institute of Child Health and Human Development Consensus Report

In addition to clarifying and reiterating the FHR definitions proposed by the 1997 NICHD consensus statement, the 2008 report recommended a simplified system for classifying FHR tracings, using

TABLE 5.1   Standardized Fetal Heart Rate Definitions

Pattern	Definition
Baseline	The mean FHR rounded to increments of 5 bpm during a 10-min segment, excluding accelerations, decelerations, and periods of marked FHR variability
	The baseline must be for a minimum of 2 min (not necessarily contiguous) in any 10-min segment, or the baseline for that segment is defined as "indeterminate"
Tachycardia	Baseline FHR >160 bpm
Bradycardia	Baseline FHR <110 bpm
Baseline variability	Fluctuations in the FHR baseline that are irregular in amplitude and frequency; variability is measured from the peak to the trough of the FHR fluctuations and is quantitated in beats per minute
	Variability is classified as follows:
	Absent: amplitude range undetectable
	Minimal: amplitude range detectable but ≤5 bpm
	Moderate: amplitude range 6–25 bpm
	Marked: amplitude range >25 bpm
	No distinction is made between short-term variability (or beat-to-beat variability or R-R wave period differences in the electrocardiogram) and long-term variability because in actual practice they are visually determined as a unit
Acceleration	A visually apparent abrupt increase (onset to peak <30 seconds) in the FHR from the baseline
	At 32 weeks' gestation and beyond, an acceleration has a peak at least 15 bpm above baseline and a duration of at least 15 seconds but <2 min
	Before 32 weeks' gestation, an acceleration has a peak at least 10 bpm above baseline and a duration of at least 10 seconds but <2 min
	Prolonged acceleration lasts ≥2 min but <10 minutes
	If an acceleration lasts ≥10 minutes, it is a baseline change
Early deceleration	In association with a uterine contraction, a visually apparent, gradual (onset to nadir ≥ 30 seconds) decrease in FHR with return to baseline
	In general, the nadir of the deceleration occurs at the same time as the peak of the contraction
Late deceleration	In association with a uterine contraction, a visually apparent, gradual (onset to nadir ≥30 seconds) decrease in FHR with return to baseline
	In general, the onset, nadir, and recovery of the deceleration occur after the beginning, peak, and end of the contraction, respectively

Continued

TABLE 5.1   Standardized FHR Definitions—cont'd

Pattern	Definition
Variable deceleration	An abrupt (onset to nadir <30 seconds), visually apparent decrease in the FHR below the baseline
	The decrease in FHR is at least 15 bpm and lasts at least 15 seconds but <2 minutes.
Prolonged deceleration	Visually apparent decrease in the FHR at least 15 bpm below the baseline lasting at least 2 minutes but <10 minutes from onset to return to baseline
Periodic deceleration	Accompanies a uterine contraction
Episodic deceleration	Does not accompany a uterine contraction
Sinusoidal pattern	Visually apparent, smooth, sine wave–like undulating pattern in FHR baseline with a cycle frequency of 3–5/min that persists for ≥20 minutes

FHR, fetal heart rate.
Adapted from G.A. Macones et al., The 2008 National Institute of Child Health and Human Development workshop report on electronic fetal monitoring: update on definitions, interpretation, and research guidelines, Obstet. Gynecol. 112 (3) (2008) 661–666.

baseline rate, variability, deceleration, and the sinusoidal pattern to group FHR tracings into one of three categories (Table 5.2). Category I includes tracings with a normal baseline rate (110 to 160), moderate variability, and no variable, late or prolonged decelerations. Category III includes tracings with absent variability and recurrent late decelerations, absent variability with recurrent variable decelerations, absent variability with bradycardia for at least 10 minutes, or a sinusoidal pattern for at least 20 minutes. Category II includes all tracings that do not meet criteria for classification as Category I or Category III. The proposed FHR categories represent a shorthand method of defining FHR tracings. Because Category II includes a wide range of FHR tracings, the categories alone do not provide sufficient information for FHR interpretation or management. The categories do not

TABLE 5.2   Three-Tier Fetal Heart Rate Classification System

Category I	
Normal	FHR tracing includes all of the following:
	Baseline rate: 110–160 bpm
	Baseline FHR variability: moderate
	Accelerations: present or absent
	Late or variable decelerations absent
	Early decelerations present or absent

TABLE 5.2   Three-Tier Fetal Heart Rate Classification System—cont'd

Category II	
Indeterminate	Includes all FHR tracings not assigned to Categories I or III
Category III	
Abnormal	FHR tracing includes at least one of the following:
	Absent variability with recurrent late decelerations
	Absent variability with recurrent variable decelerations
	Absent variability with bradycardia for at least 10 minutes
	Sinusoidal pattern for at least 20 minutes

FHR, fetal heart rate.
Adapted from G.A. Macones et al., The 2008 National Institute of Child Health and Human Development workshop report on electronic fetal monitoring: update on definitions, interpretation, and research guidelines, Obstet. Gynecol. 112 (3) (2008) 661–666.

replace a full description of baseline rate, variability, accelerations, decelerations, sinusoidal pattern, and changes or trends over time.

Evidence-Based Interpretation of Fetal Heart Rate Patterns

This chapter reviews the relationship between FHR patterns and fetal physiology with particular emphasis on the underlying scientific evidence. Principles of FHR interpretation are stratified here by supporting evidence according to the method outlined by the U.S. Preventive Services Task Force, summarized in Box 5.1. Level I evidence is considered to be the most robust and Level III the least. Specifically, Level I and II evidence is capable of establishing statistically significant relationships. Level III evidence is descriptive. As such, Level III evidence is capable of generating theories and hypotheses, but it is not capable of proving them.

As discussed previously, the primary objective of intrapartum FHR monitoring is to assess fetal oxygenation during labor. However, a number of conditions and/or exposures can influence the appearance of an FHR tracing via mechanisms unrelated to fetal oxygenation. Common maternal factors include fever, infection, medications, and thyroid disease. Common fetal factors include fever, infection, medications, prematurity, anemia, cardiac arrhythmias, anomalies, preexisting neurologic injury, and sleep cycles. Thorough assessment of an FHR tracing should take into account the factors summarized in Table 5.3. If FHR changes are thought to be related

BOX 5.1   Stratification of Scientific Evidence[a]

Level I	Evidence obtained from at least one properly designed randomized controlled trial.
Level II-1	Evidence obtained from well-designed controlled trials without randomization.
Level II-2	Evidence obtained from well-designed cohort or case-control analytic studies, preferably from more than one center or research group.
Level II-3	Evidence obtained from multiple time series with or without the intervention. Dramatic results in uncontrolled experiments also could be regarded as this type of evidence.
Level III	Opinions of respected authorities, based on clinical experience, descriptive studies, or reports of expert committees.

[a] According to method outlined by United States Preventive Services Task Force, Guide to Clinical Preventative Services. Report of the U.S. Preventive Services Task Force, second ed., Williams and Wilkins, Baltimore, MD, 1996.

TABLE 5.3   Factors Not Specifically Related to Fetal Oxygenation That May Influence Fetal Heart Rate

Factor	Reported FHR associations (most evidence Level II-3 and Level III)
Fever/infection	Increased baseline rate, decreased variability
Medications	Effects depend on specific medication and may include changes in baseline rate, frequency and amplitude of accelerations, variability, and sinusoidal pattern
Hyperthyroidism	Tachycardia, decreased variability
Prematurity	Increased baseline rate, decreased variability, reduced frequency and amplitude of accelerations
Fetal anemia	Sinusoidal pattern, tachycardia
Fetal heart block	Bradycardia, decreased variability
Fetal tachyarrhythmia	Variable degrees of tachycardia, decreased variability
Congenital anomaly	Decreased variability, decelerations
Preexisting neurologic abnormality	Decreased variability, absent accelerations
Sleep cycle	Decreased variability, reduced frequency and amplitude of accelerations

FHR, fetal heart rate.

to interrupted fetal oxygenation, management is directed at assessing the oxygen pathway and improving the transfer of oxygen from the environment to the fetus, as described in Chapter 2. However, if an FHR abnormality is related to any of the conditions summarized in Table 5.3, then individualized management is directed at the specific underlying process. During the following discussion of physiology and interpretation, FHR patterns related to interrupted fetal oxygenation are considered separately from FHR patterns caused by other mechanisms.

NATIONAL INSTITUTE OF CHILD HEALTH AND HUMAN DEVELOPMENT DEFINITIONS: GENERAL CONSIDERATIONS

The standardized definitions proposed by the NICHD in 1997 and reiterated in 2008 apply to the interpretation of FHR patterns produced by a direct fetal electrode detecting the fetal electrocardiogram (FECG) or by an external Doppler device detecting fetal cardiac motion using the autocorrelation technique. *Autocorrelation* is a computerized method of minimizing the artifact associated with Doppler ultrasound calculation of the FHR. This technology is built into all modern FHR monitors. Patterns are categorized as *baseline, periodic,* or *episodic.* Baseline patterns include baseline rate and variability. Periodic and episodic patterns include FHR accelerations and decelerations. Periodic patterns are those associated with uterine contractions, and episodic patterns are those not associated with uterine contractions. Decelerations are defined as *abrupt* if the onset to nadir (lowest point) is <30 seconds and *gradual* if the onset to nadir is ≥30 seconds. Accelerations are defined as abrupt if the onset to peak is <30 seconds and gradual if the onset to peak is ≥30 seconds. Although terms such as *beat-to-beat* variability, *short-term* variability, and *long-term* variability have been used commonly in clinical practice, the 1997 and 2008 NICHD consensus reports recommended that no distinction be made among short-term, beat-to-beat, and long-term variability because in actual practice they are visually determined as a unit. A number of FHR characteristics are dependent on gestational age, so gestational age must be considered in the full description of the pattern. In addition, the FHR tracing should be evaluated in the context of maternal medical condition, prior results of fetal assessment, medications, and other factors. Finally, it is essential to recognize that FHR patterns do not occur alone and generally evolve over time. Therefore a full description of an FHR tracing requires a qualitative and quantitative description of uterine contractions and each of the FHR components.

Five Essential Components of a Fetal Heart Rate Tracing

In addition to evaluation of uterine contractions, the five components of an FHR tracing include the following:
1. Baseline rate
2. Variability
3. Accelerations
4. Decelerations
5. Changes or trends over time

DEFINITIONS, PHYSIOLOGY, AND INTERPRETATION OF SPECIFIC FETAL HEART RATE PATTERNS

Baseline Rate

Definition

Baseline FHR is defined as the approximate mean FHR rounded to increments of 5 bpm during a 10-minute segment, excluding accelerations, decelerations, and periods of marked variability (Figs. 5.1, 5.2, 5.3). Baseline rate is defined as a single number

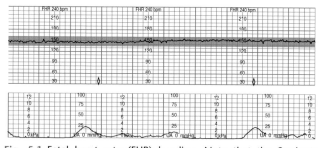

Fig. 5.1 Fetal heart rate (FHR) baseline. Note that the 2-minute minimum for identifiable baseline does not require 2 contiguous or continuous minutes; rather, it is the total identifiable baseline in the 10-minute window that must add up to 2 minutes. Also, baseline may occur (and be interpreted) ***during contractions***, as seen here. Baseline (*highlighted*) is identified over the entire 10-minute window, exceeding the 2-minute minimum. *UA*, uterine activity.

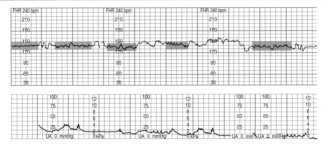

Fig. 5.2 Fetal heart rate (FHR) baseline. Note that the 2-minute minimum for identifiable baseline does not require 2 contiguous or continuous minutes; rather, it is the total identifiable baseline in the 10-minute window that must add up to 2 minutes. Also, baseline may occur (and be interpreted) during contractions, as seen in Fig. 5.1. Baseline (*highlighted*) is identified **between accelerations** or between segments differing by 25 bpm or more; identifiable baseline is approximately 5 minutes total (note the 2-minute minimum is met). *UA,* uterine activity.

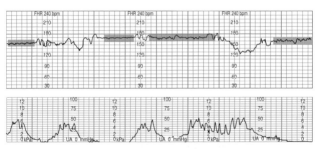

Fig. 5.3 Fetal heart rate (FHR) baseline. Note that the 2-minute minimum for identifiable baseline does not require 2 contiguous or continuous minutes; rather, it is the total identifiable baseline in the 10-minute window that must add up to 2 minutes. Also, baseline may occur (and be interpreted) during contractions, as seen in Fig. 5.1. Baseline (*highlighted*) is identified **between decelerations** or between segments differing by 25 bpm or more; identifiable baseline is approximately 5 minutes total (note the 2-minute minimum is met). *UA,* uterine activity.

(for example, 145 bpm), not as a range (for example, "140–150 bpm" or "140s"), because the definitions of other FHR components, including accelerations and decelerations, are based on the degree of deviation from the baseline rate. In any 10-minute window the minimum baseline duration must be at least 2 minutes (not necessarily contiguous), or the baseline for that period is deemed indeterminate (Fig. 5.4). If the baseline during any 10-minute segment is deemed

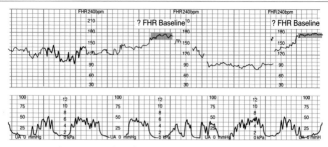

Fig. 5.4 Indeterminate baseline. Note that there are less than 2 minutes of identifiable baseline during this 10-minute window. The baseline would be labeled *indeterminate* for this portion of the tracing, and the clinician would need to refer to previous portions of the strip to determine baseline. Prior baseline was 155 bpm. *FHR,* fetal heart rate; *UA,* uterine activity.

indeterminate, it may be necessary to refer to previous 10-minute segment(s) for determination of the baseline. A normal FHR baseline ranges from 110 to 160 bpm.

Physiology

Baseline FHR is regulated by intrinsic cardiac pacemakers (sinoatrial [SA] node, atrioventricular [AV] node) and conduction pathways, autonomic innervation (sympathetic, parasympathetic), humoral factors (catecholamines), extrinsic factors (medications), and local factors (calcium, potassium). Sympathetic innervation and plasma catecholamines increase baseline FHR, whereas parasympathetic innervation reduces the baseline rate. Autonomic input regulates the FHR in response to fluctuations in Po_2, Pco_2, and blood pressure detected by chemoreceptors and baroreceptors located in the aortic arch and carotid arteries.

CATEGORIES OF BASELINE RATE

Tachycardia

Definition

Baseline FHR in excess of 160 bpm is defined as tachycardia (Fig. 5.5).

Interpretation

Fetal oxygenation: As discussed in Chapter 2, recurrent or sustained interruption of oxygen transfer from the environment to the fetus can lead to progressive deterioration of fetal oxygenation and,

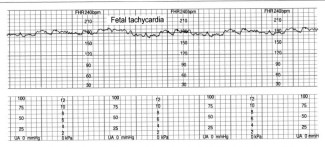

Fig. 5.5 Fetal tachycardia: fetal heart rate (FHR) >160 bpm. *UA,* uterine activity.

eventually, to fetal metabolic acidemia. In the setting of metabolic acidemia, blunting of parasympathetic cardiac stimulation can cause the FHR to rise above the normal range. Sympathetic and humoral factors may play a role as well. Because there are many possible causes of fetal tachycardia that are not directly related to interruption of fetal oxygenation, the association between fetal tachycardia and fetal oxygenation is nonspecific. The scientific evidence supporting a relationship between fetal tachycardia and interrupted fetal oxygenation primarily is Level III. Nevertheless, the observation of fetal tachycardia should prompt consideration of all possible causes, including interruption of oxygenation.

Other mechanisms: Many potential causes of fetal tachycardia are not directly related to fetal oxygenation. For example, abnormalities involving fetal cardiac pacemakers and/or the cardiac conduction system can result in sinus tachycardia, supraventricular tachycardia, atrial fibrillation, atrial flutter, and ventricular dysrhythmias. Maternal fever and infection and fetal anemia are well-known associations that likely act through the fetal autonomic nervous system and circulating catecholamines to cause fetal tachycardia. Maternal thyroid-stimulating antibodies can cause maternal hyperthyroidism and maternal tachycardia. Rarely, transplacental passage of thyroid-stimulating antibodies can result in fetal hyperthyroidism and tachycardia. Finally, many medications have been reported to cause fetal tachycardia. General categories include parasympatholytic drugs (atropine, hydroxyzine, phenothiazines) and sympathomimetic drugs (terbutaline, albuterol). Caffeine, theophylline, cocaine, and methamphetamine are other possible causes. Most of the scientific evidence regarding these mechanisms is Level II-3 and Level III. Potential causes of fetal tachycardia are summarized in Box 5.2.

BOX 5.2   Potential Causes of Fetal Tachycardia

Maternal fever
Infection
Medications/drugs
- Sympathomimetics
- Parasympatholytics
- Caffeine
- Theophylline
- Cocaine
- Methamphetamines
Fetal anemia
Maternal hyperthyroidism
Arrhythmias
- Sinus tachycardia
- Supraventricular tachycardia
- Atrial fibrillation
- Atrial flutter
- Ventricular arrhythmia
Metabolic acidemia

Bradycardia

Definition

Baseline FHR <110 bpm is defined as bradycardia (Fig. 5.6).

Interpretation

Fetal oxygenation: In the past, the term *bradycardia* has been used interchangeably with the term *prolonged deceleration*. However, this practice is imprecise and should be avoided. According to the definitions proposed by the NICHD, bradycardia is a baseline

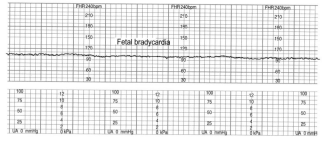

Fig. 5.6 Fetal bradycardia: fetal heart rate (FHR) <110 bpm. *UA,* uterine activity.

BOX 5.3   Potential Causes of Fetal Bradycardia

Medications, including sympatholytics
Cardiac conduction abnormalities
Heart block
Heterotaxy syndrome
Structural cardiac defects
Viral infections, for example, cytomegalovirus
Sjögren's antibodies
Fetal heart failure
Maternal hypoglycemia
Maternal hypothermia
Interruption of fetal oxygenation

rate <110 bpm for at least 10 minutes, whereas a prolonged deceleration is a periodic or episodic deceleration that interrupts the baseline. Decelerations are common and can reflect interruption of fetal oxygenation. True baseline bradycardia is uncommon and is not specifically related to fetal oxygenation.

Other mechanisms: Baseline fetal bradycardia can be caused by abnormalities at the level of the cardiac pacemakers and/or conduction system. AV dissociation or "heart block" can result from disruption of the cardiac conduction system by structural cardiac defects, viral infections (cytomegalovirus [CMV]), or maternal Sjögren's antibodies. Medications (adrenergic antagonists) do not commonly cause a reduction in baseline FHR <110 bpm. In descriptive studies that represent Level III evidence, fetal bradycardia has been reported in association with fetal heart failure, maternal hypoglycemia, and maternal hypothermia during cardiac surgery, urosepsis, and magnesium sulfate infusion. Potential causes of fetal bradycardia are summarized in Box 5.3.

Baseline Fetal Heart Rate Variability

Definition

FHR variability is defined as *fluctuations in the baseline FHR that are irregular in amplitude and frequency*. Variability is quantitated in beats per minute and is measured from the peak to the trough in beats per minute. No distinction is made between *short-term (beat-to-beat)* variability and *long-term* variability because in actual practice they are visually determined as a unit. There is no consensus whether beat-to-beat variability alone is interpretable to the unaided eye. Variability is categorized as *absent, minimal, moderate,* or *marked* as shown in Fig. 5.7.

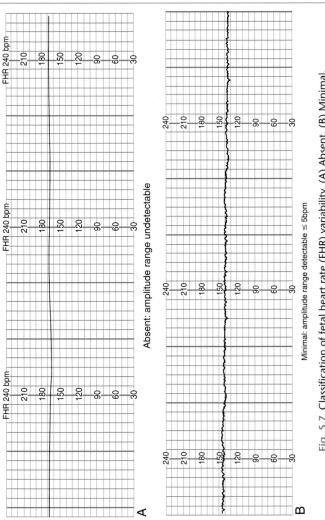

Fig. 5.7 Classification of fetal heart rate (FHR) variability. (A) Absent. (B) Minimal.

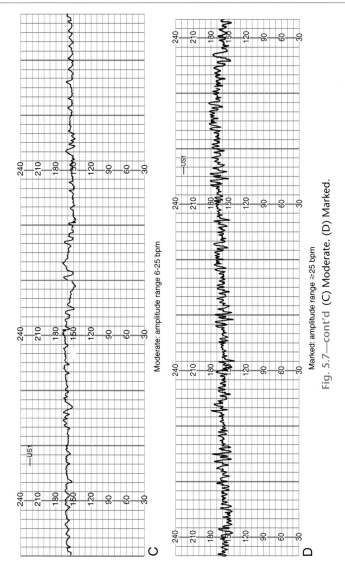

Moderate: amplitude range 6-25 bpm

Marked: amplitude range ≥25 bpm

Fig. 5.7—cont'd (C) Moderate. (D) Marked.

Physiology

Many factors interact to regulate FHR variability, including cardiac pacemakers (SA node, AV node) and the cardiac conduction system, autonomic innervation (sympathetic, parasympathetic), humoral factors (catecholamines), extrinsic factors (medications), and local factors (calcium, potassium). Fluctuations in Po_2, Pco_2, and blood pressure are detected by chemoreceptors and baroreceptors located in the aortic arch and carotid arteries. Signals from these receptors are processed in the medullary vasomotor center, possibly with regulatory input from higher centers in the hypothalamus and cerebral cortex. Sympathetic and parasympathetic signals from the medullary vasomotor center modulate the FHR in response to moment-to-moment changes in fetal Po_2, Pco_2, and blood pressure. With every heartbeat, slight corrections in the heart rate help optimize fetal cardiac output and maximize the distribution of oxygenated blood to the fetal tissues. As illustrated in Fig. 5.7, this variation is referred to as *FHR variability* and is displayed visually on the FHR graph as an irregular horizontal line. The small oscillations that represent FHR changes between each successive heartbeat have been referred to as *beat-to-beat* variability or *short-term* variability. The broader oscillations have been referred to as *long-term* variability. These terms describe two elements of FHR variability that occur together and that are evaluated as a unit. Therefore, as discussed earlier in the chapter, no distinction is made between short-term (beat-to-beat) variability and long-term variability. These terms are not included in standardized NICHD terminology. For purposes of clear and consistent communication, they should be avoided.

CATEGORIES OF BASELINE VARIABILITY

Absent Variability

Definition

As depicted in Fig. 5.7, variability is defined as *absent if the amplitude range of the FHR fluctuations is undetectable to the unaided eye.*

Interpretation

Fetal oxygenation: Recurrent or sustained interruption of oxygen transfer from the environment to the fetus can lead to progressive deterioration of fetal oxygenation, metabolic acidemia, and blunting of parasympathetic outflow that can reduce the moment-to-moment regulation of the FHR. In the FHR tracing, these changes can be seen as minimal to absent variability. Although FHR variability ≤5 bpm is relatively common, persistently absent variability (amplitude range undetectable) is not. If variability ≤5 bpm is caused by interrupted fetal oxygenation, other FHR observations may be present, including decelerations, absent accelerations, and tachycardia. There are many possible causes of FHR variability ≤5 bpm. However, when persistent absent variability (amplitude range undetectable) is observed, careful evaluation should be undertaken to exclude fetal metabolic acidemia if possible.

Other mechanisms: Decreased FHR variability can be caused by a number of mechanisms that are unrelated to fetal oxygenation, including fetal sleep cycles, fetal tachycardia, and extreme prematurity. Congenital anomalies and preexisting neurologic injury are other possible causes. Several medications have been implicated in decreased FHR variability. General categories include central nervous system depressants (narcotics, barbiturates, phenothiazines, tranquilizers, general anesthetics) and parasympatholytics (atropine). Most of the scientific evidence regarding these mechanisms is Level III. It is important to note that most studies in the literature define "decreased" variability as ≤5 bpm and do not further stratify variability as "absent" (amplitude range undetectable) or "minimal" (amplitude range detectable but ≤5 bpm). Therefore it is not possible to draw valid distinctions regarding the relative clinical significance of these two categories. Causes of decreased FHR variability are summarized in Box 5.4.

BOX 5.4   Potential Causes of Decreased Fetal Heart Rate Variability

Fetal sleep cycle
Fetal tachycardia
Medications
- Narcotics
- Barbiturates
- Phenothiazines
- Tranquilizers
- General anesthetics
- Atropine
Prematurity
Congenital anomalies
Fetal anemia
Fetal cardiac arrhythmia
Infection
Preexisting neurologic injury
Fetal metabolic acidemia

Minimal Variability

Definition

Minimal variability is defined as an *amplitude range that is detectable but ≤5 bpm.*

Interpretation

Fetal oxygenation: Interrupted fetal oxygenation leading to metabolic acidemia and blunted autonomic regulation of the FHR can result in decreased FHR variability.

The specific relationship among minimal variability, fetal oxygenation, and fetal metabolic acidemia is not known, primarily because the literature has not consistently distinguished between minimal and absent variability. In the setting of persistently minimal variability without accelerations or moderate variability, the FHR tracing alone cannot reliably exclude metabolic acidemia.

Other mechanisms: Minimal variability may be associated with mechanisms other than interruption of fetal oxygenation, including fetal sleep cycles, fetal tachycardia, prematurity, congenital anomalies, pre-existing neurologic injury, and medications, as summarized in Box 5.4. Most of the scientific evidence regarding these mechanisms is Level III.

Moderate Variability

Definition

Moderate variability (see Fig. 5.7) has an amplitude range of 6 to 25 bpm.

Interpretation

Fetal oxygenation: Moderate FHR variability indicates normal control of the FHR by cardiac pacemakers and conduction pathways, autonomic innervation, humoral, extrinsic, and local factors. Specifically, moderate variability indicates that autonomic regulation of the FHR is not blunted by interruption of fetal oxygenation that has progressed to the stage of metabolic acidemia. One of the central principles of electronic FHR monitoring is that moderate variability reliably predicts the absence of fetal metabolic acidemia and ongoing hypoxic injury at the time it is observed [3–8]. Supporting evidence is Level II-2, II-3, and III.

Other mechanisms: Moderate variability indicates normal neurologic regulation of the FHR at the time it is observed but does not exclude the possibility of preexisting neurologic injury [1,9–11].

Marked Variability

Definition

Marked variability is defined as *FHR variability that is >25 bpm in amplitude* (see Fig. 5.7).

Interpretation

The significance of marked variability is not known. In many cases, it likely represents a normal variant. It is plausible that marked variability reflects autonomic perturbation in the setting of early hypoxemia. Scientific evidence regarding this pattern is limited. All available evidence is Level III.

Sinusoidal Pattern

The sinusoidal pattern (Fig. 5.8) is defined as a smooth, sine wave–like undulating pattern in FHR baseline with a cycle frequency of 3 to 5 per minute that persists for at least 20 minutes. It is not included in the definition of FHR variability. A practical way to distinguish FHR variability from the sinusoidal pattern is to recognize that variability is defined as fluctuations in the baseline that are irregular in amplitude and frequency, whereas the sinusoidal pattern is characterized by fluctuations in the baseline that are regular in amplitude and frequency. Sinusoidal FHR is an uncommon pattern. Although the pathophysiologic mechanism is not known, this pattern classically is associated with severe fetal anemia. Variations of the pattern have

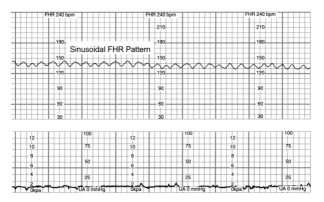

Fig. 5.8 Sinusoidal pattern. *FHR,* fetal heart rate; *UA,* uterine activity.

been described in association with chorioamnionitis, fetal sepsis, or administration of narcotic analgesics [9]. Scientific evidence regarding associated factors is Level II-2 to Level III. Evidence regarding pathophysiology is Level III.

Acceleration

Definition

Acceleration is an abrupt (onset to peak <30 seconds) increase in FHR above baseline. The peak is at least 15 bpm above baseline, and the acceleration lasts at least 15 seconds from the onset to return to baseline (Fig. 5.9). Before 32 weeks' gestation, an acceleration is defined as having a peak at least 10 bpm above baseline and a duration of at least 10 seconds. An acceleration lasting at least 2 minutes but less than 10 minutes is defined as a prolonged acceleration. An acceleration lasting 10 minutes or longer is defined as a baseline change. The amplitude of an acceleration is quantitated in beats per minute above the baseline excluding transient spikes or electronic artifact. The duration is quantitated in minutes and seconds.

Physiology

Accelerations in FHR frequently occur in association with fetal movement, probably as a result of stimulation of peripheral proprioceptors, increased catecholamine release, and autonomic stimulation of the heart. In the absence of spontaneous accelerations, fetal scalp stimulation or vibroacoustic stimulation can provoke fetal movement and FHR accelerations.

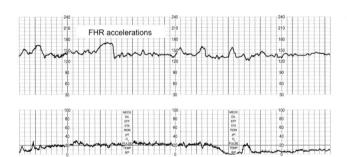

Fig. 5.9 Accelerations of fetal heart rate (FHR) in a term pregnancy. Note that the 15-bpm peak and 15-second duration criteria are met. (Courtesy Lisa A. Miller, CNM, JD.)

Interpretation

Fetal oxygenation: Accelerations, like moderate variability, reflect normal autonomic regulation of the FHR. The presence of accelerations indicates that autonomic regulation of the FHR is not blunted by interruption of oxygenation that has progressed to the stage of metabolic acidemia. A central principle of electronic FHR monitoring is that FHR accelerations are highly predictive of the absence of fetal metabolic acidemia and ongoing hypoxic injury at the time they are observed [12–15]. Supporting evidence is Level II-2, II-3, and III.

Other mechanisms: Accelerations indicate normal autonomic regulation of the FHR at the time they are observed [1,10,11,16]. However, the presence of FHR accelerations does not reliably exclude preexisting neurologic injury. Another suspected mechanism of FHR acceleration is transient compression of the umbilical vein, resulting in decreased fetal venous return and a reflex rise in heart rate. Evidence is Level III.

Decelerations

Definition

FHR decelerations are identified as early, late, variable, or prolonged. Late decelerations and early decelerations are gradual in onset and periodic in timing (associated with uterine contractions). Variable decelerations are abrupt in onset and may be periodic or episodic in timing. Prolonged decelerations may be abrupt or gradual in onset and may be periodic or episodic in timing. Decelerations are defined as recurrent if they occur with at least 50% of uterine contractions in any 20-minute segment. All decelerations are quantitated by depth in beats per minute below the baseline (excluding transient spikes or electronic artifact) and duration in minutes and seconds. Standardized NICHD terminology does not classify FHR decelerations as *mild, moderate,* or *severe* because the prognostic significance of such subclassification has not been established. The following sections review the standard definition and interpretation of each pattern.

Physiology

Early decelerations represent a reflex fetal response to fetal head compression during uterine contractions. Late, variable, and prolonged FHR decelerations represent reflex fetal responses to interruption of the oxygen pathway at one or more points. Scientific evidence supporting these mechanisms ranges from Level II-1 to Level III.

TYPES OF DECELERATIONS

Early Deceleration

Definition

Early deceleration is defined as a gradual (onset to nadir of 30 seconds or more) decrease in FHR from the baseline and subsequent return to baseline associated with a uterine contraction (Fig. 5.10). In most cases the onset, nadir, and recovery of the deceleration occur at the same time as the beginning, peak, and end of the contraction, respectively. Early decelerations are defined as recurrent if they occur with at least 50% of uterine contractions in any 20-minute segment.

Interpretation

Fetal oxygenation: Early decelerations have no known relationship to fetal oxygenation.

Other mechanisms: Although the precise physiologic mechanism is not known, early decelerations are thought to represent a fetal autonomic response to changes in intracranial pressure and/or cerebral blood flow caused by intrapartum compression of the fetal head (Fig. 5.11). These decelerations do not appear to be associated with poor outcome and therefore are considered clinically benign. Evidence is Level II-3 and Level III.

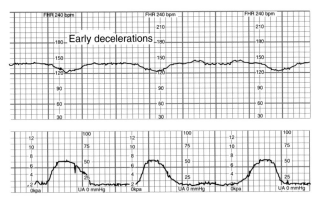

Fig. 5.10 Early decelerations. *FHR,* fetal heart rate; *UA,* uterine activity.

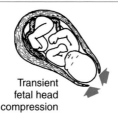

Transient
fetal head
compression

Physiologic mechanism of early deceleration

Transient fetal head compression
↓
Altered intracranial pressure and/or cerebral blood flow
↓
Reflex parasympathetic outflow
↓
Gradual slowing of the FHR
↓
Early deceleration
↓
When head compression is relieved, autonomic reflexes subside

Fig. 5.11 Physiologic mechanism of early decelerations.

Late Deceleration

Definition

Late deceleration of the FHR is defined as a gradual (onset to nadir ≥30 seconds) decrease of the FHR from the baseline and subsequent return to the baseline associated with a uterine contraction (Fig. 5.12). In most cases the onset, nadir, and recovery of the deceleration occur after the beginning, peak, and ending of the contraction, respectively. Late decelerations are defined as recurrent if they occur with at least 50% of uterine contractions in any 20-minute segment. They are defined as intermittent if they occur with <50% of contractions in any 20-minute segment.

Interpretation

Fetal oxygenation: A late deceleration is a reflex fetal response to transient hypoxemia during a uterine contraction. Myometrial contractions can compress maternal blood vessels traversing the uterine wall and disrupt maternal perfusion of the intervillous

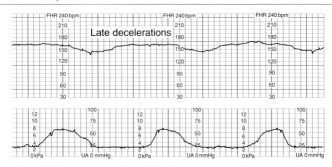

Fig. 5.12 Late decelerations. *FHR*, fetal heart rate; *UA*, uterine activity.

space of the placenta. Reduced delivery of oxygenated blood to the intervillous space can reduce the diffusion of oxygen into the fetal capillary blood in the chorionic villi, leading to a decline in fetal Po_2 below the normal range of approximately 15 to 25 mm Hg. If the fetal Po_2 falls below a critical threshold, chemoreceptors detect the change and signal medullary vasomotor centers to initiate a protective reflex response. Sympathetic outflow causes peripheral vasoconstriction and centralization of blood volume, favoring perfusion of the brain, heart, and adrenal glands. The resulting increase in peripheral resistance causes a rise in mean arterial blood pressure and a subsequent baroreceptor-mediated reflex slowing of the heart rate to reduce cardiac output and return the blood pressure to normal. This mechanism has been elucidated elegantly in a number of animal studies [2,17–25]. It is summarized in Fig. 5.13. If disruption of fetal oxygenation is recurrent or sustained, it may progress to the stage of metabolic acidemia. In the setting of metabolic acidemia, a late deceleration can reflect a direct myocardial depressant effect of hypoxia. In that event, other FHR abnormalities would be expected, such as fetal tachycardia, absent variability, and absent accelerations. For the purpose of standardized interpretation of intrapartum FHR patterns, a late deceleration reflects transient interruption of oxygen transfer from the environment to the fetus during a uterine contraction, resulting in transient fetal hypoxemia. The scientific evidence supporting the physiologic basis of a typical late deceleration is Level II-1 and II-2.

Other mechanisms: No other mechanisms are known to cause late decelerations.

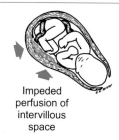

Impeded
perfusion of
intervillous
space

Physiologic mechanism of late deceleration

Uterine contraction impedes
maternal perfusion of the
placental intervillous space
↓
Transient fetal hypoxemia ⟶
↓
Chemoreceptor stimulation
↓
Reflex sympathetic outflow
↓
Peripheral vasoconstriction, preferentially
shunting oxygenated blood away from the
peripheral tissues and toward central vital
organs: brain, heart, adrenal glands
↓
Increase in fetal peripheral resistance
and blood pressure
↓
Baroreceptor stimulation
↓
Reflex parasympathetic outflow
↓
Gradual slowing of the FHR
↓
Late deceleration ⟵
↓
After the contraction, these reflexes subside

Note: In the presence
of fetal metabolic
acidemia, transient
hypoxemia may result
in myocardial hypoxia
and a late deceleration
secondary to direct
myocardial depression

Fig. 5.13 Physiologic mechanism of late decelerations. *FHR,* fetal heart rate.

Variable Deceleration

Definition

Variable deceleration of the FHR is defined as an abrupt (onset to nadir <30 seconds) decrease in FHR below the baseline, calculated from the most recent determined portion of the baseline (Fig. 5.14). The decrease in FHR below the baseline is at least 15 bpm, and the

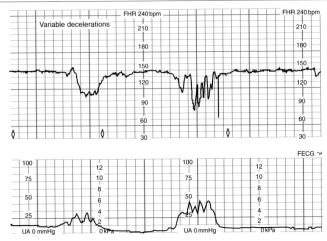

Fig. 5.14 Variable decelerations. *FECG,* fetal electrocardiogram; *FHR,* fetal heart rate; *UA,* uterine activity.

deceleration lasts at least 15 seconds and <2 minutes from onset to return to baseline. Variable decelerations are not necessarily associated with uterine contractions. However, when they are, the onset, depth, and duration commonly vary with successive uterine contractions. In addition, if they are associated with uterine contractions, variable decelerations are defined as recurrent if they occur with at least 50% of uterine contractions in any 20-minute segment.

Interpretation

Fetal oxygenation: Variable decelerations result from transient mechanical compression of umbilical blood vessels within the umbilical cord (Fig. 5.15) [26–35]. Initially, compression of the umbilical cord occludes the thin-walled, compliant umbilical vein, decreasing fetal venous return and triggering a baroreceptor-mediated reflex rise in FHR (commonly described as a "shoulder"). Further compression of the umbilical cord results in occlusion of the umbilical arteries, causing an abrupt increase in fetal peripheral resistance and blood pressure. Baroreceptors detect the abrupt rise in blood pressure and signal the medullary vasomotor center, which, in turn, triggers an increase in parasympathetic outflow along the vagus nerve and an abrupt decrease in heart rate. Parasympathetic stimulation of the heart may result in a junctional or idioventricular rhythm that appears as a relatively stable rate of 60 to 80 bpm at the base of a variable

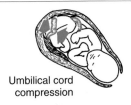

Umbilical cord
compression

Physiologic mechanism of variable deceleration

Umbilical cord compression
↓
Initial compression of umbilical vein
↓
Transient decreased fetal venous return
↓
Transient reduction in fetal cardiac output and blood pressure
↓
Baroreceptor stimulation
↓
Transient reflex rise in FHR
↓
Umbilical artery compression
↓
Abrupt rise in fetal peripheral resistance and blood pressure
↓
Baroreceptor stimulation
↓
Reflex parasympathetic outflow
↓
Abrupt slowing of the FHR
↓
Variable deceleration
↓
When umbilical cord compression is relieved, this process
occurs in reverse

Fig. 5.15 Physiologic mechanism of variable decelerations. *FHR,* fetal
heart rate.

deceleration. As the cord is decompressed, this sequence of events
occurs in reverse. A shoulder is common after a variable deceleration. It is important to note that the term *shoulder* is not included
in the standard NICHD definitions of FHR patterns. This term, and
others lacking standard definitions, are addressed in a separate section of this chapter. Umbilical cord compression results in transient
interruption of normal oxygen transfer from the environment to
the fetus. During a variable deceleration, the fetal Po_2 may or may
not fall below the normal range of 15 to 25 mm Hg. Regardless

of the effect on fetal Po_2, a variable deceleration is transient by definition (duration <2 min), and occasional compression of the umbilical cord usually has little clinical significance. Recurrent variable decelerations, on the other hand, can result in recurrent disruption of fetal oxygenation and lead to a cascade of progressive physiologic changes including hypoxemia, hypoxia, metabolic acidosis, and eventually metabolic acidemia. In that event, associated FHR observations may include a rising baseline rate, minimal to absent variability, absent accelerations, and slow return to baseline after decelerations. The latter has been referred to as a *variable with a late component.* This term is not defined by the NICHD and is addressed later in the chapter. For the purposes of FHR interpretation, a variable deceleration reflects transient interruption of oxygen transfer from the environment to the fetus at the level of the umbilical cord. Supporting evidence is Level II-1, II-2, II-3, and III.

Other mechanisms: Other suggested physiologic mechanisms resulting in variable deceleration include a fetal vagal response to umbilical cord stretching and reflex vagal response to head compression. The former mechanism may be similar to the mechanism underlying umbilical cord compression. The latter likely is similar to the mechanism underlying early decelerations. Supporting evidence is limited (Level III).

Prolonged Deceleration

Definition

Prolonged deceleration (Fig. 5.16) of the FHR is defined as a decrease (either gradual or abrupt) in FHR at least 15 bpm below the baseline lasting at least 2 minutes from onset to return to baseline.

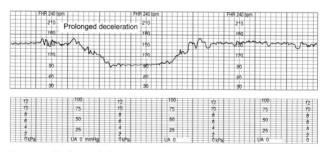

Fig. 5.16 Prolonged decelerations. *FHR,* fetal heart rate; *UA,* uterine activity.

According to NICHD terminology, a prolonged deceleration lasting 10 minutes or longer is defined as a baseline change. Under no
circumstances should this statement be interpreted to suggest that
a prolonged deceleration turns into a benign baseline change after
10 minutes.

Interpretation

Fetal oxygenation: A prolonged deceleration reflects disrupted oxygen transfer from the environment to the fetus at one or more points
along the oxygen pathway. As described in the introduction to FHR
decelerations, there are two basic physiologic mechanisms:

1. Reflex autonomic response
2. Direct myocardial depression

A prolonged deceleration usually begins as a reflex autonomic
response to disruption of the oxygen pathway. If the oxygen pathway is disrupted by mechanical compression of the umbilical cord,
the FHR deceleration begins as a reflex autonomic response to
fetal hypertension. Alternatively, an acute event such as placental
abruption or uterine rupture can cause an abrupt fall in fetal Po_2.
Reflex peripheral vasoconstriction centralizes blood volume and
increases blood pressure. The resulting FHR deceleration begins
as a reflex autonomic response to the rise in blood pressure trig-
gered by falling Po_2. Regardless of the cause, sustained disruption
of oxygen transfer can lead to progressive physiologic changes,
including fetal hypoxemia, hypoxia, metabolic acidosis, and metabolic acidemia. Eventually, tissue hypoxia and acidosis can lead
to failure of peripheral vascular smooth muscle contraction. The
resultant fetal hypotension reduces diastolic blood pressure and
compromises coronary blood flow, leading to myocardial hypoxia,
direct myocardial depression, and slowing of the FHR. If this process is not corrected, the heart may stop beating altogether. It is
likely that both mechanisms (autonomic reflex and direct myocardial depression) contribute to the underlying physiology of a
prolonged FHR deceleration; however, their precise relative roles
are not known. In general, autonomic reflexes appear to predomi-
nate initially, and hypoxic myocardial depression appears to be
a later mechanism. Supporting evidence is Level II-1, II-2, II-3,
and III. For the purposes of standard FHR interpretation, a prolonged deceleration reflects interruption of oxygen transfer from
the environment to the fetus at one or more points along the oxygen pathway.

Other mechanisms: Other proposed mechanisms of prolonged decelerations can overlap with those causing fetal bradycardia. Examples include fetal heart failure, maternal hypoglycemia, and hypothermia. Supporting evidence is Level III.

FETAL CARDIAC ARRHYTHMIAS

Precise characterization of fetal cardiac arrhythmias can challenge the clinical skills of the most experienced specialist, even with the benefit of direct, magnified visualization of the fetal heart using state-of-the-art sonographic equipment with color, pulse-wave, and M-mode Doppler capability. Therefore any attempt to classify fetal cardiac arrhythmias using electronic FHR monitoring alone is destined to result in a tentative diagnosis at best. This imprecision is compounded by the fact that rates >240 bpm may be halved or not printed at all by the monitor. This severely limits the ability of the FHR monitor to distinguish between fetal conditions such as supraventricular tachycardia, atrial fibrillation, and atrial flutter, all of which can result in FHRs >240 bpm (the upper limit of the FHR graph on standard paper). Electronic FHR monitoring cannot determine whether a fetal heartbeat is initiated by an electrical impulse originating in the atrium or in the ventricle. In other words, an electronic monitor cannot reliably distinguish an atrial arrhythmia from a ventricular arrhythmia. Nevertheless, electronic FHR monitoring can offer some clues to the presence of an abnormal fetal heart rhythm. For example, dropped beats might appear on the FHR monitor as sharp downward spikes that nadir at approximately half of the baseline rate. A premature beat with a compensatory pause might appear as a sharp upward spike followed immediately by a downward spike. Bradycardia caused by heart block can appear persistently or intermittently as a baseline rate that is half of the normal rate. Sinus bradycardia should be suspected if the baseline rate is <110 bpm but higher than half of the normal rate. Any FHR baseline of <110 bpm requires thorough evaluation before it can be attributed to a benign condition. If the fetal heart is not generating electrical activity, as in the case of fetal demise, a fetal scalp electrode may detect the electrical impulses from the maternal heart and record the maternal heart rate. If there is any question about the clinical significance of any unusual fetal heart rhythm that is seen on the fetal monitor or detected audibly, further evaluation with other modalities is necessary to establish an accurate diagnosis.

TERMS AND CONCEPTS NOT SUPPORTED BY EVIDENCE OR CONSENSUS

Several terms and concepts that may be encountered in practice or in the medicolegal arena are not supported by scientific evidence and are not included in standard NICHD recommendations. Some of these are discussed next.

Wandering Baseline

An FHR baseline that is within the normal range (110–160 bpm) but is not stable at a single rate for long enough to define a mean has been described as a *wandering baseline.* Absent variability and absent accelerations are prominent features. Decelerations can be present or absent. This combination of FHR findings has been suggested to indicate preexisting neurologic injury and impending fetal death. The physiologic mechanism is not known, and published data are limited (Level III). If this pattern is observed, it should be interpreted in the context of other FHR observations and clinical factors.

Lambda Pattern

The *lambda* FHR pattern is characterized by a brief acceleration followed by a small deceleration [36]. Common during early labor, this pattern has no known clinical significance. The underlying physiologic mechanism is not known (Level III).

Shoulder

As discussed earlier in the chapter, variable decelerations result from transient mechanical compression of umbilical blood vessels within the umbilical cord. Initial compression of the umbilical vein reduces fetal venous return and triggers a baroreceptor-mediated reflex rise in FHR that commonly is described as a shoulder. As the cord is decompressed, a second shoulder frequently follows the deceleration and likely reflects the same underlying mechanism. The precise mechanism has not been confirmed. There is no known association with adverse newborn outcome. On the other hand, there is no firm evidence that the observation reflects normal fetal oxygenation. It is considered a clinically benign observation. Supporting evidence is Level III.

Checkmark Pattern

The *checkmark pattern* is an unusual FHR pattern that has been described in association with neurologic injury, neonatal convulsions, and possible in utero fetal seizure activity. Unlike most FHR patterns described in association with neurologic injury, the checkmark pattern is not necessarily accompanied by absent baseline variability. All evidence related to the visual appearance of the pattern and the putative clinical significance is Level III.

End-Stage Bradycardia and Terminal Bradycardia

Standardized NICHD FHR terminology clearly indicates that the term *bradycardia* applies to the baseline FHR. The term specifically does not apply to a "prolonged deceleration" that interrupts the baseline. The terms *end-stage bradycardia* and *terminal bradycardia* have been used to describe a prolonged deceleration observed at the end of the second stage of labor. Such decelerations are common in the course of normal vaginal delivery and usually are of little clinical significance. The precise cause is unknown; however, suggested mechanisms include umbilical cord compression, umbilical cord stretching, fetal head compression, and transient fetal hypoxemia caused by excessive uterine activity and/or maternal expulsive efforts. The effect on immediate newborn outcome is variable and depends on a number of interacting factors, including but not limited to the physiologic cause of the deceleration, prior condition of the fetus, and duration of the deceleration. Consistent with NICHD terminology, end-stage bradycardia and terminal bradycardia should be discarded in favor of the more precise term *prolonged deceleration.* Evidence is Level III.

Uniform Accelerations

Various terms have been used to describe FHR accelerations. Examples include uniform sporadic accelerations, variable sporadic accelerations, uniform periodic accelerations, sporadic periodic accelerations, and crown accelerations. These terms are not included in standardized NICHD definitions, and there is no documented physiologic basis for such classification.

Atypical Variable Decelerations

Overshoot

The term *overshoot* has been used to describe an FHR pattern characterized by persistently absent variability, absent accelerations, and a variable deceleration followed by a smooth, prolonged rise in the FHR above the previous baseline with gradual return [37–41]. As with the wandering baseline, essential elements of this uncommon pattern include the persistent absence of variability and the absence of accelerations. The overshoot pattern has been attributed to a range of conditions, including "mild fetal hypoxia above the deceleration threshold," "chronic fetal distress," and "repetitive transient central nervous system ischemia." However, all of these associations are speculative and none has been substantiated by available scientific evidence. The physiologic mechanisms responsible for the overshoot pattern are not known. However, the pattern has been described in association with abnormal neurologic outcome with or without metabolic acidemia, suggesting that it might indicate preexisting neurologic injury. Because of the wide variation in reported associations and the lack of agreement regarding the definition and clinical significance of overshoot, it is best to avoid the use of this term in favor of specific terminology. All evidence regarding the overshoot pattern in humans is Level III.

Variable Deceleration With a Late Component

Variable deceleration with a late component describes a deceleration with an abrupt onset and a gradual return to baseline. The abrupt onset suggests that the deceleration begins as a reflex autonomic response to an abrupt rise in blood pressure caused by umbilical cord compression (the "variable" component of the pattern). The gradual return to baseline suggests a gradual reduction of autonomic outflow on resolution of transient hypoxemia, as occurs in a late deceleration (the "late" component of the pattern). A plausible explanation of the pattern would be initial umbilical cord compression causing a reflex fall in FHR and a transient decline in fetal Po_2. The Po_2 probably drops below the threshold that triggers the reflex sympathetic outflow and peripheral vasoconstriction characteristic of a late deceleration. Decompression of the umbilical cord brings about rapid resolution of the variable deceleration; however, the physiologic mechanisms responsible for late deceleration resolve more slowly, causing the FHR to return slowly to the previous baseline. Although the specific physiologic mechanism has not been studied systematically, this explanation is a reasonable extrapolation from known mechanisms. Scientific evidence regarding the underlying physiologic mechanism is limited to Level III. Second-stage variable decelerations with slow recovery have been reported to increase the likelihood of operative delivery; however, no consistent effect on newborn outcome has been described [42]. In the absence of a standard definition of this pattern, its use is best avoided in favor of standard terminology, for example, *variable deceleration with gradual return to baseline.*

Mild, Moderate, and Severe Variable Decelerations

The depth and duration of variable decelerations have been suggested as predictors of newborn outcome. Kubli and colleagues proposed three categories of variable decelerations based on these characteristics [43]. According to this classification system, a *mild variable deceleration* was defined by a duration less than 30 seconds regardless of depth, a depth no lower than 80 bpm, or a depth of 70 to 80 bpm lasting less than 60 seconds. A *moderate variable deceleration* was defined by a depth <70 bpm lasting 30 to 60 seconds or a depth of 70 to 80 bpm lasting more than 60 seconds. A *severe deceleration* was defined as a deceleration <70 bpm lasting more than 60 seconds. There is no conclusive evidence in the literature that the depth of any type of deceleration (early, variable, late, or prolonged) is predictive of fetal metabolic acidemia or newborn outcome independent of other important FHR characteristics such as baseline rate, variability, accelerations, and frequency of decelerations. Therefore *mild, moderate,* and *severe* categories are not included in standard NICHD definitions of FHR decelerations. Consistent with NICHD terminology, all decelerations are quantitated by depth in beats per minute and duration in minutes and seconds.

V-Shaped Variables and W-Shaped Variables

The visual appearance of a variable deceleration has been suggested to predict the underlying cause. For example, a *V-shaped* variable deceleration has been suggested to indicate umbilical cord compression caused by oligohydramnios, whereas a *W-shaped* variable deceleration has been suggested to reflect umbilical cord compression caused by a nuchal cord. There is no evidence in the literature to confirm this distinction. These terms are not included in standardized NICHD terminology.

Good Variability Within the Deceleration

At the nadir of a variable or late deceleration, the FHR frequently appears irregular, similar to the appearance of moderate variability. The visual similarity has led some to suggest that "variability" during a deceleration has the same clinical significance as baseline variability. Although the concept is physiologically plausible, it has never been studied or confirmed. In addition, it is inconsistent with standard terminology. Variability is a characteristic of the FHR baseline. The term *variability* is not used to qualify periodic or episodic decelerations that interrupt the baseline. In the absence of evidence, the safest approach is to avoid assigning undue significance to this observation.

Other Mechanisms That Lack Scientific Basis

Fetal Head Compression

Early deceleration of the FHR has long been recognized as a benign reflex response to transient compression of the fetal head during a uterine contraction. The innocuous nature of this phenomenon is underscored by the inclusion of early decelerations in NICHD Category I (2008), indicating normal fetal oxygenation. However, some have suggested that intrapartum fetal head compression can cause hypoxic-ischemic brain injury, even in a normally oxygenated fetus [44]. This notion contends that uterine contractions compress the fetal head against the maternal pelvis with such force that fetal intracranial pressure exceeds cerebral perfusion pressure, reducing intracranial blood flow to the point of regional cerebral ischemia, focal hypoxic-ischemic brain injury, and cerebral palsy (CP). Descriptive studies have reported that fetal head pressures during uterine contractions can be more than twice as high as intraamniotic pressures [45]. Other studies have demonstrated changes in fetal cerebral perfusion pressure, cerebral blood flow, and cerebral oxygen consumption during fetal head pressure [46–48]. However, no published Level I or Level II evidence has demonstrated that these changes translate to histologic or clinical evidence of neurologic injury. On the contrary, observations in fetal sheep suggest that the reflex Cushing response to head compression may be protective against such injury [49,50]. Level II evidence, in the form of case-control studies, has identified several perinatal risk factors for CP, including prematurity, infection, hemorrhage, maternal thyroid disease, and congenital malformations. However, no Level I or II evidence has demonstrated a link between any measure of uterine activity and the later development of CP. The notion that localized fetal brain injury can be caused by the mechanical forces of labor is further challenged by Level II evidence from a large cohort study including more than 380,000 spontaneous vaginal deliveries and more than 33,000 cesarean deliveries without labor [51]. Neonates exposed to uterine contractions and maternal expulsive efforts of sufficient frequency, intensity, and duration to result in spontaneous vaginal delivery had no higher rates of mechanical brain injury, in the form of intracranial hemorrhage, than did neonates who were exposed to no uterine contractions. No analytic evidence in the literature has identified any objective measure of uterine activity or maternal expulsive effort as a risk factor for CP. On the contrary, analytic studies have failed to identify an association between uterine activity and CP, much less as a causal relationship. A systematic review of the literature regarding intrapartum fetal head compression concluded that "fetal intracranial pressure is well protected from extracranial forces. Available data do not support intrapartum fetal extracranial pressure as a cause of fetal brain injury" [52]. Finally, there is no evidence in the literature that this hypothetical mechanism of injury could be prevented or mitigated by any known obstetric intervention. In the absence of supporting scientific evidence, this theory should not be used as a foundation for intrapartum management decisions.

Prediction and Prevention of Fetal Stroke

An extension of the theory just described is the notion that FHR and uterine activity monitoring can be used to predict and prevent perinatal arterial ischemic stroke (PAIS). A meta-analysis of four studies reported a possible relationship between abnormal intrapartum FHR patterns and the later diagnosis of PAIS [53]. One of the four studies included only preterm deliveries, did not specify the FHR "abnormalities" that were observed in the control and study groups, and did not control for known confounding factors such as baseline rate; presence or absence of moderate variability; presence or absence of accelerations; or the type, number, duration, or frequency of FHR "abnormalities" [54]. The other three studies included only term deliveries, and none of these demonstrated an independent link between FHR abnormalities and PAIS [55–57]. There is no published evidence supporting a causal relationship between FHR abnormalities and PAIS at any gestational age. There is no published evidence that intrapartum electronic fetal monitoring or uterine activity monitoring is capable of detecting or predicting PAIS or that any form of obstetric intervention is capable of preventing PAIS. There is no

Level I or II evidence linking PAIS independently with any measure of uterine activity or labor duration [12]. This is consistent with the 2007 consensus report of the National Institute of Neurologic Disorders and Stroke and the NICHD, which concluded that "there are no reliable predictors of perinatal ischemic stroke upon which to base prevention or treatment strategies" [19].

The "Fetal Reserve Index"

Some authors have suggested that intrapartum fetal brain injury can be predicted by a proprietary scoring system including maternal and fetal risk factors and certain features of FHR and uterine activity [58]. The authors named their scoring system the "Fetal Reserve Index," and claimed that it identified intrapartum fetal neurologic injury better than a Category III FHR pattern. However, their study did not include a matched control group, did not standardize the diagnosis of intrapartum neurologic injury, did not attempt to ascertain neurologic outcomes in the controls, and failed to control for significant confounding and ascertainment bias in the identification of "cases." Studies of the Fetal Reserve Index do not include Level I or Level II scientific evidence, and they do not permit meaningful conclusions regarding the relationship between maternal–fetal observations and subsequent neurologic outcomes. In the absence of such evidence, the Fetal Reserve Index should not be used as the basis for critical decisions regarding obstetric care.

SUMMARY

The three basic elements of FHR monitoring are (1) definitions, (2) interpretation, and (3) management. A standardized, evidence-based approach to each element facilitates effective communication, promotes patient safety, and helps ensure optimal outcomes.

Standardized definitions have been endorsed by all major professional organizations in the United States representing providers of obstetric care. The simple agreement to adopt a common language sets the stage for the next essential step. Standardized FHR interpretation requires a critical assessment of the scientific evidence underlying the relationships between FHR patterns and fetal physiology. This chapter has reviewed in detail the relationships between specific FHR patterns and fetal physiology with particular emphasis on evidence-based interpretation. Regarding the relationship between FHR patterns and fetal oxygenation, evidence-based FHR interpretation can be distilled into two basic concepts. These concepts are illustrated in Fig. 5.17.

The concepts developed in this chapter form the basis of systematic management of FHR patterns discussed in Chapter 6.

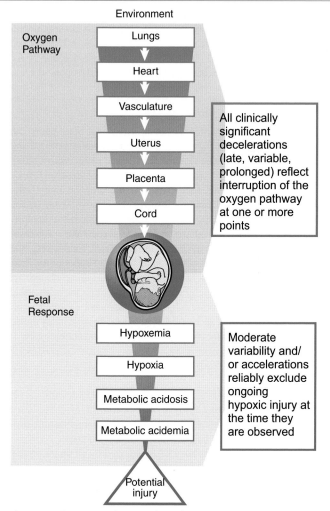

Fig. 5.17 Two central principles of intrapartum fetal heart rate interpretation.

References

[1] Electronic fetal heart rate monitoring: research guidelines for interpretation. National Institute of Child Health and Human Development Research Planning Workshop, Am. J. Obstet. Gynecol. 177 (1997) 1385–1390.

[2] J. Itskovitz, E.F. LaGamma, A.M. Rudolph, Effect of cord compression on fetal blood flow distribution and O_2 delivery, Am. J. Physiol. 252 (1987) H100–H109.

[3] American College of Obstetricians and Gynecologists, Intrapartum fetal heart rate monitoring. ACOG Practice Bulletin No.70, Obstet. Gynecol. 106 (2005) 1453–1461.

[4] A. Fleischer, H. Schulman, N. Jagani, J. Mitchell, G. Randolph, The development of fetal acidosis in the presence of an abnormal fetal heart rate tracing. I. The average for gestational age fetus, Am. J. Obstet. Gynecol. 144 (1982) 55–60.

[5] J.A. Low, R.S. Galbraith, D.W. Muir, H.L. Killen, E.A. Pater, E.J. Karchmar, Factors associated with motor and cognitive deficits in children after intrapartum fetal hypoxia, Am. J. Obstet. Gynecol. 148 (1982) 533–539.

[6] I. Ingemarsson, A. Herbst, K. Thorgren-Jerneck, Long term outcome after umbilical artery acidemia at term birth: influence of gender and fetal heart rate abnormalities, Br. J. Obstet. Gynaecol. 104 (1997) 1123–1127.

[7] J.T. Parer, T. King, S. Flanders, M. Fox, S.J. Kilpatrick, Fetal acidemia and electronic fetal heart rate patterns: is there evidence of an association? J. Matern. Fetal Neonatal Med. 19 (2006) 289–294.

[8] J.T. Parer, T. Ikeda, A framework for standardized management of intrapartum fetal heart rate patterns, Am. J. Obstet. Gynecol. 197 (2007) 26e1–26e6.

[9] C.G. Hatjis, P.J. Meis, Sinusoidal fetal heart rate pattern associated with butorphanol administration, Obstet. Gynecol. 67 (1986) 377–380.

[10] M. Hallak, J. Martinez-Poyer, M.L. Kruger, S. Hassan, S.C. Blackwell, Y. Sorokin, The effect of magnesium sulfate on fetal heart rate parameters: a randomized, placebo-controlled trial, Am. J. Obstet. Gynecol. 181 (1999) 1122–1127.

[11] G. Giannina, E.R. Guzman, Y.L. Lai, M.F. Lake, M. Cernadas, A.M. Vintzileos, Comparison of the effects of meperidine and nalbuphine on intrapartum fetal heart rate tracings, Obstet. Gynecol. 86 (1995) 441–445.

[12] S.L. Clark, M.L. Gimovski, F.C. Miller, Fetal heart rate response to scalp blood sampling, Am. J. Obstet. Gynecol. 144 (1982) 706–708.

[13] C.V. Smith, H.N. Nguyen, J.P. Phelan, R.H. Paul, Intrapartum assessment of fetal well-being: a comparison of fetal acoustic stimulation with acid base determinations, Am. J. Obstet. Gynecol. 155 (1986) 726–728.

[14] J.A. Read, F.C. Miller, Fetal heart rate aceleration in response to acoustic stimulation as a measure of fetal well-being, Am. J. Obstet. Gynecol. 129 (1997) 512–517.

[15] A. Elimian, R. Figueroa, N. Tejani, Intrapartum assessment of fetal well being: a comparison of scalp stimulation with scalp blood pH sampling, Obstet. Gynecol. 89 (1997) 373–376.

[16] E.A. Kopecky, M.L. Ryan, J.F. Barrett, P.G. Seaward, G. Ryan, G. Koren, et al., Fetal response to maternally administered morphine, Am. J. Obstet. Gynecol. 183 (2000) 424–430.

[17] C.B. Martin Jr., J. de Haan, B. van der Wildt, H.W. Jongsma, A. Dieleman, T.H. Arts, Mechanisms of late decelerations in the fetal heart rate. A study with autonomic blocking agents in fetal lambs, Eur. J. Obstet. Gynecol. Reprod. Biol. 9 (6) (1979) 361–373.

[18] H.E. Cohn, E.J. Sacks, M.A. Heymann, A.M. Rudolph, Cardiovascular response to hypoxemia and acidemia in fetal lambs, Am. J. Obstet. Gynecol. 120 (1974) 817–824.

[19] L.L. Peeters, R.D. Sheldon, M.D. Jones, E.L. Makowski, G. Meschia, Blood flow to fetal organs as a function of arterial oxygen content, Am. J. Obstet. Gynecol. 135 (1979) 637–646.

[20] B.S. Richardson, D. Rurak, J.E. Patrick, J. Homan, L. Carmichael, Cerebral oxidative metabolism during prolonged hypoxemia, J. Dev. Physiol. 11 (1989) 37–43.

[21] D.R. Field, J.T. Parer, R.A. Auslander, D.B. Cheek, W. Baker, J. Johnson, Cerebral oxygen consumption during asphyxia in fetal sheep, J. Dev. Physiol. 14 (1990) 131–137.

[22] D.L. Reid, J.T. Parer, K. Williams, D. Darr, T.M. Phermaton, J.H.H. Rankin, Effects of severe reduction in maternal placental blood flow on blood flow distribution in the sheep fetus, J. Dev. Physiol. 15 (1991) 183–188.

[23] A. Jensen, C. Roman, A.M. Rudolph, Effects of reducing uterine blood flow on fetal blood flow distribution and oxygen delivery, J. Dev. Physiol. 15 (1991) 309–323.

[24] R.H. Ball, M.I. Expinoza, J.T. Parer, Regional blood flow in asphyxiated fetuses with seizures, Am. J. Obstet. Gynecol. 170 (1994) 156–161.

[25] R.H. Ball, J.T. Parer, L.E. Caldwell, J. Johnson, Regional blood flow and metabolism in ovine fetuses during severe cord occlusion, Am. J. Obstet. Gynecol. 171 (1994) 1549–1555.

[26] J. Barcroft, Researches in Prenatal Life, Blackwell Scientific Publications, Oxford, UK, 1946.

[27] M.D. Towell, H.S. Salvador, Compression of the umbilical cord, in: P. Crasignoni, G. Pardi (Eds.), An Experimental Model in the Fetal Goat, Fetal Evaluation during Pregnancy and Labor, Academic Press, New York, 1971, pp. 143–156.

[28] S.T. Lee, E.H. Hon, Fetal hemodynamic response to umbilical cord compression, Obstet. Gynecol. 22 (1963) 553–562.

[29] M.N. Yeh, H.O. Morishima, W.E. Niemann, L.S. James, Myocardial conduction defects in association with compression of the umbilical cord. Experimental observations on fetal baboons, Am. J. Obstet. Gynecol. 121 (1975) 951–957.

[30] B. Siassi, P.Y. Wu, C. Blanco, C.B. Martin, Baroreceptor and chemoreceptor responses to umbilical cord occlusion in fetal lambs, Biol. Neonate. 35 (1979) 66–73.

[31] J. Itskovitz, E.F. LaGamma, A.M. Rudolph, Heart rate and blood pressure responses to umbilical cord compression in fetal lambs with special reference to the mechanism of variable deceleration, Am. J. Obstet. Gynecol. 147 (1983) 451–457.

[32] J. Itskovitz, E.F. LaGamma, A.M. Rudolph, The effect of reducing umbilical blood flow on fetal oxygenation, Am. J. Obstet. Gynecol. 145 (1983) 813–818.

[33] L.S. James, M.N. Yeh, H.O. Morishima, S.S. Daniel, S.N. Caritis, W.H. Niemann, et al., Umbilical vein occlusion and transient acceleration of the fetal heart rate. Experimental observations in subhuman primates, Am. J. Obstet. Gynecol. 126 (1976) 276–283.

[34] E. Mueller-Heubach, A.F. Battelli, Variable heart rate decelerations and transcutaneous Po_2 during umbilical cord occlusion in fetal monkeys, Am. J. Obstet. Gynecol. 144 (1982) 796–802.

[35] C.Y. Lee, P.C. Di Loreto, J.M. O'Lane, A study of fetal heart rate acceleration patterns, Obstet. Gynecol. 45 (1975) 142–146.

[36] K. Brubaker, T.J. Garite, The lambda fetal heart rate pattern: an assessment of its significance in the intrapartum period, Obstet. Gynecol. 72 (1988) 881–885.

[37] J.A. Westgate, L. Bennet, H.H. de Haan, A.J. Gunn, Fetal heart rate overshoot during repeated umbilical cord occlusion in sheep, Obstet. Gynecol. 97 (2001) 454–459.

[38] J.R. Shields, B.S. Schifrin, Perinatal antecedents of cerebral palsy, Obstet. Gynecol. 71 (1988) 899–905.

[39] J. Saito, K. Okamura, K. Akagi, S. Tanigawara, Y. Shintaku, T. Watanabe, et al., Alteration of FHR pattern associated with progressively advanced fetal acidemia caused by cord compression, Nippon Sanka Fujinka Gakkai Zasshi 40 (1988) 775–780.

[40] B.S. Schifrin, T. Hamilton-Rubinstein, J.R. Shield, Fetal heart rate patterns and the timing of fetal injury, J. Perinatol. 14 (1994) 174–181.

[41] R.C. Goodlin, E.W. Lowe, A functional umbilical cord occlusion heart rate pattern. The significance of overshoot, Obstet. Gynecol. 43 (1974) 22–30.

[42] C.Y. Spong, C. Rasul, J.Y. Collea, G.S. Eglinton, A. Ghidini, Characterization and prognostic significance of variable decelerations in the second stage of labor, Am. J. Perinatol. 15 (1998) 369–374.

[43] F.W. Kubli, E.H. Hon, A.F. Khazin, H. Takemura, Observations on heart rate and pH in the human fetus during labor, Am. J. Obstet. Gynecol. 104 (1969) 1190–1206.

[44] B.S. Schifrin, S. Ater, Fetal hypoxic and ischemic injuries, Curr. Opin. Obstet. Gynecol. 18 (2006) 112–122.

[45] L. Svenningsen, R. Lindemann, K. Eidal, Measurements of fetal head compression pressure during bearing down and their relationship to the

condition of the newborn, Acta Obstet. Gynecol. Scand. 67 (2) (1988) 129–133.

[46] L.I. Mann, A. Carmichael, S. Duchin, The effect of head compression on FHR, brain metabolism, and function, Obstet. Gynecol. 39 (1972) 721–726.

[47] W.F. O'Brien, S.E. Davis, M.P. Grissom, R.R. Eng, S.M. Golden, Effect of cephalic pressure on fetal cerebral blood flow, Am. J. Perinatol. 1 (1984) 223–226.

[48] C.J. Aldrich, D. D'Antona, J.A. Spencer, et al., The effect of maternal pushing on fetal cerebral oxygenation and blood volume during the second stage of labour, Br. J. Obstet. Gynaecol. 102 (1995) 448–453.

[49] A.P. Harris, R.C. Koehler, C.A. Gleason, M.D. Jones Jr., R.J. Traystman, Cerebral and peripheral circulatory responses to intracranial hypertension in fetal sheep, Circ. Res. 64 (5) (1989) 991–1000.

[50] A.P. Harris, S. Helou, R.J. Traystman, M.D. Jones Jr., R.C. Koehler, Efficacy of the Cushing response in maintaining cerebral blood flow in premature and near-term fetal sheep, Pediatr. Res. 43 (1) (1998 Jan) 50–56.

[51] D. Towner, M.A. Castro, E. Eby-Wilkens, W.M. Gilbert, Effect of mode of delivery in nulliparous women on neonatal intracranial injury, N. Engl. J. Med. 341 (1999) 1709–1714.

[52] K.D. Heybourne, A systematic review of intrapartum fetal head compression: what is the impact on the fetal brain? Am. J. Perinatol. Rep. 7 (2017) e79–e85.

[53] L. Luo, D. Chen, Y. Qu, J. Wu, X. Li, D Mu, Association between hypoxia and perinatal arterial ischemic stroke: a meta-analysis, PLoS One 9 (2) (2014) e90106. http://dx.doi.org/10.1371/journal.pone.0090106.

[54] M.J. Benders, F. Groenendaal, C.S. Uiterwaal, P.G. Nikkels, H.W. Bruinse, et al., Maternal and infant characteristics associated with perinatal arterial stroke in the preterm infant, Stroke 38 (6) (2007) 1759–1765.

[55] J. Lee, L.A. Croen, K.H. Backstrand, C.K. Yoshida, L.H. Henning, C. Lindan, D.M. Ferriero, H.J. Fullerton, A.J. Barkovich, Y.W. Wu, Maternal and infant characteristics associated with perinatal arterial stroke in the infant, JAMA 293 (6) (2005) 723–729.

[56] V. Darmency-Stamboul, C. Chantegret, C. Ferdynus, N. Mejean, C. Durand, P. Sagot, M. Giroud, Y. Bejot, J.B. Gouyon, Antenatal factors associated with perinatal arterial ischemic stroke, Stroke 43 (9) (2012) 2307–2312.

[57] J.C. Harteman, F. Groenendaal, A. Kwee, P.M. Welsing, M.J. Benders, L.S. de Vries, Risk factors for perinatal arterial ischaemic stroke in full-term infants: a case-control study, Arch. Dis. Child. Fetal Neonatal Ed. 97 (6) (2012) F411–F416.

[58] R.D. Eden, M.I. Evans, S.M. Evans, B.S. Schifrin, The "Fetal Reserve Index": re-engineering the interpretation and responses to fetal heart rate patterns, Fetal Diagn. Ther. 43 (2) (2018) 90–104.

CHAPTER 6

Intrapartum Management of the Fetal Heart Rate Tracing

Chapters 2 and 4 provided the physiologic basis for fetal heart rate (FHR) monitoring and evaluation of uterine activity. Chapter 5 reviewed the standardized National Institute of Child Health and Human Development (NICHD) definitions and introduced an evidence-based approach to the interpretation of FHR patterns. This chapter incorporates those previously developed concepts and presents a systematic, comprehensive, and multidisciplinary approach to management of intrapartum FHR tracings.

FUNDAMENTAL PRINCIPLES

As introduced in Chapter 5, fetal oxygenation involves the transfer of oxygen from the environment to the fetus along the oxygen pathway, and the potential consequences of interruption of this pathway. Two central principles of evidence-based FHR interpretation provide the foundation for a systematic approach to FHR management. Fig. 6.1 illustrates these principles. They are as follows:

1. All clinically significant decelerations (late, variable, prolonged) reflect interruption of the oxygen pathway at one or more points
2. Moderate variability and/or accelerations reliably exclude ongoing hypoxic injury at the time they are observed.

A standardized approach to intrapartum FHR management does not replace individual clinical judgment. On the contrary, standardized intrapartum FHR management is intended to encourage the timely application of individual clinical judgment and to serve as a systematic reminder of potential sources of preventable error in an effort to optimize outcomes and minimize risk. The model described in this chapter uses the standardized FHR definitions and categories proposed by the NICHD in 2008 [1]. It does not include adjunctive tests of fetal status such as fetal scalp blood sampling, fetal pulse oximetry, and fetal ST segment analysis that are currently unavailable for general clinical use in the United States. These techniques are reviewed at the end of the chapter.

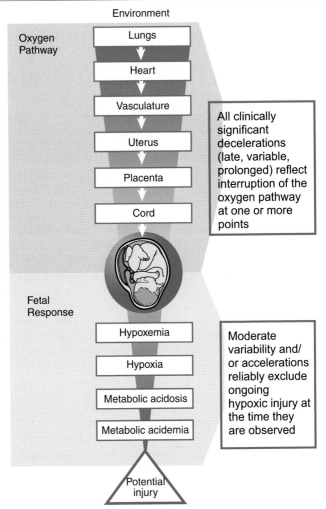

Fig. 6.1 Two central principles of intrapartum fetal heart rate interpretation.

Standard of Care

The standard of care mandates that practitioners provide patient care that is reasonable. Reasonableness derives from credibility, which in turn is founded on factual accuracy and the ability to articulate a clear and understandable rationale for the care that is proposed. Standard definitions and interpretation help ensure factual accuracy. A standardized approach to management provides a framework for organized, evidence-based planning that can minimize variation, reduce the potential for preventable error, and be articulated clearly and understandably.

Confirm Fetal Heart Rate and Uterine Activity

Reliable information is vital to the success of intrapartum FHR monitoring. Therefore the first step in standardized management is to confirm that the monitor is recording the FHR and uterine activity accurately (Fig. 6.2). If external monitoring is not adequate for definition and interpretation, a fetal scalp electrode and/or intrauterine pressure catheter might provide useful information. Under certain circumstances, the FHR monitor can inadvertently record the maternal heart rate. For example, if the fetus is not alive, an internal fetal scalp electrode will record the maternal heart rate. An external Doppler device can record the maternal heart rate even if the fetus is alive. Particularly in the setting of maternal tachycardia, the maternal heart rate can appear deceptively similar to a normal FHR. At times the monitor can alternately record the fetus and the mother. When switching from one to the other, the tracing does not necessarily demonstrate discontinuity; therefore continuity of the tracing alone should not be relied on to exclude this phenomenon. Unless the monitor is recording the FHR, it cannot provide information regarding the condition of the fetus. Thus it is essential to distinguish between the heart rates of the mother and the fetus. If there is any question, consider other methods such as ultrasound, palpation of the maternal pulse, fetal scalp electrode, or maternal pulse oximetry.

Evaluate Fetal Heart Rate Components

Thorough, systematic evaluation of an FHR tracing includes assessment of uterine contractions along with the FHR components defined by the NICHD: baseline rate, variability, accelerations, decelerations, sinusoidal pattern, and changes or trends in the tracing over time. The 2008 NICHD consensus report defined three categories of FHR tracings as summarized in Table 6.1 [1]. If all FHR components are normal (Category I), then the FHR tracing reliably predicts the absence of fetal metabolic acidemia and ongoing hypoxic injury. The American College of Obstetrics and Gynecology (ACOG) Practice Bulletin 106 and ACOG American Academy of Pediatrics (AAP) Guidelines for Perinatal Care recommend that, in low-risk patients, the FHR tracing should be reviewed at least every 30 minutes during the active phase of the first stage of labor and at least every 15 minutes

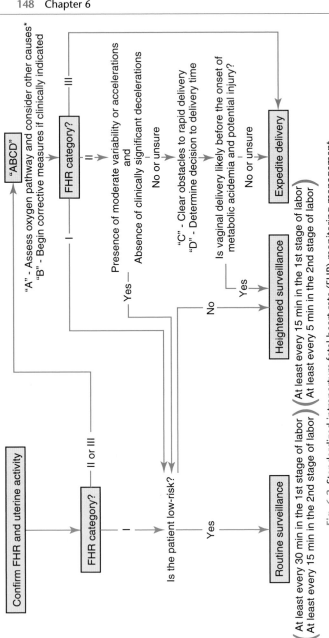

Fig. 6.2 Standardized intrapartum fetal heart rate (FHR) monitoring management.

TABLE 6.1   Three-Tier Fetal Heart Rate Classification System

Category I	
Normal	FHR tracing includes all of the following:
	Baseline rate: 110–160 bpm
	Baseline FHR variability: moderate
	Accelerations: present or absent
	Late or variable decelerations absent
	Early decelerations present or absent
Category II	
Indeterminate	Includes all FHR tracings not assigned to Categories I or III
Category III	
Abnormal	FHR tracing includes at least one of the following:
	Absent variability with recurrent late decelerations
	Absent variability with recurrent variable decelerations
	Absent variability with bradycardia for at least 10 minutes
	Sinusoidal pattern for at least 20 minutes

FHR, fetal heart rate.

Adapted from G.A. Macones et al., The 2008 National Institute of Child Health and Human Development workshop report on electronic fetal monitoring: update on definitions, interpretation, and research guidelines, Obstet. Gynecol. 112 (2008) 661–666.

during the second stage [2,3]. In high-risk patients, the FHR tracing should be reviewed at least every 15 minutes during the active phase of the first stage of labor and at least every 5 minutes during the second stage (see Fig. 6.2). As reasonably feasible, nursing documentation should comply with hospital policies and procedures. Physician and midwife documentation should be performed periodically. The timing and content of documentation should be guided by the clinical scenario and reasonable clinical judgment. Documentation and risk management issues are discussed in detail in Chapter 10.

A Standardized "ABCD" Approach to Fetal Heart Rate Management

As reviewed in previous chapters, FHR tracings in Category I reflect normal fetal oxygenation. If assessment of FHR components indicates that the tracing is not Category I, further evaluation is warranted. A practical, systematic "ABCD" approach to management is as follows:

A: Assess the oxygen pathway (and consider other possible causes of FHR changes)

B: Begin conservative corrective measures as needed

C: Clear obstacles to rapid delivery

D: Delivery plan

This approach is summarized in Table 6.2.

TABLE 6.2   ABCD Fetal Heart Rate Management

	"A" Assess Oxygen Pathway	"B" Begin Corrective Measures[a]		"C" Clear Obstacles to Rapid Delivery	"D" Determine Decision to Delivery Time
Lungs	Respiration	Oxygen	Facility	Consider OR availability Equipment	Facility response time
Heart	Heart rate	Position changes Fluid bolus Correct hypotension	Staff	Consider notifying Obstetrician Surgical assistant Anesthesiologist Neonatologist Pediatrician Nursing staff	Consider staff: Availability Training Experience
Vasculature	Blood pressure		Mother	Consider Informed consent Anesthesia options Laboratory tests Blood products Intravenous access Urinary catheter Abdominal prep Transfer to OR	Surgical considerations (prior surgery) Medical considerations (obesity, diabetes) Obstetric considerations (parity, pelvimetry)

TABLE 6.2 ABCD Fetal Heart Rate Management—cont'd

	"A" Assess Oxygen Pathway	"B" Begin Corrective Measures[a]		"C" Clear Obstacles to Rapid Delivery	"D" Determine Decision to Delivery Time
Uterus	Contraction strength Contraction frequency Contraction duration Baseline uterine tone Exclude uterine rupture	Reduce stimulant Uterine relaxant	Fetus	Consider Fetal number Fetal weight Gestational age Presentation Position Anomalies	Consider Fetal number Estimated fetal weight Gestational age Presentation Position Anomalies
Placenta Cord	Check for bleeding Exclude cord prolapse	Amnioinfusion	Labor	Confirm that contraction monitoring is adequate to allow appropriately informed management decisions	Consider factors such as: Protracted labor Previous uterine relaxant Remote from delivery Poor expulsive efforts

[a]Conservative corrective measures should be guided by clinical circumstances. For example, amnioinfusion may be appropriate in the presence of variable decelerations but would not be expected to result in resolution of late decelerations.

Examples of clinical factors to be considered in a systematic fashion. Institutions may modify to individual circumstances.

OR, operating room.

A: Assess the Oxygen Pathway and Consider Other Causes of Fetal Heart Rate Changes

Rapid, systematic assessment of the pathway of oxygen transfer from the environment to the fetus can identify potential sources of interrupted oxygenation. Assessment of the maternal lungs can be as simple as checking the respiratory rate. The heart and the vasculature usually can be assessed by checking the maternal pulse and blood pressure. Uterine activity can be assessed by palpation or by review of the information obtained from a tocodynamometer or intrauterine pressure catheter. In the appropriate clinical setting, evaluation for the possibility of uterine rupture may be warranted. The possibility of placental separation can be assessed by checking for vaginal bleeding. Finally, the possibility of umbilical cord prolapse can be assessed by visual examination or by a vaginal examination. If rapid evaluation of these steps suggests that further investigation is warranted, it should be undertaken as deemed necessary. Chapter 5 identified a number of maternal and fetal factors that can influence the appearance of the FHR tracing by mechanisms other than interruption of fetal oxygenation (Box 6.1). If the FHR changes are thought to be caused by any condition not directly related to fetal oxygenation, then individualized management should be directed at the specific cause. Enhancement of fetal oxygenation cannot reasonably be expected to resolve FHR abnormalities that are not related to oxygenation. For example, supplemental oxygen, maternal position changes, and intravenous fluid boluses are unlikely to correct

---

BOX 6.1   Causes of Fetal Heart Rate Changes Not Directly Related to Fetal Oxygenation

Maternal
- Fever
- Infection
- Medication
- Hyperthyroidism

Fetal
- Sleep cycle
- Infection
- Anemia
- Arrhythmia
- Heart block
- Congenital anomaly
- Preexisting neurologic injury
- Extreme prematurity

fetal tachycardia that is secondary to fetal arrhythmia or severe fetal anemia caused by parvovirus infection or Rh isoimmunization. Corrective interventions for conditions such as fetal arrhythmias or severe fetal anemia can be extremely complex and usually require subspecialty consultation. Diagnosis and management of conditions such as these is beyond the scope of this chapter.

B: Begin Corrective Measures as Indicated

At each point along the oxygen pathway, conservative corrective measures are initiated, if indicated, to optimize fetal oxygenation (see Table 6.2). Scientific evidence supporting the efficacy of each of these measures is detailed in an excellent review by Simpson and James [4]. These conservative corrective measures are summarized next.

Supplemental Oxygen

Fetal oxygenation is dependent on the oxygen content of maternal blood perfusing the intervillous space of the placenta, as discussed in Chapter 2. Administration of supplemental oxygen increases the Po_2 of inspired air, increasing both the partial pressure of oxygen dissolved in maternal blood and the amount of oxygen bound to hemoglobin. This can increase the oxygen concentration gradient across the placental blood–blood barrier and lead to increased fetal Po_2 and oxygen content. Several studies have reported resolution of FHR decelerations after administration of supplemental oxygen to the mother, providing indirect evidence of improved fetal oxygenation [4]. Direct evidence is provided by fetal pulse oximetry studies demonstrating increased fetal hemoglobin saturation after maternal administration of oxygen. Although the optimal method and duration of oxygen administration have not been established definitively, available data support the use of a nonrebreather face mask to administer oxygen at a rate of 10 L/min for approximately 15 to 30 minutes [4].

Maternal Position Changes

There are sound physiologic reasons to avoid the supine position during labor. Supine positioning increases the likelihood that pressure on the inferior vena cava will impair venous return, cardiac output, perfusion of the uterine, and perfusion of the intervillous space of the placenta. It also increases the likelihood that pressure on the descending aorta and/or iliac vessels will impede the delivery of oxygenated blood to the uterus and placenta. Prospective fetal pulse oximetry data confirm that maternal left or right lateral positioning results in higher fetal hemoglobin saturation levels than does supine positioning [4]. In the setting of suspected umbilical cord compression, maternal position changes may result in fetal position changes and relief of pressure on the umbilical cord.

Intravenous Fluid Administration

Optimal uterine perfusion depends on optimal cardiac output and intravascular volume. Normal blood pressure does not necessarily reflect optimal intravascular volume, venous return, preload, or cardiac output. An intravascular bolus of isotonic fluid can improve cardiac output not only by increasing circulating volume but also by increasing venous return, left ventricular end diastolic pressure, ventricular preload, and, ultimately, stroke volume in accordance with the Frank–Starling mechanism. In this way, a relatively small increase in intravascular volume can have a significant effect on cardiac output and uterine perfusion. An intravenous fluid bolus of 500 to 1000 mL can result in improved fetal oxygenation even in an apparently euvolemic patient [4]. Excessive fluid administration can have serious consequences, and caution must be exercised in patients at risk for volume overload, pulmonary edema, or both. The optimal rate of intravenous fluid administration during labor has not been established definitively. Potential maternal and fetal complications argue against routine administration of large-volume intravenous boluses of glucose-containing fluids.

Correct Maternal Blood Pressure

A number of factors predispose laboring women to transient episodes of hypotension. These include inadequate hydration, insensible fluid losses, supine position resulting in compression of the inferior vena cava, decreased venous return and reduced cardiac output, and peripheral vasodilation caused by sympathetic blockade during regional anesthesia. Maternal hypotension can reduce uterine perfusion and fetal oxygenation. Hydration and lateral or Trendelenburg positioning usually correct the blood pressure. If these measures do not achieve the desired result, medication may be necessary. Ephedrine is a sympathomimetic amine with weak α- and β-agonist activity. The primary mechanism of action is the release of norepinephrine from presynaptic vesicles, resulting in stimulation of postsynaptic adrenergic receptors. Ephedrine has no known adverse effect on fetal outcome.

Reduce Uterine Activity

As discussed in previous chapters, excessive uterine activity is a common cause of interrupted fetal oxygenation. It is also a common source of medicolegal liability. Clinicians have used a number of terms to describe excessive uterine activity. Examples include *hyperstimulation, hypercontractility, tachysystole, hypertonus,* and *tetanic contraction.* These terms are defined inconsistently in the literature and are used inconsistently by clinicians. The 2008 NICHD consensus statement recommended using the term *tachysystole* to describe uterine contraction frequency in excess of five contractions in 10 minutes averaged over 30 minutes [1]. Normal contraction frequency is defined as five or fewer contractions in 10 minutes averaged over 30 minutes. The report specifically noted that other features of uterine activity are clinically important as well, including contraction duration, intensity, resting tone, and time between contractions. For the purposes of FHR management, if an abnormal FHR pattern is thought to be related to excessive uterine activity, options include position changes, intravenous hydration, reduction in dose or discontinuation of uterine stimulants, and/or administration of uterine relaxants. The evaluation and management of uterine activity are discussed in detail in Chapter 4.

Alter Second-stage Pushing Technique

During the second stage of labor, maternal expulsive efforts can be associated with FHR decelerations. Suggested corrective approaches include open-glottis rather than Valsalva-style pushing, fewer pushing efforts per contraction, shorter individual pushing efforts, pushing with every other or every third contraction, and, in patients with regional anesthesia, pushing only with perceived urge [4].

Amnioinfusion

Intrapartum amnioinfusion involves infusion of isotonic fluid through an intrauterine catheter into the amniotic cavity to restore the amniotic fluid volume to normal or near-normal levels. The procedure is intended to relieve intermittent umbilical cord compression, variable FHR decelerations, and transient fetal hypoxemia and to dilute thick meconium in an attempt to prevent meconium aspiration syndrome. Amnioinfusion performed for the indication of oligohydramnios and umbilical cord compression can reduce the occurrence of variable decelerations and lower the rate of cesarean delivery. It has no known effect on late decelerations. Routine amnioinfusion for meconium-stained amniotic fluid without variable decelerations is not recommended by ACOG [5]. A procedure for amnioinfusion is described in Appendix A. A systematic approach to FHR management does not require the use of all of these measures in every situation. It simply helps to ensure that important considerations are not overlooked and that decisions are made in a timely manner. In addition, it provides a framework to help clinicians articulate a thoughtful, organized plan of management, a key element of reasonableness and the standard of care.

Reevaluate the Fetal Heart Rate Tracing

After assessing the oxygen pathway and beginning corrective measures that are deemed appropriate, the tracing is reevaluated. The time frame for reevaluation is based on reasonable clinical judgment and usually ranges from 5 to 30 minutes, in accordance with ACOG-AAP guidelines [2,3]. If the FHR tracing returns to Category I, continued surveillance is likely appropriate. The decision to perform routine or heightened surveillance is based on reasonable clinical judgment, taking into account the entire clinical situation. If the FHR tracing progresses to Category III despite appropriate conservative corrective measures, delivery is usually expedited. Tracings that remain in Category II warrant additional evaluation. Category II is extremely broad. It includes some FHR tracings for which continued surveillance may be appropriate; however, it also includes some tracings that may require preparations for rapid delivery. If a Category II FHR tracing reveals clinically insignificant interruption of fetal oxygenation (absent or infrequent decelerations) and excludes fetal metabolic acidemia and ongoing hypoxic injury (moderate variability and/or accelerations), continued surveillance likely is reasonable. Category II tracings that do not meet these criteria require further measures. If there is any question regarding the clinical significance of any decelerations, the presence of moderate variability or the presence of accelerations, the safest and easiest approach is to take the next step in the ABCD management model.

C: Clear Obstacles to Rapid Delivery

If conservative corrective measures do not result in moderate variability (and/or accelerations) and resolution of clinically significant decelerations, it is prudent to plan ahead for the possible need for rapid delivery. Planning ahead does not constitute a commitment to a particular time or method of delivery. Instead, it serves as a systematic reminder of common sources of unnecessary delay so that important factors are not overlooked and decisions are made in a timely manner. This can be accomplished by systematically gathering necessary information and communicating proactively with other members of the team. Potential sources of unnecessary delay can be grouped into five major categories. Organized in nonrandom order, from largest to smallest, these five categories include the facility, staff, mother, fetus, and labor. Table 6.2 identifies some examples of potential sources of unnecessary delay at each level. Standardized intrapartum FHR management does not mandate that each of these measures is performed. It simply provides a practical checklist of factors to consider under common circumstances. The checklist approach promotes team communication, encourages timely decision-making, and minimizes preventable errors.

D: Delivery Plan

After appropriate conservative measures have been implemented, it is sensible to take a moment to estimate the time needed to accomplish delivery in the event of a sudden deterioration of the FHR tracing. The anticipated decision-to-delivery time must be taken into consideration when weighing the risks and benefits of continued expectant management versus expeditious delivery. This step can be facilitated by systematically considering individual characteristics of the facility, staff, mother, fetus, and labor (see Table 6.2).

Management steps A, B, C, and D are largely uncontroversial. They are readily amenable to standardization and represent the majority of decisions that must be made during labor. However, once they are exhausted, further management decisions rely on the reasonable clinical judgment of the care provider who is ultimately responsible for the timing and method of delivery.

Expectant Management Versus Delivery

If conservative measures are unsuccessful, the clinician must decide whether to await spontaneous vaginal delivery or to expedite delivery by other means. This decision demands reasonable clinical judgment, weighing the estimated time until vaginal delivery against the estimated time until the onset of potential injury. In 2013 Clark and colleagues proposed a standardized approach to the management of persistent Category II FHR tracings [6]. The authors recommended that, in the setting of moderate variability or accelerations and normal progress in the active phase or second stage of labor, expectant management with close observation is reasonable in most cases, regardless of the presence of decelerations.

One exception is a prolonged deceleration, which requires prompt evaluation and intervention. Another is the setting in which vaginal bleeding and/or previous cesarean delivery(ies) introduce the risks of placental abruption or uterine rupture. If moderate variability and accelerations are absent and recurrent significant decelerations fail to respond to corrective measures for approximately 30 minutes, the algorithm suggests that delivery should be considered regardless of the stage of labor. If moderate variability and accelerations are absent *without* recurrent decelerations, the authors recommended consideration of delivery after approximately 60 minutes. These recommendations reflect the consensus of 18 authors regarding one reasonable approach to persistent Category II FHR patterns. No single approach to such patterns has been demonstrated to be superior to all others. However, there is a growing body of evidence supporting the concept that the adoption of one appropriate management plan, by virtue of standardization alone, will yield results superior to those achieved by random application of several individually equivalent approaches [6].

In 2018, Shields and colleagues described a standardized algorithm for the management of Category II FHR tracings with recurrent "significant" FHR decelerations [7]. Significant decelerations were defined as late decelerations, prolonged decelerations, or variable decelerations lasting at least 60 seconds and reaching a nadir of ≤60 bpm, or at least 60 bpm below baseline. Six hospitals in a large health system participated in a cohort study comparing maternal and neonatal outcomes before and after the introduction of a standardized management algorithm. Fetal monitor tracings that demonstrated moderate (or marked) variability and significant decelerations with >50% of contractions for 30 minutes were managed as follows. If cervical dilation was <4 cm and recurrent decelerations did not resolve with conservative corrective measures, delivery was accomplished. If cervical dilation was ≥4 cm, labor was permitted to continue only in the presence of normal progress. Normal labor progress in the first stage was defined as cervical dilation ≥1 cm/hr. Normal labor progress in the second stage required descent with pushing, and the total duration of the second stage was limited to 90 minutes. If criteria for normal labor progress were not met, delivery was warranted. If the FHR tracing demonstrated a persistent pattern of minimal-absent variability, delivery was indicated regardless of labor progress. Before introduction of the standardized management algorithm, the rate of primary cesarean birth among eligible deliveries was 19.8%. After introduction of the standardized algorithm, the rate of primary cesarean birth was 18.3%, a statistically significant difference ($P < 0.05$). Introduction of the algorithm was associated with a statistically significant reduction in low 5-minute Apgar scores (from 2.3% to 1.7%). In addition, the authors reported a statistically significant reduction (from 1.6% to 1.2%) in severe newborn complications, defined as a composite of severe respiratory complications, sepsis, birth trauma, neonatal shock, or neurologic injury. During the same time period, the 23 hospitals that did not use the standardized management algorithm experienced a reduction in primary cesarean births from 19% to 18.2% ($P = 0.02$), but no improvements in Apgar scores or newborn complications. Importantly, the authors noted that nearly 98% of screened patients were managed according to the recommendations of the algorithm. If the results of this study can be replicated in other clinical settings, they may provide valuable guidance in the management of some of the most difficult FHR tracings. In the meantime, it seems reasonable to consider adopting more conservative expectations for normal labor progress, such as those described in this study, in a subset of patients with significant recurrent decelerations or minimal-absent variability that persist despite appropriate conservative corrective measures.

In the setting of a persistent Category II FHR tracing, a common, preventable error in management is to postpone a difficult decision in the hope that the situation will resolve on its own. It is highly advisable in this setting to resist the urge to delay an indicated decision. Instead, the clinician should use discipline and individual clinical judgment to make and document a plan based on the best information available. If the clinician decides to expedite delivery, the rationale should be documented, and the plan should be implemented. If the clinician decides to continue to wait for vaginal delivery, the rationale and plan should be documented, and the decision should be revisited after a reasonable period of time. It is critical to recognize that, both medically and legally, "deciding to wait" is distinctly different from "waiting to decide." The former reflects the application of clinical judgment, whereas the latter can be construed as procrastination. As long as reasonable judgment is exercised, "deciding to wait" is likely to be defensible. "Waiting to decide," however, puts the clinician in the difficult position of trying to explain why he or she neglected to make a medically necessary decision in a timely fashion.

The standardized management algorithms detailed in this chapter summarize an organized, systematic framework that can help clinicians at all levels of training and experience formulate a care plan that is factually accurate and articulate.

OTHER METHODS OF FETAL MONITORING

One of the major shortcomings of electronic fetal monitoring is a high rate of false-positive results. Even the most abnormal patterns are poorly predictive of neonatal morbidity. This has led to exploration of alternative methods of evaluating fetal status, including fetal scalp pH determination, scalp stimulation or vibroacoustic stimulation, computer analysis of FHR, fetal pulse oximetry, and ST segment analysis. In assessing the immediate condition of the newborn, umbilical cord acid–base determination is an adjunct to the Apgar score.

Intrapartum Fetal Scalp pH and Lactate Determination

Intermittent sampling of scalp blood for pH determination was described in the 1960s and studied extensively in the 1970s. However, its use has been limited by many factors, including the requirements for cervical dilation and membrane rupture, technical difficulty of the procedure, the need for serial pH determinations, and uncertainty regarding interpretation and application of results. It is used infrequently in the United States but remains a common practice in many other countries. A meta-analysis revealed that fetal scalp lactate determination was accomplished successfully more frequently than scalp pH determination. However, there were no differences in maternal, fetal, neonatal, or infant outcomes [8].

Fetal Scalp Stimulation and Vibroacoustic Stimulation

A number of studies in the 1980s reported that an FHR acceleration in response to fetal scalp stimulation or vibroacoustic stimulation was highly predictive of normal scalp blood pH [9–15]. A literature review and meta-analysis by Skupski and colleagues confirmed the utility of various methods of intrapartum fetal stimulation, including scalp puncture, atraumatic stimulation with an Allis clamp, vibroacoustic stimulation, and digital stimulation [16]. It is crucial for clinicians to recognize that fetal scalp stimulation and vibroacoustic stimulation are diagnostic tools used to provoke FHR accelerations to exclude the presence of fetal metabolic acidemia and ongoing fetal hypoxic injury. As noted previously, fetal stimulation procedures should be performed at times when the FHR is at baseline. Neither fetal scalp stimulation nor vibroacoustic stimulation is intended for use during FHR decelerations or bradycardia.

Computer Analysis of Fetal Heart Rate

Subjective interpretation of FHR tracings by visual analysis has been hampered by inconsistency and imprecision. In an attempt to overcome this limitation, Dawes and others derived a system of numeric analysis of FHR [17]. Computer analysis of intrapartum FHR records has been reported to be more precise than visual assessment [18,19]. However, intrapartum computer analysis has not been shown to improve prediction of neonatal outcome. Keith and colleagues reported the results of a multicenter trial of an intelligent computer system using clinical data in addition to FHR data [20]. In 50 cases analyzed, the system's performance was indistinguishable from that of 17 expert clinicians. The authors reported that the system was highly consistent, recommended no unnecessary intervention, and performed better than all but two of the experts.

Fetal Pulse Oximetry

Intrapartum reflectance fetal pulse oximetry is a modification of transmission pulse oximetry that indirectly measures the oxygen saturation of hemoglobin in fetal blood. An intrauterine sensor placed in contact with fetal skin uses the differential absorption of red and infrared light by oxygenated and deoxygenated fetal hemoglobin to provide continuous estimation of fetal oxygen saturation. A number of studies have examined the utility of intrapartum fetal pulse oximetry [21–32].

Although the technology appears to reduce the incidence of cesarean delivery for fetal indications, no consistent effect on overall cesarean rates or newborn outcomes has been demonstrated. The results of a number of randomized trials led the manufacturer to announce that it would no longer distribute the sensors, effectively withdrawing the product from the market.

ST Segment Analysis

Study of the fetal electrocardiogram produced promising initial results. In sheep, FHR decelerations that accompanied hypoxemia were associated with characteristic changes in the fetal P-R interval.

In 2000 Strachan and colleagues compared standard electronic fetal monitoring with electronic fetal monitoring plus P-R interval analysis in 1038 women [33]. The groups demonstrated statistically similar rates of operative intervention for presumed fetal distress and no differences in newborn outcomes. The ST segment of the fetal electrocardiogram represents myocardial repolarization. Myocardial hypoxia can lead to elevation of the ST segment and T wave secondary to catecholamine release, β-adrenoceptor activation, glycogenolysis, and tissue metabolic acidosis [34,35]. These observations have led to the development of technology to analyze the fetal electrocardiogram plus the ST waveform (STAN; Neoventa Medical, Göteborg, Sweden) [29,36]. One randomized trial in 2434 patients demonstrated a 46% reduction in operative intervention for fetal distress when ST segment analysis was added to standard electronic fetal monitoring [37]. Operative interventions for dystocia and other indications were not increased. Fewer cases of metabolic acidemia and low 5-minute Apgar scores were observed in the group with electronic fetal monitoring plus ST segment analysis; however, these differences did not reach statistical significance. Another trial using newer technology included 4966 women randomized to electronic fetal monitoring alone versus electronic fetal monitoring plus ST segment analysis [36]. When analyzed according to intention to treat, the incidence of umbilical artery acidemia was 53% lower in the electronic fetal monitoring plus ST segment analysis group. In the electronic fetal monitoring plus ST segment analysis group, the incidence of cesarean delivery for fetal distress was 8%, compared with 9% in the group monitored with electronic fetal monitoring alone ($P = 0.047$). After excluding patients with inadequate FHR recordings and fetal malformations, these differences were slightly more pronounced.

A meta-analysis of four studies, including 9829 women, concluded that adjunctive ST segment analysis was associated with significantly fewer cases of severe metabolic acidemia at birth, fewer cases of neonatal encephalopathy, and fewer operative vaginal deliveries [38]. There were no significant differences in cesarean delivery rates, low 5-minute Apgar scores, or neonatal intensive care unit (NICU) admissions. One large multicenter trial randomized 5681 women to intrapartum electronic FHR monitoring alone versus electronic monitoring plus ST segment analysis [39]. No significant difference was observed in the primary outcome of metabolic acidosis, defined as an umbilical artery pH <7.05 with a base deficit of >12 mmol/L in the extracellular fluid. In the group with electronic monitoring plus ST analysis, there were statistically fewer cases of fetal blood sampling during labor (10.6% vs. 20.4%, relative risk 0.52, 95% confidence interval 0.46–0.59), umbilical artery pH <7.05 and base deficit >12 mmol/L (1.6% vs. 2.6%, relative risk 0.63, 95% confidence interval 0.42–0.97) and fewer cases of umbilical artery pH <7.05 (1.9% vs. 2.7%, relative risk 0.67, 95% confidence interval 0.46–0.97). Total operative deliveries, cesarean deliveries, and instrumented vaginal deliveries occurred with statistically similar frequency in both groups. There were no differences in operative deliveries for fetal distress. There were no other statistically significant differences in newborn outcome. The NICHD Maternal Fetal Medicine Units Network published a Phase III trial of the STAN monitor as an adjunct to electronic fetal monitoring in the United States. The multicenter trial randomized 11,108 women to undergo standard FHR monitoring with or without ST segment analysis. There were no significant differences between the two groups in the rates of operative vaginal delivery, cesarean delivery, NICU admission, meconium aspiration, or shoulder dystocia. The authors concluded that the use of STAN as an adjunct to conventional intrapartum electronic FHR monitoring did not improve perinatal outcomes or decrease operative deliveries in hospitals in the United States [40].

Umbilical Cord Blood Gas Analysis

Umbilical cord blood gas and pH assessment is a useful adjunct to the Apgar score in assessing the immediate condition of the newborn. There are no contraindications to obtaining cord gases.

ACOG [41] suggested obtaining cord gases in the following clinical situations:

- Cesarean delivery for fetal compromise
- Low 5-minute Apgar score
- Severe growth restriction
- Abnormal FHR tracing
- Maternal thyroid disease
- Intrapartum fever
- Multifetal gestations

Umbilical arterial values reflect fetal condition, whereas umbilical venous values reflect placental function. Normal findings preclude the presence of acidemia at, or immediately before, delivery.

Approximate normal values for cord blood are summarized in the following chart [42–45].

Approximate Normal Values for Cord Blood

Vessel	pH	P_{CO_2}	P_{O_2}	Base Deficit
Artery	7.2–7.3	45–55	15–25	<12
Vein	7.3–7.4	35–45	25–35	<12

The base deficit reflects utilization of buffer bases to help stabilize pH, usually in the setting of peripheral tissue hypoxia, anaerobic metabolism, and accumulation of lactic acid. An umbilical artery pH <7.20 usually is considered to define acidemia. Note that a much lower pH (7.0) is used to define the threshold of potential injury.

Acidemia is categorized as respiratory, metabolic, or mixed. Isolated respiratory acidemia is diagnosed when the umbilical artery pH is less than 7.20, the P_{CO_2} is elevated, and the base deficit is <12 mmol/L. This reflects interrupted exchange of blood gases, usually as a transient phenomenon related to umbilical cord compression. Isolated respiratory acidemia is not associated with fetal neurologic injury. Isolated metabolic acidemia is diagnosed when the pH is less than 7.20, the P_{CO_2} is normal, and the base deficit is at least 12 mmol/L. Metabolic acidemia can result from recurrent or prolonged interruption of fetal oxygenation that has progressed to the stage of peripheral tissue hypoxia, anaerobic metabolism, and lactic acid production in excess of buffering capacity. Although most cases of fetal metabolic acidemia do not result in injury, the risk is increased in the setting of significant metabolic acidemia (umbilical artery pH <7.0 and base deficit ≥12 mmol/L). Mixed (respiratory and metabolic) acidemia is diagnosed when the pH is below 7.20, the P_{CO_2} is elevated, and the base deficit is 12 mmol/L or greater. The clinical significance of mixed acidemia is similar to that of isolated metabolic acidemia. The types of acidemias (respiratory, metabolic, or mixed) are summarized in the following chart.

Types of Acidemia

Value	Respiratory	Metabolic	Mixed
pH[a]	<7.20	<7.20	<7.20
P_{CO_2}	Elevated	Normal	Elevated
Base deficit[a]	<12 mmol/L	≥12 mmol/L	≥12 mmol/L

[a]Threshold for potentially significant metabolic acidemia: pH ≤7.0 and base deficit ≥12 mmol/L.

The procedure for obtaining umbilical cord blood consists of double-clamping a 10- to 20-cm segment of the umbilical cord immediately after delivery. A specimen should be drawn with a 1-mL plastic syringe that has been flushed with heparin solution (1000 U/mL). Using separate syringes, draw blood from an umbilical artery first and then from the umbilical vein.

SUMMARY

Progress toward consensus in FHR monitoring makes it possible to construct a practical, standardized approach to FHR interpretation and management. The intrapartum FHR management model described in this chapter is not intended to dictate actions that must be taken in response to specific FHR patterns. Instead, it is intended to serve as a reminder of common sources of preventable error and an indicator of actions that should be considered to ensure that management decisions are made in a timely fashion. FHR definition, interpretation, and management should be guided by a few basic principles:

1. Simplicity is the key to consistent communication: *Unnecessary complexity predisposes to error.*
2. "Deciding to wait" is distinctly different from "waiting to decide": *The former reflects the application of clinical judgment; the latter can be construed as procrastination.*
3. The standard of care requires factual accuracy and the ability to articulate clearly and understandably: *Factual accuracy can be achieved by adhering to standardized FHR definitions and interpretation. A standardized "ABCD" approach to FHR management provides a framework that can help clinicians articulate a thorough, thoughtful, consistent plan of management.*

References

[1] G.A. Macones, G.D. Hankins, C.Y. Spong, J. Hauth, T. Moore, The 2008 National Institute of Child Health and Human Development workshop report on electronic fetal monitoring: update on definitions, interpretation, and research guidelines, Obstet. Gynecol. 112 (3) (2008) 661–666.
[2] American College of Obstetricians and Gynecologists, ACOG Practice Bulletin No. 106: Intrapartum fetal heart rate monitoring: nomenclature, interpretation, and general management principles, Obstet. Gynecol. 114 (2009) 192–202.
[3] American Academy of Pediatrics, American College of Obstetricians and Gynecologists: Guidelines for Perinatal Care (L.E. Riley, A.R. Stark, S.J. Kilpatrick, L.A. Papile, Eds.), seventh ed., Washington, DC, 2012.

[4] K.R. Simpson, D.C. James, Efficacy of intrauterine resuscitation techniques in improving fetal oxygen status during labor, Obstet. Gynecol. 105 (6) (2005) 1362–1368.

[5] American College of Obstetricians and Gynecologists, ACOG Committee Opinion No. 346. Amnioinfusion does not prevent meconium aspiration syndrome, ACOG, Washington, DC, 2006.

[6] S.L. Clark, M.P. Nageotte, T.J. Garite, R.K. Freeman, D.A. Miller, K. Rice-Simpson, et al., Intrapartum management of category II fetal heart rate tracings–towards standardization of care, Am. J. Obstet. Gynecol. 209 (2) (2013) 89–97.

[7] LE Shields, S Wiesner, C Klein, B Pelletreau, HL Hedriana, A standardized approach for category II fetal heart rate with significant decelerations: maternal and neonatal outcomes, Am. J. Perinatol. 35 (14) (2018) 1405–1410.

[8] C.E. East, L.R. Leader, P. Sheehan, N.E. Henshall, P.B. Colditz, Intrapartum fetal scalp lactate sampling for fetal assessment in the presence of a non-reassuring fetal heart rate trace, Cochrane Database Syst. Rev. (3) (2010) CD006174. doi:http://dx.doi.org/10.1002;14651858.CD006174.pub2.

[9] S.L. Clark, M.L. Gimovsky, F.C. Miller, The scalp stimulation test: a clinical alternative to fetal scalp blood sampling, Am. J. Obstet. Gynecol. 148 (3) (1984) 274–277.

[10] T.G. Edersheim, J.M. Hutson, M.L. Druzin, E.A. Kogut, Fetal heart rate response to vibratory acoustic stimulation predicts fetal pH in labor, Am. J. Obstet. Gynecol. 157 (6) (1987) 1557–1560.

[11] A. Elimian, R. Figueroa, N. Tejani, Intrapartum assessment of fetal well-being: a comparison of scalp stimulation with scalp blood pH sampling, Obstet. Gynecol. 89 (3) (1997) 373–376.

[12] I. Ingemarsson, S. Arulkumaran, Reactive fetal heart rate response to VAS in fetuses with low scalp blood pH, Br. J. Obstet. Gynaecol. 96 (5) (1989) 562–565.

[13] G.B. Polzin, K.J. Blakemore, R.H. Petrie, E. Amon, Fetal vibro-acoustic stimulation: magnitude and duration of fetal heart rate accelerations as a marker of fetal health, Obstet. Gynecol. 72 (4) (1988) 621–626.

[14] C.V. Smith, H.N. Nguyen, J.P. Phelan, R.H. Paul, Intrapartum assessment of fetal well-being: a comparison of fetal acoustic stimulation with acid-base determinations, Am. J. Obstet. Gynecol. 155 (4) (1986) 726–728.

[15] J.A. Spencer, Predictive value of a fetal heart rate acceleration at the time of fetal blood sampling in labour, J. Perinat. Med. 19 (3) (1991) 207–215.

[16] D.W. Skupski, C.R. Rosenberg, G.S. Eglington, Intrapartum fetal stimulation tests: a meta-analysis, Obstet. Gynecol. 99 (1) (2002) 129–134.

[17] G.S. Dawes, Computerised analysis of the fetal heart rate, Eur. J. Obstet. Gynecol. Reprod. Biol. 42 (Suppl.) (1991) S5–S8.

[18] G.S. Dawes, M. Moulden, O. Sheil, C.W.G. Redman, Approximate entropy, a statistic of regularity, applied to fetal heart rate data before and during labor, Obstet. Gynecol. 80 (5) (1992) 763–768.

[19] L.C. Pello, B.M. Rosevear, G.S. Dawes, M. Moulden, C.W. Redman, Computerized fetal heart rate analysis in labor, Obstet. Gynecol. 78 (4) (1991) 602–610.

[20] R.D.F. Keith, S. Beckly, J.M. Garibaldi, J.A. Westgate, E.C. Ifeachor, K.R. Greene, A multicentre comparative study of 17 experts and an intelligent computer system for managing labour using the cardiotoco-gram, Br. J. Obstet. Gynaecol. 102 (9) (1995) 688–700.

[21] S.L. Bloom, C.Y. Spong, E. Thom, M.W. Varner, D.J. Rouse, S. Weininger, et al., National Institute of Child Health and Human Development Maternal-Fetal Medicine Units Network: fetal pulse oximetry and cesarean delivery, N. Engl. J. Med. 355 (21) (2006) 2195–2202.

[22] G.A. Dildy, J.A. Thorp, J.D. Yeast, S.L. Clark, The relationship between oxygen saturation and pH in umbilical blood: implications for intrapar-tum fetal oxygen saturation monitoring, Am. J. Obstet. Gynecol. 175 (3 Pt 1) (1996) 682–687.

[23] G.A. Dildy, P.P. van den Berg, M. Katz, S.L. Clark, H.W. Jongsma, J.G. Nijhuis, et al., Intrapartum fetal pulse oximetry: fetal oxygen saturation trends during labor and relation to delivery outcome, Am. J. Obstet. Gynecol. 171 (3) (1994) 679–684.

[24] G.A. Dildy, S.L. Clark, C.A. Loucks, Preliminary experience with intra-partum fetal pulse oximetry in humans, Obstet. Gynecol. 81 (4) (1993) 630–635.

[25] G.A. Dildy, S.L. Clark, C.A. Loucks, Intrapartum fetal pulse oximetry: past, present, and future, Am. J. Obstet. Gynecol. 175 (1) (1996) 1–9.

[26] C.E. East, S.P. Brennecke, J.F. King, F.Y. Chan, P.B. Colditz, The effect of intrapartum fetal pulse oximetry, in the presence of a nonreassuring fetal heart rate pattern, on operative delivery rates: a multicenter, randomized, controlled trial (the FOREMOST trial), Am. J. Obstet. Gynecol. 194 (3) (2006) 606.e1–606.e16.

[27] T.J. Garite, G.A. Dildy, H. McNamara, M.P. Nageotte, F.H. Boehm, E.H. Dellinger, et al., A multicenter controlled trial of fetal pulse oxim-etry in the intrapartum management of nonreassuring fetal heart rate patterns, Am. J. Obstet. Gynecol. 183 (5) (2000) 1049–1058.

[28] C.K. Klauser, E.E. Christensen, S.P. Chauhan, L. Bufkin, E.F. Magann, J.A. Bofill, et al., Use of fetal pulse oximetry among high-risk women in labor: a randomized clinical trial, Am. J. Obstet. Gynecol. 192 (16) (2005) 1810–1819.

[29] M. Kuhnert, G. Seelbach-Goebel, M. Butterwegge, Predictive agree-ment between the fetal arterial oxygen saturation and fetal scalp pH: results of the German multicenter study, Am. J. Obstet. Gynecol. 178 (2) (1998) 330–335.

[30] R. Nijland, H.W. Jongsma, J.G. Nijhuis, P.P. van den Berg, B. Oese-burg, Arterial oxygen saturation in relation to metabolic acidosis in fetal lambs, Am. J. Obstet. Gynecol. 172 (3) (1995) 810–819.

[31] B. Oeseburg, B.E.M. Ringnalda, J. Crevels, H.W. Jongsma, P. Mannheimer, J. Menssen, et al., Fetal oxygenation in chronic maternal hypoxia: what's critical? Adv. Exp. Med. Biol. 317 (1992) 499–502.

[32] B. Seelbach-Gobel, M. Butterwegge, M. Kuhnert, M. Heupel, Fetal reflectance pulse oximetry. Experiences—prognostic significance and consequences—goals, Z. Geburtshilfe Perinatol. 198 (1994) 67–71.

[33] B.K. Strachan, W.J. van Wijngaarden, D. Sahota, A. Chang, D.K. James, Cardiotocography only versus cardiotocography plus PR-interval analysis in intrapartum surveillance: a randomized, multicentre trial, Lancet 355 (9202) (2000) 456–459.

[34] K.H. Hökegård, B.O. Eriksson, I. Kjellemer, R. Magno, K.G. Rosén, Myocardial metabolism in relation to electrocardiographic changes and cardiac function during graded hypoxia in the fetal lamb, Acta Physiol. Scand. 113 (1) (1981) 1–7.

[35] C. Widmark, T. Jansson, K. Lindecrantz, K.G. Rosén, ECG waveform, short term heart rate variability and plasma catecholamine concentrations in response to hypoxia in intrauterine growth retarded guinea pig fetuses, J, Dev. Physiol. 15 (3) (1991) 161–168.

[36] I. Amer-Wåhlin, C. Hellsten, H. Norén, H. Hagberg, A. Herbst, I. Kjellmer, et al., Cardiotocography only versus cardiotocography plus ST analysis of fetal electrocardiogram for intrapartum fetal monitoring: a Swedish randomised controlled trial, Lancet 358 (9281) (2001) 534–538.

[37] J. Westgate, M. Harris, J.S. Curnow, K.R. Greene, Plymouth randomized trial of cardiotocogram only versus ST waveform plus cardiotogram for intrapartum monitoring in 2400 cases, Am. J. Obstet. Gynecol. 169 (5) (1993) 1151–1160.

[38] J.P. Neilson, Fetal electrocardiogram (ECG) for fetal monitoring during labour, Cochrane Database Syst. Rev. (3) (2006) CD000116.

[39] M.E.M.H. Westerhuis, G.H.A. Visser, K.G.M. Moons, E. van Beck, et al., Cardiotography plus AS analysis of fetal electrocardiogram compared with cardiotocography only for intrapartum monitoring: a randomized trial, Obstet. Gynecol. 115 (2010) 1173–1180.

[40] M.A. Belfort, G.R. Saade, E. Thom, S.C. Blackwell, U.M. Reddy, J.M. Thorp, A.T. Tita, R.S. Miller, A.M. Peaceman, D.S. McKenna, E.K. Chien, D.J. Rouse, R.S. Gibbs, Y.Y. El-Sayed, Y. Sorokin, S.N. Caritis, J.P. VanDorsten, A randomized trial of intrapartum fetal ECG ST-segment analysis, N. Engl. J. Med. 373 (7) (2015) 632–641.

[41] American College of Obstetricians, ACOG Committee Opinion. Umbilical cord blood gas and acid–base analysis, Obstet. Gynecol. 108 (5) (2006) 1319–1322.

[42] A. Nodwell, L. Carmichael, M. Ross, B. Richardson, Placental compared with umbilical cord blood to assess fetal blood gas and acid-base status, Obstet. Gynecol. 105 (1) (2005) 129–138.

[43] B. Richardson, A. Nodwell, K. Webster, M. Alshimmiri, R. Gagnon, R. Natale, Fetal oxygen saturation and fractional extraction at birth and the relationship to measures of acidosis, Am. J. Obstet. Gynecol. 178 (3) (1998) 572–579.

[44] J.T. Helwig, J.T. Parer, S.J. Kilpatrick, R.K. Laros, Umbilical cord blood acid-base state: what is normal?, Am. J. Obstet. Gynecol. 174 (6) (1996) 1807–1812.

[45] R. Victory, D. Penava, O. Da Silva, R. Natale, B. Richardson, Umbilical cord pH and base excess values in relation to adverse outcome events for infants delivering at term, Am. J. Obstet. Gynecol. 191 (6) (2004) 2021–2028.

Influence of Gestational Age on Fetal Heart Rate

Clinicians are increasingly reliant on electronic fetal monitoring to identify fetal heart rate (FHR) characteristics that are demonstrative of adequate oxygenation and specific patterns that represent an oxygenation pathway interruption pointing to deterioration of the fetal status. When changes in oxygenation occur, the fetus initiates a physiologic defense to hypoxia to commence cardiorespiratory and metabolic adaptations, which attempt to balance oxygen delivery with metabolic demand [1,2]. This highly organized sequence of events includes acute compensation when there is maximal cardiovascular response. This is followed by an adaptive response to limit injury followed by subsequent slow decompensation to prevent cardiovascular failure if adequate oxygenation is not restored [3]. Gestational age plays a significant role in this critical process. Refer to Table 7.1 for definitions of gestational categories [4–6].

As pregnancy progresses through each trimester, a sophisticated homeostatic process, with complex physiologic changes, leads to a variety of FHR characteristics. These fluctuations are under the influence of basal sympathetic and parasympathetic tone, the central nervous system, hormones, and fetal diurnal states [7]. A key element in pattern interpretation is understanding how gestational age can influence FHR characteristics including baseline rate, variability, accelerations, and the appearance of periodic and episodic changes. Regardless of gestation, FHR patterns cannot be interpreted without a standardized approach and a clear understanding of applicable gestational age used for communication, data collection, and research purposes. This chapter reviews available literature regarding physiologic characteristics noted along the range of gestational ages with emphasis on fetal monitoring data interpretation and assessment of fetal status.

THE PRETERM FETUS

Internationally, preterm birth (PTB) accounts for approximately 15 million infants being born before 37 weeks' gestation [5]. This includes spontaneous births and those that occur for medical or

TABLE 7.1   Gestational Age Classifications

Preterm	Less than 37 0/7 weeks' gestation
Subcategories	
Extremely preterm	Less than 28 0/7 weeks' gestation[a]
Very preterm	28–31 6/7 weeks' gestation
Moderate preterm (may be further divided to include late preterm)	32–36 6/7 weeks' gestation *34–36 6/7 weeks' gestation*
Term	37 0/7 week's gestation and greater
Subcategories	
Early term	37 0/7–38 6/7 weeks' gestation
Full term	39 0/7–40 6/7 weeks' gestation
Late term	41 0/7–41 6/7 weeks' gestation
Postterm	42 0/7 week's gestation or more

[a] Periviability is included in this subcategory and is defined as 20 0/7 to 25 6/7 weeks.

Adapted from American College of Obstetricians and Gynecologists, Definition of Term Pregnancy (ACOG Committee Opinion No. 579), ACOG, Washington, DC, 2013; World Health Organization. <https://www.who.int/news-room/fact-sheets/detail/preterm-birth>; American College of Obstetricians and Gynecologists and Society for Maternal-Fetal Medicine, Periviable birth (Obstetric Care Consensus No. 6), Obstet. Gynecol. 130 (2017) e187–e199.

obstetric indications such as those associated with hypertension or diabetes. Greater than 60% of PTBs occur in Africa and South Asia, although the United States continues to remain one of the top 10 countries with the greatest prematurity rates [5]. Premature birth is one of the leading causes of mortality in children aged 5 and under. Among those who survive, there is an increased risk of short-term problems attributed to immature organ systems [8]. There is a higher likelihood of serious morbidities and severe life-long complications and neurodevelopmental disabilities including cerebral palsy and cognitive, behavioral, visual, and hearing problems [9,10].

Evidence of the pathogenesis of spontaneous PTB remains unclear. Contemporary literature is suggestive that PTB is a complex syndrome with several, often interrelated, antecedents and causes such as intraamniotic infection after preterm prelabor rupture of membranes [8,11]. Preterm and term labor share a mutual pathway related to cervical ripening and uterine activity that results in birth [8,11]. This pathway is activated physiologically in term labor, whereas several conditions or processes can activate one or more elements along this route with preterm labor. An appreciation of the complexity of FHR interpretation in this context is necessary when making clinical management decisions. For example, when preterm labor is caused by an underlying infection, management of the FHR may be different than a pattern that is interpreted in a pregnancy complicated by uterine distention and hydramnios.

Preterm fetuses have the capacity to respond and adapt to hypoxic challenges in accordance with the basic metabolic demands required for growth and development [3]. However, compared with a term fetus, a preterm fetus may have a remarkably different FHR response to hypoxia or acidosis if there are underlying conditions such as intrauterine growth restriction, making preterm fetuses susceptible to potential injury [12–18]. This may be related to either an absent or reasonably small fetal cardiovascular response caused by an immature autonomic nervous system or chemoreceptor sensitivity [19–23]. In addition, a normal FHR tracing displaying the absence of metabolic acidemia may progress more quickly to a pattern with indeterminate or abnormal FHR characteristics in a compromised preterm fetus compared with a term fetus [8,24]. These findings underscore how vital clinical expertise is when interpreting preterm FHR patterns.

Quantitative data are limited concerning preterm FHR characteristics compared with the term fetus. In general, antepartum and intrapartum FHR characteristics include the following:

- Baseline FHR frequently at the higher end of a normal range.
- Minimal variability may be observed in extremely preterm fetuses, especially those considered periviable.
- Lower acceleration frequency and amplitude until approximately 32 week's gestation.
- Variable decelerations with shorter depth and duration often unrelated to uterine contractions or periods of hypoxemia.

Baseline Fetal Heart Rate in the Preterm Fetus

The baseline FHR decreases as gestational age increases [25–29]. In a preterm fetus, a baseline rate close to 155 to 160 bpm can be normal. This is caused by an immature fetal autonomic nervous system in which the baseline FHR is the result of resistance between the parasympathetic and sympathetic systems [30]. With advancing gestation, the parasympathetic system becomes more dominant, resulting in a gradual decrease of the baseline [7]. A higher baseline rate must be interpreted with caution because this may indicate progressive fetal hypoxia, infection, or maternal pyrexia. Early studies found preterm fetal tachycardia to be more prognostic of acidemia, low Apgar scores, and adverse neonatal outcomes compared with the term fetus [30,31]. The combination of tachycardia and decelerations is a strong predictor of acidemia in the preterm fetus [32]. Tachycardia (FHR baseline >160) should always be evaluated using a systematic approach (described in Chapter 6) regardless of gestational age.

Baseline Variability in the Preterm Fetus

Similar to FHR baseline, variability within the baseline rate changes with advancing gestational age [28,29,33]. In the preterm fetus variability may be less than the term fetus based on the immature vagal and sympathetic branches of the autonomic nervous system [34–36]. The baseline variability typically increases with fetal growth, although the exact amount has not been quantified in the literature.

Periodic and Episodic Heart Rate Changes in the Preterm Fetus

Accelerations

Accelerations of the FHR in association with fetal movement begin in the second trimester of pregnancy. These accelerations are a result of the fetal somatic nervous system, which connects the central nervous system to muscle, allowing the fetus to perform specific movements and behaviors [24,37]. An FHR acceleration before 32 weeks' gestation is defined as an abrupt increase from the baseline of ≥10 bpm with a duration of ≥10 seconds from onset to offset [38] (Fig. 7.1). Prior to 32 weeks' gestation the preterm fetus may not have the physiologic maturity to generate accelerations that meet these criteria [39,40]. Similar to FHR baseline and variability, there is an increase in the number, amplitude, and duration of FHR accelerations, especially between 26 and 28 weeks' gestation and 30 to 32 weeks' gestation as the physiologic mechanisms responsible for FHR accelerations mature [26,41]. After 32 weeks' gestation FHR accelerations are defined as abrupt increases from the baseline of at least ≥15 bpm, lasting ≥15 seconds from onset to offset [38]. However, a number of fetuses with gestations <32 weeks, particularly those after 24 to 26 weeks' gestation, may meet the criteria for ≥15 bpm lasting ≥15 seconds [42,43].

Decelerations

Between 20 and 30 weeks' gestation, spontaneous decelerations occur. Typically, these are variable decelerations and are characteristically associated with fetal activity and the absence of uterine contractions. These decelerations are generally minimal in depth and

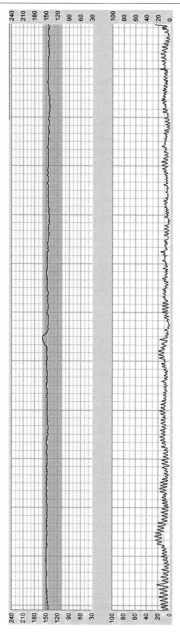

Fig. 7.1 Preterm fetal heart rate acceleration.

short in duration [37,40] (Fig. 7.2). During antepartum fetal surveillance, variable decelerations have been observed in up to 50% of
nonstress tests [44]. There is no association with fetal compromise as
long as these decelerations do not become recurrent and are less than
30 seconds in duration [44,45]. Furthermore, these decelerations do
not require corrective measures. Comparatively, when three or more
variable decelerations are present in a 20-minute period during the
antepartum period, there is an increased risk of cesarean birth related
to these tracing findings [46]. If additional information is needed
regarding fetal status in the antepartum period, testing methods such
as a biophysical profile (BPP), contraction stress test, or Doppler flow
studies may be used. Refer to Chapter 9 for additional information.

Throughout labor in the preterm population, approximately 70%
of patients between 28 and 33 weeks' gestation and 55% between 34
and 36 weeks' gestation will have variable decelerations [30] compared with an occurrence rate of 20% to 30% in the term pregnancy
[47]. There is speculation that preterm variable decelerations are
related to decreased amounts of Wharton's jelly around the umbilical
cord, oligohydramnios, or an immature fetal myocardium leading to
reduced contractility of the heart [24]. Early decelerations are rarely
observed with the majority occurring in gestations over 35 weeks
[30]. Late decelerations do not occur more or less frequently in PTB,
but clinical conditions that are associated with late decelerations (i.e.,
fetal growth restriction in the setting of hypertension) are more likely
to occur in the preterm fetus.

This has the potential to cause adverse perinatal and neonatal outcomes, including acidosis and long-term neurologic deficits [30,47].

Behavioral States in the Preterm Fetus

Many types of fetal behavior, such as the presence of fetal movement,
have been associated with a nonacidotic fetus. Spontaneous fetal
movement takes place by 7 to 8 weeks' gestation [48,49]. Maternal
perception of fetal movement, referred to as *quickening*, occurs
sometime between 14 and 20 weeks [50]. Fetal activity becomes
more coordinated and defined by the third trimester as the central
nervous system matures [49,51,52]. Four fetal behavioral states have
been defined and verified by ultrasound [53,54]. These include quiet
sleep or quiescence, active sleep, quiet awake, and active awake. The
behavior and associated FHR patterns of each of these four states
are described in Table 7.2. The fetus may cycle among these states.
Prior to 32 weeks only periods of fetal activity and quiescence are

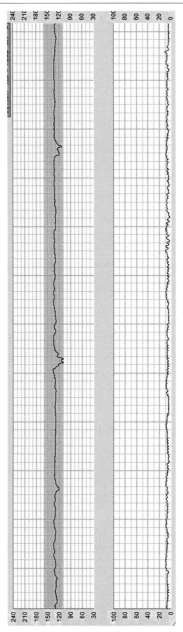

Fig. 7.2 Preterm variable decelerations.

TABLE 7.2   Fetal Behavioral States

State	Behavior	Associated FHR Pattern
1F: Quiet sleep or quiescence	Absence of REM Infrequent body and startle movement Rhythmic fetal breathing and mouthing movement	Regular/stable FHR baseline Minimal to absent variability Rare accelerations with FM
2F: Active sleep	Frequent body movement Abrupt head and limb movement REM Irregular fetal breathing and mouthing movement	Wider variation in FHR baseline Minimal to moderate variability Frequent accelerations with FM
3F: Quiet awake	Infrequent to absent body movement REM Irregular mouthing movement	Stable FHR baseline Moderate variability Absent accelerations
4F: Active awake	Continuous and vigorous movement REM Irregular fetal breathing and mouthing movement	Unstable FHR baseline Moderate to marked variability Frequent prolonged accelerations fusing into tachycardic rate

FHR, fetal heart rate; *FM,* fetal movement; *REM,* rapid eye movement.

Adapted from J.I. de Vries, G.H. Visser, E.J. Mulder, et al., Diurnal and other variations in fetal movement and heart rate patterns at 20-22 weeks, Early Hum. Dev. 15 (6) (1987) 33–348; C.B. Martin, Behavioral states in the human fetus, J. Reprod. Med. 26(8) (1981) 425–432.

distinguishable. As the fetus matures quiet sleep and active sleep are the dominant patterns [54,55].

Preterm Uterine Activity

Preterm uterine activity monitoring may be technically challenging. The smaller uterus may not accommodate effective placement of both toco and ultrasound transducers. Low-amplitude, high-frequency (LAHF) uterine contractions, frequently called *uterine irritability,* are not uncommon before term. LAHF contractions have been defined as measuring <5 mm in amplitude on the toco transducer and occurring at 1- to 2-minute intervals [56] (Fig. 7.3). In most cases, these contractions are clinically benign; however, occasionally LAHF may progress to preterm labor, resulting in cervical effacement and dilation [57], or may signal evolving placental abruption. Contractions that do not resolve must be evaluated and treated in the context of the clinical presentation and FHR observations.

Short-Term Tocolytic Therapy and Effect on Fetal Heart Rate

Tocolytics are medications that inhibit myometrial uterine activity. First-line tocolytic agents, such as prostaglandin synthase inhibitors, calcium channel blockers, and beta-sympathetic mimetics, may be given in the setting of acute preterm labor [58]. These medications often temporarily reduce or eliminate uterine activity for a brief time, but do not remove or reverse the underlying etiology. Additionally, each tocolytic agent has efficacy and safety issues. Therefore each drug's effectiveness, maternal–fetal and neonatal risks, and side effects should be considered when selecting the appropriate medication [59]. Data support short courses of tocolytics to assist with delaying birth for up to 48 hours, which allows for administration of antenatal corticosteroids to accelerate fetal lung maturation, magnesium sulfate for fetal neuroprotection, and transport to a higher level of maternal–fetal care [58–60]. There is no evidence to support that long-term or maintenance tocolysis prevents PTB or has a favorable effect on neonatal outcomes [58].

Indomethacin

Cyclooxygenase (COX), or prostaglandin synthase, is an enzyme that physiologically converts arachidonic acid to prostaglandins, which subsequently results in a coordinated uterine activity pattern [59,60]. Indomethacin is the main prostaglandin synthase inhibitor (also known as a *COX inhibitor*) and is used to inhibit prostaglandin synthesis during preterm labor episodes. Typical dosing is a 50- to 100-mg loading dose administered orally or rectally followed by 25 to 50 mg every 4 to 6 hours [59]. Therapy is generally limited to 48 hours and is not recommended after 32 weeks' gestation [59].

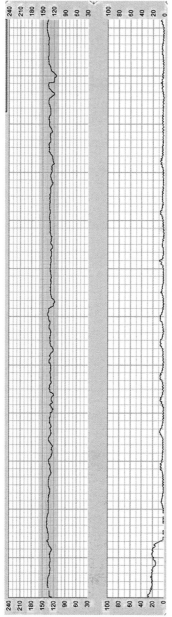

Fig. 7.3 Low-amplitude, high-frequency contractions.

The use of indomethacin beyond 48 hours is associated with fetal adverse outcomes including, but not limited to, premature closure or constriction of the ductus arteriosus and fetal renal insufficiency resulting in oligohydramnios [61]. Therefore amniotic fluid volume and fetal renal anatomy should be assessed before initiating therapy. Treatment beyond 48 hours requires intensive surveillance of amniotic fluid volume and ductal flow [59]. If oligohydramnios develops, the FHR tracing may demonstrate variable decelerations, reflecting transient umbilical cord compression.

Nifedipine

Calcium channel blockers, such as nifedipine (Procardia), also may be used as a first-line tocolytic agent. Pharmacokinetically, this medication impairs calcium channels, inhibiting the inflow of calcium into the smooth muscle cells. Along with other processes, this allows for myometrial relaxation and decreased uterine activity [59,60]. The ideal oral dosing regimen for treatment of preterm labor has not been established. The literature mentions initial dosing ranges from 10 to 40 mg followed by 10 to 20 mg every 4 to 6 hours, with titration based on the contraction pattern [62]. Maternal side effects are related to smooth muscle relaxation, resulting in peripheral vasodilation, which causes maternal hypotension and a compensatory rise in heart rate and stroke volume. Peripheral dilation and maternal hypotension can lead to hypoperfusion of the uterus and placenta [63]. Any medication that reduces maternal blood pressure has the potential to interfere with normal maternal perfusion of the intervillous space. As discussed in Chapter 5, recurrent or sustained disruption of fetal oxygenation can result in FHR changes ranging from decelerations to loss of variability, loss of accelerations, and changes in baseline rate.

Beta-Mimetics (Beta-Agonists)

Beta-mimetics such as terbutaline (Brethine) continue to be used in the preterm setting for tocolysis. The mechanism of action includes acting as an agonist for beta-2 receptors that are found in the smooth muscle. This tocolytic agent also stimulates the beta-2 receptors through a cyclic process leading to a decrease in intracellular calcium, resulting in uterine quiescence [59]. The administration of beta-mimetics for preterm labor has become less popular as a tocolytic agent mostly because of the significant maternal side effects, which include cardiac arrhythmias and maternal mortality, and the availability of other medications with fewer risks.

Generally, 0.25 mg is given subcutaneously and repeated in 15 to 30 minutes for up to four doses (if there is inadequate uterine response and no significant side effects). A U.S. Food and Drug Administration safety announcement states that injectable terbutaline should not be used beyond 48 to 72 hours because of potential adverse outcomes [64]. Oral terbutaline is not advised related to similar safety concerns and lack of evidence to support a role in preterm labor prevention [58,64]. The most common maternal side effect is tachycardia, which may be associated with increased oxygen consumption. Beta-mimetics cross the placental barrier and may result in a fetal tachyarrhythmia [59]. Prolonged periods of fetal tachycardia may be associated with loss of variability caused by the increased cardiac workload and oxygen demand. Furthermore, there is also a risk for misinterpretation of the FHR baseline because of signal ambiguity when a tachycardic rate is recorded at half the rate of the true baseline [65].

Magnesium Sulfate

Magnesium sulfate also has been historically used as a tocolytic agent to inhibit preterm uterine activity. The exact mechanism of action of magnesium sulfate's effect on uterine activity is unknown [59]. Although this medication continues to be used as a tocolytic, systematic reviews and comparative trials have indicated that intravenous magnesium sulfate is ineffective at delaying or preventing PTB or improving neonatal and maternal outcomes [66]. More contemporary cumulative evidence has demonstrated a link in the medication's role in providing fetal neuroprotective benefits when given before an anticipated PTB. Specifically, magnesium sulfate reduces the risk of neurologic morbidity, including cerebral palsy rates, when birth occurs between 23 0/7 weeks and 31 6/7 weeks' gestation [67,68]. Several neuroprotection treatment regimens have been described in the literature including a 6-g loading dose followed by 2 g/hr for up to 12 hours or a 4-g loading dose followed by 1 g/hr for up to 24 hours [67]. Magnesium sulfate crosses the placenta, and fetal serum magnesium concentrations often correlate with maternal serum levels [69]. The use of magnesium sulfate has been associated with decreasing baseline, decreased rate of variability, and loss of accelerations [70–74] (Fig. 7.4). Pathologic causes should be excluded before these changes are attributed to magnesium sulfate therapy. Exposure to magnesium sulfate does not increase the incidence of bradycardia or category change [73].

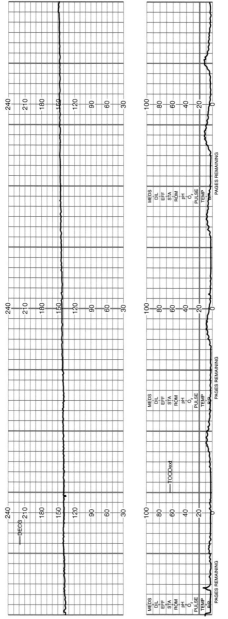

Fig. 7.4 Preterm fetus and fetal heart rate during therapy with magnesium sulfate.

As discussed in Chapters 6 and 9, vibroacoustic stimulation can provoke accelerations and may improve variability, although a blunted response may be elicited when magnesium sulfate is infusing [75]. BPPs and Doppler flow studies may also provide useful information regarding interpretation and management of the FHR tracing [76–78].

Antenatal Corticosteroid Therapy

Corticosteroid administration is among one of the most important and widely used interventions to improve outcomes for preterm infants [68,79]. This class of medication enhances fetal lung maturity, reduces the risk of respiratory distress syndrome, and lowers neonatal morbidity and mortality rates in preterm pregnancies [79]. Current guidelines recommend administration of a single course of either betamethasone or dexamethasone to women who are between 23 0/7 to 24 0/7 weeks' gestation and 33 6/7 week's gestation at risk of a PTB within 7 days. A single repeat course can be considered in women who are less than 34 0/7 weeks' gestation whose prior course of antenatal corticosteroids was administered more than 14 days previously. Based on the clinical scenario, this repeat corticosteroid dose may be given as early as 7 days from the prior dose. Furthermore, a single course of betamethasone is recommended for women between 34 0/7 weeks and 36 6/7 weeks of gestation at risk of PTB within 7 days, and who have not received a previous course of antenatal corticosteroids. Single-course betamethasone therapy consists of two doses of 12 mg given intramuscularly 24 hours apart or dexamethasone four doses of 6 mg given intramuscularly 12 hours apart [79].

No long-term negative effects from a single course of corticosteroids have been reported. There are direct, transient effects on fetal movement, FHR, and variability that typically return to baseline within 4 days of administration [80,81]. Betamethasone has been associated with an increase in FHR baseline, decreasing variability, and loss of accelerations [82,83]. There is limited data on dexamethasone's effect on the FHR. Most experts have concluded that the effect on FHR characteristics is similar to betamethasone, although other experts dispute this stating there is no significant change [80,81]. Neither of these medications has been associated with altered Doppler flow in the fetal middle cerebral artery and umbilical artery. Transient periods of suppression of biophysical characteristics (movement, fetal breathing, and reactivity) may be noted in patients receiving betamethasone. By 48 hours, the BPP score (see Chapter 9) may be as low as 6 of 10 when the maximum peak of the steroid has been reached [81,84]. These observations may be misinterpreted as a deteriorating fetal oxygenation status. Knowledge of these changes should be considered to avoid an iatrogenic preterm delivery. In these situations, Doppler flow studies in conjunction with BPPs may assist with interpretation and management of the FHR after steroid administration.

Monitoring the Preterm Fetus

Antepartum Fetal Assessment

Antepartum fetal assessment is an integral part of assessing fetuses at risk for an injury that is a result of a disrupted oxygenation pathway. The goal is to improve perinatal outcomes, specifically stillbirth and long-term neurologic impairments, while avoiding unnecessary interventions and unwarranted preterm delivery [8,45,85]. Fetal assessment is reviewed in Chapter 9.

Triage and Inpatient Antepartum Monitoring

During the antepartum period, FHR monitoring is often initiated during an outpatient triage encounter or on admission for patient evaluation or management of high-risk conditions such as but not limited to preterm labor, fetal growth restriction, or severe preeclampsia. This decision, whether short term or continuous, can produce a clinical dilemma for healthcare clinicians [24]. There is a risk that a false-positive indeterminate or abnormal FHR tracing will prompt unnecessary birth of a normal uncompromised fetus when FHR monitoring is performed prior to term. The earlier in gestation this occurs, the higher the likelihood of serious iatrogenic sequelae of prematurity. This risk must be weighed carefully against anticipated benefits of data that are obtained electronically. Implementing fetal monitoring may be beneficial in that early detection of an interruption in fetal oxygenation will prompt timely performance of corrective measures or possibly an operative intervention. Regardless of gestational age, several corrective measures, such as maternal lateral positioning, can be implemented for indeterminate or abnormal FHR patterns, which are discussed in Chapter 6. Using a shared decision-making process with a patient who is an active participant, decisions to initiate or discontinue fetal monitoring or perform continuous versus intermittent monitoring in a preterm gestation is individualized to each woman's clinical situation [86]. An objective assessment of the anticipated risks, benefits, limitations, and alternatives are presented to each patient in conjunction with an opportunity for questions to be answered thoroughly.

Intrapartum Monitoring

Depending on the gestational age, intrapartum management may include intermittent monitoring, time-specific prolonged monitoring, or continuous monitoring until birth. As previously discussed, interruption in the oxygenation pathway in a preterm fetus may progress more rapidly to metabolic acidemia and potential injury [16,47]. In addition, the possibility of infection must be considered in cases of preterm labor and/or premature membrane rupture. The effects of infection and/or inflammation on the FHR tracing are not completely understood, but limited evidence supports the observations that inflammation results in abnormal fetal cardiac function [8,87]. In preterm gestations the FHR tracing may be less reliable in excluding metabolic acidemia and predicting outcome because of the differences in FHR characteristics between preterm and term fetuses. All these factors must be taken into consideration when planning intrapartum management of the preterm fetus.

The periviable gestation is even more unique in regard to electronic fetal monitoring because FHR characteristics such as minimal variability or variable decelerations may be reflective of an immature central nervous system, not an interruption in the oxygenation pathway. Because the initial assessment for neonatal resuscitation of a potentially liveborn neonate has decreased to a threshold of 22 0/7 weeks, electronic fetal monitoring may be considered a part of a clinical management plan [68]. The decision to proceed with cesarean birth for fetal indications is based on a woman's individual and shared considerations and perspectives in conjunction with an interdisciplinary team [86]. If a woman chooses not to have a cesarean birth but elects to have neonatal resuscitation for a potentially viable liveborn fetus, electronic fetal monitoring may be considered in those situations when corrective measures are thought to affect neonatal outcome.

THE LATE-TERM AND POSTTERM FETUS

In a majority of pregnancies, there is sufficient placental function to support appropriate interval fetal growth and act as a safeguard from the normal hypoxic stressors of labor. As gestational age progresses to term or later, placental function decreases and the placenta may no longer be able to meet the fetal demands of an advanced pregnancy. Vital statistics collected from birth certificate data show that approximately 6% of infants are born late term. This statistic drops significantly to less than 0.4% in pregnancies that are 42 weeks and greater [88]. Despite advances in antepartum and intrapartum care, fetal and neonatal morbidity and mortality rates increase as pregnancy advances beyond 39 to 40 weeks' gestation [89,90].

The risk of stillbirth at term increases exponentially with each gestational age with the highest risk at 42 weeks or greater [91,92]. Additionally induction of labor at 41 weeks or greater is associated with an increased risk of cesarean birth, chorioamnionitis, labor dystocia, uterine rupture, oligohydramnios, and meconium-stained fluid [93].This has led to a shift in offering women elective induction of labor at 39 weeks based on more current data demonstrating a significantly lower risk of cesarean birth, maternal peripartum infection, and perinatal adverse outcomes, including respiratory morbidity, intensive care unit admission, and mortality [94,95].

Fetal Assessment

Antepartum and intrapartum surveillance related to definitions and interpretation in this population is similar to those in the preterm fetus. One exception is acceleration amplitude. Because there is an increase in perinatal mortality in these advanced gestational ages, antepartum fetal assessment is recommended. Antepartum fetal assessment is reviewed in Chapter 9.

Risks Associated with Postterm Pregnancy

Postmaturity or Dysmaturity Syndrome

A sequela of pregnancies that extends beyond a term gestation is *postmaturity or dysmaturity* syndrome. These terms are used to describe specific clinical characteristics that are assessed at the initial newborn physical examination. Clinical findings include reduced subcutaneous tissue; dry, wrinkled, peeling skin; meconium staining; hypothermia; hypoglycemia, polycythemia, and hyperviscosity [96,97]. These assessment findings are thought to reflect disruption of normal placental transfer of oxygen and nutrients caused by altered surface area and inadequate exchange within the placenta. In turn, this leads to decreased blood flow, nutritional deprivation, fetal wasting, decreased fat and glycogen stores, oligohydramnios, and chronic hypoxemia with compensatory hematopoiesis [98–100].

Oligohydramnios

The term pregnancy has an estimated amniotic fluid volume of 700 to 800 mL, which declines at a rate of 8% per week after 40 weeks' gestation [101]. Abnormalities in amniotic fluid volume are associated with adverse perinatal outcomes, particularly oligohydramnios, which is observed with increased frequency in late-term and post-term gestations. Sonographic descriptions of decreased fluid volume are outlined in Chapter 9. As the placenta ages uteroplacental function reduces, eliciting a physiologic response in which blood flow is preferentially directed to the fetal brain, heart, and adrenal glands and diverted away from the kidneys, resulting in decreased fetal urine production and eventually oligohydramnios. Low amniotic fluid volume in term gestations is associated with higher rates of perinatal and neonatal morbidity and mortality. These include but are not limited to intrauterine fetal death, meconium-stained amniotic fluid, meconium aspiration syndrome, umbilical cord compression resulting in variable decelerations, labor induction, cesarean birth for fetal indications, and low Apgar scores and umbilical artery pH values [89,100–106].

Intrapartum amnioinfusion may reduce the frequency of variable and prolonged decelerations, decrease the incidence of cesarean birth for fetal indications, and improve Apgar scores and cord pH values [107].

Meconium

The nature of the relationship between fetal well-being and meconium-stained fluid remains unclear [108]. As the fetus matures and pregnancy advances past 36 weeks' gestation, there is a higher incidence of meconium-stained fluid [108–110]. However, meconium passage may also signify that there has been stimulation of the vagal system by umbilical cord compression and hypoxia-related stress or an infectious process such as an intraamniotic infection [111,112]. The literature has described an increased risk of neonatal morbidity when meconium is associated with fetal heart tracings displaying indeterminate characteristics [113,114]. Additionally, postterm gestations have a higher incidence of meconium aspiration syndrome compared with earlier gestational ages. This type of neonatal respiratory distress syndrome is a result of aspiration of meconium resulting in pulmonary disease. In severe forms, meconium aspiration syndrome is associated with persistent pulmonary hypertension, hypoxic ischemic encephalopathy, and death [115].

Management of Postterm Pregnancy

The optimal management for late-term and postterm pregnancies, including the type of intervention and timing of delivery, is unclear. At a minimum, most experts agree that some form of antepartum fetal surveillance, including fetal movement counting, is indicated especially at or beyond 41 weeks' gestation [45,85,89]. The presence of clinically significant decelerations or oligohydramnios warrants consideration of labor induction. At 42 0/7 weeks and by 42 6/7 weeks' gestation induction of labor is recommended because of the increased perinatal morbidity and mortality rates [89]. The decision for induction of labor versus expectant management is dependent on a variety of factors, such as the gestational age, fetal surveillance results, Bishop score of the cervix, and shared decision-making. Clinicians should strive for a balanced conversation that includes maternal preferences related to pregnancy management in addition to providing evidence-driven risk, benefits, and treatment options [86].

SUMMARY

Maturation of the physiologic mechanisms responsible for regulation of the FHR is associated with characteristic changes in the FHR tracing. In addition, many factors associated with preterm and late-term or postterm pregnancy can influence the appearance of the FHR tracing, including medications, infection, placental function, and oligohydramnios. All these factors must be taken into consideration when interpreting the FHR tracing and planning management of pregnancies before and after term.

References

[1] A.J. Gunn, L. Bennet, Fetal hypoxia insults and patterns of brain injury: insights from animal models, Clin. Perinatol. 36 (3) (2009) 579–593.

[2] D.A Giussani, The fetal brain sparing response to hypoxia: physiological mechanisms, J. Physiol. 594 (5) (2016) 1215–1230.

[3] L. Bennet, Sex, drugs and rock and roll: tales from preterm fetal life, J. Physiol. 595 (6) (2017) 1865–1881.

[4] American College of Obstetricians and Gynecologists and Society for Maternal-Fetal Medicine, Definition of term pregnancy. Committee Opinion No. 579, Obstet. Gynecol. 122 (5) (2013; reaffirmed 2019) 1139–1140.

[5] World Health Organization Preterm Birth. https://www. who. int/news-room/fact-sheets/detail/preterm-birth. Accessed December 20, 2019.

[6] American College of Obstetricians and Gynecologists and Society for Maternal-Fetal Medicine, Periviable birth (Obstetric Care Consensus No. 6), Obstet. Gynecol. 130 (2017) e187–e199.

[7] C.J. Shaw, B.J. Allison, N. Itani, et al., Altered autonomic control of heart rate variability in the chronically hypoxic fetus, J. Physiol. 596 (23) (2018) 6105–6119.

[8] R. Romero, S.K. Dey, S.J. Fisher, Preterm labor: one syndrome, many causes, Science 345 (6198) (2014) 760–765.

[9] C. Lee, H. Blencowe, J.E. Lawn, Small babies, big numbers: global estimates of preterm birth, Lancet Glob Health 7 (1) (2019) e2–e3.

[10] L. Liu, S. Oza, D. Hogan, et al., Global, regional, and national causes of under-5 mortality in 2000-15: an updated systematic analysis with implications for the Sustainable Development Goals, Lancet 388 (10063) (2016) 3027–3035.

[11] M.S. Esplin, The importance of clinical phenotype in understanding and preventing spontaneous preterm birth, Am. J. Perinatol. 33 (3) (2016) 236–244.

[12] J.M. Ayoubi, F. Audibert, C. Boithias, et al., Perinatal factors affecting survival and survival without disability of extreme premature infants at two years of age, Eur. J. Obstet. Gynecol. Reprod. Biol. 105 (2) (2002) 124–131.

[13] M. Ayoubi, F. Audibert, M. Vial, et al., Fetal heart rate and survival of the very premature newborn, Am. J. Obstet. Gynecol. 187 (4) (2002) 1026–1030.

[14] P. Holmes, L.W. Oppenheimer, A. Gravelle, M. Walker, M. Blayney, The effect of variable heart rate decelerations on intraventricular hemorrhage and other perinatal outcomes in preterm infants, J. Matern. Fetal Med. 10 (4) (2001) 264–268.

[15] M. Westgren, S. Holmquist, N.W. Venningsen, I. Ingemarsson, Intrapartum fetal monitoring in preterm deliveries: prospective study, Obstet. Gynecol. 60 (1) (1982) 99–106.

[16] M. Westgren, P. Hormquist, I. Ingemarsson, N. Svenningsen, Intrapartum fetal acidosis in preterm infants: fetal monitoring and long-term morbidity, Obstet. Gynecol. 63 (3) (1984) 355–359.

[17] S. Eventov-Friedman, E.S. Shinwell, E. Barnea, et al., Correlation between fetal heart rate reactivity and mortality and severe neurological morbidity in extremely low birth weight infants, J. Matern. Fetal Neonatal Med. 25 (6) (2012) 654–655.

[18] L. Bennet, S. Dhillon, C.A. Lear, et al., Chronic inflammation and impaired development of the preterm brain, J. Reprod. Immunol. 125 (2018) 45–55.

[19] M. Walker, J.P. Cannata, M.H. Dowling, B.C. Ritchie, J.E. Maloney, Age-dependent pattern of autonomic heart rate control during hypoxia in fetal and newborn lambs, Biol. Neonate 35 (3) (1979) 198–208.

[20] H.S. Iwamoto, T. Kaufman, L.C. Keil, A.M. Rudolph, Responses to acute hypoxemia in fetal sheep at 0. 6–0. 7 gestation, Am. J. Physiol. 256 (3 Pt 2) (1989) H613–H620.

[21] C.A. Gleason, C. Hamm, M.D. Jones, Effect of acute hypoxemia on brain blood flow and oxygen metabolism in immature fetal sheep, Am. J. Physiol. 258 (4 Pt 2) (1990) H1064–H1069.

[22] Jensen, R. Berger, Fetal circulatory responses to oxygen lack, J. Dev. Physiol. 16 (4) (1991) 181–207.

[23] Y. Matsuda, J. Patrick, L. Carmichael, J. Challis, B. Richardson, Effects of sustained hypoxemia on the sheep fetus at midgestation: endocrine, cardiovascular, and biophysical responses, Am. J. Obstet. Gynecol. 167 (2) (1992) 531–540.

[24] K. Afors, E. Chandraharan, Use of continuous electronic fetal monitoring in a preterm fetus: clinical dilemmas and recommendations for practice, J. Pregnancy 2011 (2011) 1–7.

[25] R.D. Eden, L.S. Seifert, J. Frese-Gallo, et al., Effect of gestational age on baseline fetal heart rate during the third trimester of pregnancy, J. Reprod. Med. 32 (4) (1987) 285–286.

[26] T. Wheeler, A. Murrills, Patterns of fetal heart rate during normal pregnancy, Br. J. Obstet. 85 (1) (1978) 18–27.

[27] V. Serra, J. Bellver, M. Moulden, C.W. Redman, Computerized analysis of normal fetal heart rate pattern throughout gestation, Ultrasound in Obstet. Gynecol. 34 (1) (2009) 74–79.

[28] L.C. Shuffrey, M.M. Myers, H.J. Odendaal, Fetal heart rate, heart rate variability, and heart rate/movement coupling in the Safe Passage Study, J. Perinatol. 39 (5) (2019) 608–618.

[29] C. Amorim-Costa, C. Costa-Santos, D. Ayres-de-Campos, J. Bernardes, Longitudinal evaluation of computerized cardiotocographic parameters throughout pregnancy in normal fetuses: a prospective cohort study, Acta obstetricia et gynecologica Scandinavica 95 (10) (2016) 1143–1152.

[30] M. Westgren, S. Holmquist, N.W. Venningsen, I. Ingemarsson, Intrapartum fetal monitoring in preterm deliveries: prospective study, Obstet. Gynecol. 60 (1) (1982) 99–106.

[31] D.R. Burrus, T.M. O'Shea, J.C. Veille, E. Mueller-Heubach, The predictive value of intrapartum fetal heart rate abnormalities in the extremely premature infant, Am. J. Obstet. Gynecol. 171 (4) (1994) 1128–1132.

[32] M. Holzmann, S. Wretler, S. Cnattingius, L Nordström, Cardiotocography patterns and risk of intrapartum fetal acidemia, J. Perinat. Med. 43 (4) (2015) 473–479.

[33] G.H. Visser, G.S. Dawes, C.W. Redman, Numerical analysis of the normal human antenatal fetal heart rate, Br. J. Obstet. Gynaecol. 88 (8) (1981) 792–802.

[34] U. Schneider, E. Schleussner, A. Fiedler, et al., Fetal heart rate variability reveals differential dynamics in the intrauterine development of the sympathetic and parasympathetic branches of the autonomic nervous system, Physiol. Meas. 30 (2) (2009) 215–226.

[35] P. Van Leeuwen, D. Cysarz, F. Edelhäuser, D. Grönemeyer, Heart rate variability in the individual fetus, Auton. Neurosci. 178 (1) (2013) 24–28.

[36] D. Hoyer, J. Żebrowski, D. Cysarz, et al., Monitoring fetal maturation— objectives, techniques and indices of autonomic function, Physiol. Meas. 38 (5) (2017) R61–R88.

[37] Y. Sorokin, L.J. Kierker, S. Pillay, et al., The association between fetal heart rate patterns and fetal movements in pregnancies between 20 and 30 weeks' gestation, Am. J. Obstet. Gynecol. 143 (3) (1982) 243–249.

[38] G.A. Macones, G.D. Hankins, C.Y. Spong, et al., The 2008 National Institute of Child Health and Human Development workshop report on electronic fetal monitoring: update on definitions, interpretation, and research guidelines, Obstet. Gynecol. 112 (3) (2008) 661–666.

[39] R.A. Castillo, L.D. Devoe, M. Arthur, et al., The preterm nonstress test: effects of gestational age and length of study, Am. J. Obstet. Gynecol. 160 (1) (1989) 172–175.

[40] M. Pillai, D. James, The development of fetal heart rate patterns during normal pregnancy, Obstet. Gynecol. 76 (5) (1990) 812–816.

[41] R. Gagnon, K. Campbell, C. Hunse, J. Patrick, Patterns of human fetal heart rate accelerations from 26 weeks to term, Am. J. Obstet. Gynecol. 157 (3) (1987) 743–748.

[42] L.D. Devoe, Antepartum fetal heart rate testing in preterm pregnancy, Obstet. Gynecol. 60 (4) (1982) 431–436.

[43] J.P. Lavin, M. Miodovnik, T.P. Barden, Relationship of nonstress test reactivity and gestational age, Obstet. Gynecol. 63 (3) (1984) 338–344.

[44] P.J. Meis, J.R. Ureda, M. Swain, et al., Variable decelerations during nonstress tests are not a sign of fetal compromise, Am. J. Obstet. Gynecol. 154 (3) (1986) 586–590.

[45] American College of Obstetricians and Gynecologists, Antepartum fetal surveillance. Practice Bulletin No. 145, Obstet. Gynecol. 124 (2014) 182–192.

[46] Anyaegbunam, L. Brustman, M. Divon, O. Langer, The significance of antepartum variable decelerations, Am. J. Obstet. Gynecol 155 (4) (1986) 707–710.

[47] B. Zanini, R.H. Paul, J.R. Huey, Intrapartum fetal heart rate: correlation with scalp pH in the preterm fetus, Am. J. Obstet. Gynecol. 136 (1) (1980) 43–47.

[48] E. Borsani, A.M. Della Vedova, R. Rezzani, L.F. Rodella, C. Cristini, Correlation between human nervous system development and acquisition of fetal skills: An overview, Brain Dev. 41 (3) (2019) 225–233.

[49] J.L. De Vries, G.H. Visser, H.F. Prechtl, The emergence of fetal behaviour. I. Qualitative aspects, Early Hum. Dev. 7 (4) (1982) 301–322.

[50] J.L. Engstrom, Quickening and auscultation of fetal heart tones as estimators of the gestational interval: a review, J. Nurse Midwifery 30 (1) (1985) 25–32.

[51] J.L. De Vries, G.H. Visser, H.F. Prechtl, The emergence of fetal behaviour. II. Quantitative aspects, Early Hum. Dev. 12 (2) (1985) 99–120.

[52] P.J Roodenburg, J.W. Wladimiroff, A. Van Es, H.F. Prechtl, Classification and quantitative aspects of fetal movements during the second half of normal pregnancy, Early Hum. Dev. 25 (1) (1991) 19–35.

[53] J.G. Nijhuis, H.F. Prechtl, C.B. Martin Jr, R.S. Bots, Are there behavioural states in the human fetus? Early Hum. Dev. 6 (2) (1982) 177–195.

[54] M. Pillai, D. James, Behavioural states in normal mature human fetuses, Arch. Dis. Child 65 (1) (1990) 39–43.

[55] M. Pillai, D. James, Development of human fetal behavior: a review, Fetal Diagn. Ther. 5 (1) (1990) 15–32.

[56] R.B. Newman, P.J. Gill, S. Campion, et al., Antepartum ambulatory tocodynamometry: the significance of low-amplitude, high-frequency contractions, Obstet. Gynecol. 70 (5) (1987) 701–705.

[57] M. Katz, R.B. Newman, P.J. Gill, Assessment of uterine activity in ambulatory patients at high risk of preterm labor and delivery, Am. J. Obstet. Gynecol. 154 (1) (1986) 44–47.

[58] American College of Obstetricians and Gynecologists, Management of preterm labor. Practice Bulletin No. 171, Obstet. Gynecol. 128 (4) (2016) e155–e163.

[59] S.S. Patel, J. Ludmir, Drugs for the treatment and prevention of preterm labor, Clin. Perinatol. 46 (2) (2019) 159–172.

[60] R. Navathe, V. Berghella, Tocolysis for acute preterm labor: where have we been, where are we now, and where are we going? Am. J. Perinatol. 33 (03) (2016) 229–235.

[61] D. Doni, G. Paterlini, et al., Effects of antenatal indomethacin on ductus arteriosus early closure and on adverse outcomes in preterm neonates, J. Matern. Fetal. Neonatal Med. 33 (4) (2020) 645–650.

[62] H. Nassar, J. Aoun, I.M. Usta, Calcium channel blockers for the management of preterm birth: a review, Am. J. Perinatol. 28 (01) (2011) 57–66.

[63] Abramovici, J. Cantu, S.M. Jenkins, Tocolytic therapy for acute preterm labor, Obstet. Gynecol. Clin. North Am. 39 (1) (2012) 77–87.

[64] Food Drug Administration, FDA drug safety communication: New warnings against use of terbutaline to treat preterm labor. Available from: http://www.fda.gov/drugs/drugsafety/ucm243539.htm (accessed 2.28.20).

[65] R.L. Cypher, When Signals Become Crossed: Maternal-Fetal Signal Ambiguity, J. Perinat. Neonatal Nurs. 33 (2) (2019) 105–107.

[66] C.A. Crowther, J. Brown, C.J.D. McKinlay, P. Middleton, Magnesium sulphate for preventing preterm birth in threatened preterm labour, Cochrane Database of Systematic Reviews (8) (2014). Art. No.: CD001060.

[67] American College of Obstetricians and Gynecologists, Magnesium sulfate before anticipated preterm birth for neuroprotection. Committee Opinion No. 455, Obstet. Gynecol. 115 (2010) 669–671.

[68] American College of Obstetricians and Gynecologists and Society for Maternal-Fetal Medicine, Periviable birth (Obstetric Care Consensus No. 6), Obstet. Gynecol. 130 (2017) e187–e199.

[69] M. Hallak, S.M. Berry, F. Madincea, R. Romero, M.I. Evans, D.B. Cotton, Fetal serum and amniotic fluid magnesium concentrations with maternal treatment, Obstet. Gynecol. 81 (1993) 185–188.

[70] M. Hallack, J. Martinez-Poyer, M.L. Kruger, et al., The effect of magnesium sulfate on fetal heart rate parameters: a randomized, placebo-controlled trial, Am. J. Obstet. Gynecol. 181 (5) (1999) 1122–1127.

[71] D. Nensi, De Silva, P. von Dadelszen, et al., Effect of magnesium sulphate on fetal heart rate parameters: a systematic review, J. Obstet. Gynaecol. Can. 36 (12) (2014) 1055–1064.

[72] K.M. Verdurmen, A.D. Hulsenboom, J.O. van Laar, S.G. Oei, Effect of tocolytic drugs on fetal heart rate variability: a systematic review, J. Matern. Fetal Neonatal Med. 30 (2) (2017) 2387–2394.

[73] A.M. Stewart, G.A. Macones, A.O. Odibo, R. Colvin, A.G. Cahill, Changes in fetal heart tracing characteristics after magnesium exposure, Am. J. Perinatol. 31 (10) (2014) 869–874.

[74] M.W. Atkinson, M.A. Belfort, G. Saade, K.J. Moise, The relation between magnesium sulfate therapy and fetal heart rate variability, Obstet. Gynecol. 83 (6) (1984) 967–970.

[75] D.M. Sherer, Blunted fetal response to vibroacoustic stimulation associated with maternal intravenous magnesium sulfate therapy, Am. J. Perinatol. 11 (6) (1994) 401–403.

[76] S. Carlan, W. O'Brien, The effect of magnesium sulfate on the biophysical profile of normal term fetuses, Obstet. Gynecol. 77 (5) (1991) 681–684.

[77] P.S. Ramsey, D.J. Rouse, Magnesium sulfate as a tocolytic agent, Semin. Perinatol. 25 (4) (2001) 236–247.

[78] D.M. Twickler, D.D. McIntire, J.M. Alexander, et al., Effects of magnesium sulfate on preterm fetal cerebral blood flow using doppler analysis, Obstet. Gynecol. 115 (1) (2010) 21–25.

[79] American College of Obstetricians and Gynecologists, Antenatal corticosteroid therapy for fetal maturation. Committee Opinion No. 713, Obstet. Gynecol. 130 (2) (2017) e102–e109.

[80] V. Mariotti, A.M. Marconi, G. Pardi, Undesired effects of steroids during pregnancy, J. Matern. Fetal Neonatal Med. 16 (2) (2004) 5–7.

[81] K.M. Verdurmen, J. Renckens, J.O. van Laar, S.G. Oei, The influence of corticosteroids on fetal heart rate variability: a systematic review of the literature, Obstet. Gynecol. Surv. 68 (12) (2013) 811–824.

[82] L. Noben, K.M. Verdurmen, G.J. Warmerdam, et al., The fetal electrocardiogram to detect the effects of betamethasone on fetal heart rate variability, Early Hum. Dev. 130 (2019) 57–64.

[83] J. Weyrich, A. Setter, A. Müller, et al., Longitudinal progression of fetal short-term variation and average acceleration and deceleration capacity after antenatal maternal betamethasone application, Eur. J. Obstet. Gynecol. Reprod. Biol. 212 (2017) 85–90.

[84] O. Deren, C. Karaer, L. Onderoglu, et al., The effect of steroids on the biophysical profile and Doppler indices of umbilical and middle cerebral arteries in healthy preterm fetuses, Eur. J. Obstet. Gynecol. Reprod. Biol. 99 (1) (2001) 72–76.

[85] C. Signore, R.K. Freeman, C.Y. Spong, Antenatal testing: a reevaluation, Obstet. Gynecol. 113 (3) (2009) 687–701.

[86] R.L. Cypher, Shared Decision-Making: A Model for Effective Communication and Patient Satisfaction, J. Perinat. Neonatal Nurs. 33 (4) (2019) 285–287.

[87] R. Galinsky, G.R. Polglase, S.B. Hooper, M.J. Black, T.J. Moss, The consequences of chorioamnionitis: preterm birth and effects on development, J. Pregnancy 2013 (2013) 1–11.

[88] J.A. Martin, B.E. Hamilton, M.J.K. Osterman, A.K. Driscoll, Births: Final data for 2018. National Vital Statistics Reports; vol 68, no 13. Hyattsville, MD: National Center for Health Statistics. 2019.

[89] American College of Obstetricians and Gynecologists, Management of late-term and postterm pregnancies, Practice Bulletin No. 146, Obstet. Gynecol. 124 (2) (2014) 390–396.

[90] B.D. Einerson, W.A. Grobman, Elective induction of labor: friend or foe? Semin. Perinatol. 44 (2) (2019) 151214.

[91] M.J. Rosenstein, Y.W. Cheng, J.M Snowden, J.M. Nicholson, A.B. Caughey, Risk of stillbirth and infant death stratified by gestational age, Obstet. Gynecol. 120 (1) (2012) 76–82.

[92] J. Muglu, H. Rather, D. Arroyo-Manzano, et al., Risks of stillbirth and neonatal death with advancing gestation at term: A systematic review and meta-analysis of cohort studies of 15 million pregnancies, PLoS Medicine 16 (7) (2019).

[93] E. Rydahl, L. Eriksen, M. Juhl, Effects of induction of labor prior to post-term in low-risk pregnancies: a systematic review, JBI Database System Rev. Implement Rep. 17 (2) (2019) 170–208.

[94] W.A. Grobman, A.B. Caughey, Elective induction of labor at 39 weeks compared to expectant management: a meta-analysis of cohort studies, Am. J. Obstet. Gynecol. 221 (4) (2019) 304–310.

[95] R.G. Sinkey, C.T. Blanchard, J.M. Szychowski, et al., Elective Induction of Labor in the 39th Week of Gestation Compared With Expectant Management of Low-Risk Multiparous Women, Obstet. Gynecol. 134 (2) (2019) 282–287.

[96] L. Ballard, K.K. Novak, M. Driver, A simplified score for assessment of fetal maturation of newly born infants, J. Pediatr. 95 (5) (1979) 769–774.

[97] S.H. Clifford, Postmaturity, with placental dysfunction: clinical syndromes and pathologic findings, J. Pediatr. 44 (1) (1954) 1–13.

[98] N. Walker, J.H. Gan, Prolonged pregnancy, Obstet. Gynaecol. Reprod. Med. 25 (3) (2015) 83–87.

[99] F. Mannino, Neonatal complications of postterm gestation, J. Reprod. Med. 33 (3) (1988) 271–276.

[100] H. Vorherr, Placental insufficiency in relation to postterm pregnancy and fetal postmaturity: evaluation of fetoplacental function; management of the postterm gravida, Am. J. Obstet. Gynecol. 123 (1) (1975) 67–103.

[101] T.R. Moore, Amniotic fluid dynamics reflect fetal and maternal health and disease, Obstet. Gynecol. 116 (3) (2010) 759–765.

[102] C.J. Bochner, A.L. Medearis, J. Davis, et al., Antepartum predictors of fetal distress in postterm pregnancy, Am. J. Obstet. Gynecol. 157 (2) (1987) 353–358.

[103] P.F. Chamberlain, F.A. Manning, I. Morrison, C.R. Harman, I.R. Lange, Ultrasound evaluation of amniotic fluid volume: I. The relationship of marginal and decreased amniotic fluid volumes to perinatal outcome, Am. J. Obstet. Gynecol. 150 (3) (1984) 245–249.

[104] G. Shrem, S.S. Nagawkar, M. Hallak, A. Walfisch, Isolated oligohydramnios at term as an indication for labor induction: a systematic review and meta-analysis, Fetal Diagn. Ther. 40 (3) (2016) 161–173.

[105] R.K. Morris, C.H. Meller, J. Tamblyn, Association and prediction of amniotic fluid measurements for adverse pregnancy outcome: systematic review and meta-analysis, BJOG 121 (6) (2014) 686–699.

[106] H. Miremberg, E. Grinstein, H.G. Herman, et al., The association between isolated oligohydramnios at term and placental pathology in correlation with pregnancy outcomes, Placenta. 90 (2020) 37–41.

[107] G.J. Hofmeyr, T.A. Lawrie, Amnioinfusion for potential or suspected umbilical cord compression in labour, Cochrane Database Syst. Rev. 1 (2012) CD000013.

[108] I. Balchin, J.C. Whittaker, R.F. Lamont, P.J. Steer, Maternal and fetal characteristics associated with meconium-stained amniotic fluid, Obstet. Gynecol. 117 (4) (2011) 828–835.

[109] Y. Oyelese, A. Culin, C.V. Ananth, L.M. Kaminsky, A. Vintzileos, J.C. Smulian, Meconium-stained amniotic fluid across gestation and neonatal acid–base status, Obstet. Gynecol. 108 (2) (2006) 345–349.

[110] G. Murzakanova, S. Räisänen, A.F. Jacobsen, et al., Adverse perinatal outcomes in 665,244 term and post-term deliveries—a Norwegian population-based study, Eur. J. Obstet. Gynecol. Reprod. Biol. 247 (2020) 212–218.

[111] L. Monen, T.H. Hasaart, S.M. Kuppens, The aetiology of meconium-stained amniotic fluid: pathologic hypoxia or physiologic foetal ripening? Early Hum. Dev. 90 (7) (2014) 325–328.

[112] S. Mitchell, E. Chandraharan, E. Meconium-stained amniotic fluid. Obstetrics, Gynaecology & Reproductive Medicine 28 (4) (2018) 120–124.

[113] H.A. Frey, M.G. Tuuli, A.L.G.A. Macones, A.G. Cahill, Interpreting category II fetal heart rate tracings: does meconium matter? Am. J. Obstet. Gynecol. 211 (6) (2014) 644 -e1.

[114] H. Xu, M. Mas-Calvet, S.Q. Wei, Z.C. Lu, W.D. Fraser, Abnormal fetal heart rate tracing patterns in patients with thick meconium staining of the amniotic fluid: association with perinatal outcomes, Am. J. Obstet. Gynecol. 200 (3) (2009) 283–287.

[115] P.D. Thornton, R.T. Campbell, M.F. Mogos, Meconium aspiration syndrome: Incidence and outcomes using discharge data, Early Hum. Dev. 136 (2019) 21–26.

CHAPTER 8

Fetal Assessment in Non-Obstetric Settings

MATERNAL TRAUMA ALGORITHM

Fetal assessment and care of a pregnant woman can occur in a variety of locations, including the surgical setting, critical care unit, emergency department, or a separate obstetric-gynecologic triage environment, which is gaining hold as an alternative healthcare access point for obstetric patients. These areas function similarly to emergency departments in that these units can evaluate and treat presenting symptoms, prioritize care, improve utilization of staffing and patient services, and create a plan that incorporates maternal–fetal well-being [1]. Patients seek care outside an obstetric setting for a variety of reasons. These include but are not limited to a pregnancy below the viability threshold, a situation requiring surgical or medical expertise, or a lack of patient knowledge on where to present for care. Also, as rural and critical access hospitals permanently close obstetric service lines, women are compelled to seek care in an emergency department. The focus of this chapter is maternal–fetal assessment and management in the non-obstetric setting.

A CULTURE OF PATIENT SAFETY

Collaboration and ongoing communication among an interdisciplinary healthcare team caring for obstetric patients are essential in demonstrating a commitment to patient safety. Furthermore, pregnant women require the *right* healthcare clinicians at the *right* time and in the *right* setting. Regardless of the healthcare setting or gestational age, the fetus should not be overlooked. The healthcare team must have the requisite skills and expertise to be qualified to evaluate the obstetric patient.

Patient handoffs that occur between departments, such as an emergency department and an obstetric unit, have a higher likelihood of error and inefficiency [2]. Communication between service lines and healthcare team members must be clear and timely to ensure that the maternal–fetal dyad receives appropriate care by the most appropriate staff member. One initiative that may improve response time to a maternal and fetal evaluation in a trauma situation is implementing an interdisciplinary emergency response team for nontrauma specialists when a pregnant patient presents for care [3].

PREGNANCY ANATOMY AND PHYSIOLOGY

Evaluation of an obstetric patient brings a unique set of dilemmas, but a systematic approach to patient evaluations should be conducted in the same manner as with the nonpregnant patient, beginning with a comprehensive history and physical [4]. Considerable anatomic, physiologic, and biochemical changes occur during a pregnancy [5–7]. Comprehension and integration of these fundamental anatomic and physiologic changes are required so that the evaluation and management of these complex patients are optimized. Although many of these changes are normal, anatomic and physiologic changes are occasionally interpreted as a non-obstetric disease process. These changes may also reveal or exacerbate a preexisting condition such as hypertension or gallbladder disease. Prompt recognition of clinical symptoms and non-obstetric emergencies may be distorted, and normal discomforts may contribute to a confusing clinical picture. Some pregnancy adaptations are substantial and would be considered pathologic in the nonpregnant woman (Box 8.1). For example, the symphysis pubis protects the bladder. In pregnancy the bladder shifts to an intraabdominal position, making this area more susceptible to injury [8]. Laboratory values may be altered in the pregnant patient as opposed to a nonpregnant patient related to adaptations required by the body to support the pregnancy [4,8]. Not only does the pregnant woman present with unique challenges, but the fetus also requires assessment and possible intervention. Fetal stability depends on maternal stability. If caregivers do not understand and support pregnancy adaptations, then there is a potential for adverse maternal and fetal outcomes.

OBSTETRIC PATIENTS IN THE EMERGENCY DEPARTMENT

One of the leading diagnoses for an emergency department visit in women of childbearing age is a pregnancy-related complaint, many being nonurgent conditions that could have potentially been addressed in an outpatient setting [9,10]. Although some women access healthcare through emergency departments for urgent or

BOX 8.1   Physiologic Adaptations to Pregnancy

Cardiovascular
- Physiologic anemia, hypervolemia (expansion of plasma volume greater than expansion of red cell mass)
- Blood volume increases by 30% to 40% (1200–1500 mL higher than prepregnant state)
- Plasma increases 70%, cells 30%
- Hematocrit of 32% to 34% is not unusual
- Cardiac output increases 30% to 50% (a result of increased blood volume)
- Heart rate and stroke volume increase
- Systemic vascular resistance decreases, with resultant decrease in blood pressure and mean arterial pressure
- Uteroplacental vascular bed is dilated; passive low resistance system
- Uteroplacental unit receives 20% of cardiac output
- Peripheral edema, dyspnea, presence of third heart sound
- Pelvic venous congestion

Hematologic
- Increased clotting factors VII–X and fibrinogen (hypercoagulable)
- Decreased serum albumin may lower colloid osmotic pressure (predisposing to pulmonary edema)

Renal
- Smooth muscle relaxation, increased urinary stasis, hydronephrosis, hydroureter; increased susceptibility to urinary tract infection
- Increased creatinine clearance
- Decrease in serum creatinine and urea nitrogen (BUN)

Respiratory
- Tidal volume increases by 30% to 40%; respiratory rate unchanged
- Oxygen consumption increases by 20%
- Diaphragm elevated by the growing fetus
- Arterial Pco_2 decreases as a result of hyperventilation, resulting in a "compensated" respiratory alkalosis

Gastrointestinal
- Smooth muscle relaxes, increasing gastric emptying time
- Gastric motility decreases, sphincters relax, higher likelihood of aspiration

Musculoskeletal
- Increased risk of ligament injury secondary to relaxin and progesterone
- Shifting center of gravity with growth of fetus, diastasis of the rectus abdominus
- Symphyseal separation
  BUN, blood urea nitrogen.

Adapted from references [4–7,32].

trauma situations, others present because of a lack of readily accessible primary or obstetric care, an inability to schedule an appointment, or for convenience [1]. Regardless of the intention, a *primary* survey occurs when a woman first presents and is asked, "Why are you here?" A quick initial assessment can be completed and is crucial to determining triage and treatment priorities. This evaluation is predicated on a woman's ability to communicate effectively with a healthcare team. For example, if English is not the primary language, a translation service is used. A *secondary* survey includes obtaining detailed information about signs, symptoms, the mechanism of injury if applicable, and a thorough head-to-toe physical assessment [8,11]. Findings from the primary and secondary survey and pregnancy confirmation and determination of gestational age are key factors for identifying the specific department in which the woman's care would be most appropriately managed. Additional emergency department screening questions, regardless of the presenting problem, include but are not limited to the presence or absence of

- Fetal movement (if appropriate for gestational age, usually ≥18–20 weeks)
- Cramping, pelvic pressure, backache, or uterine contractions
- Vaginal bleeding
- Leaking of fluid

An assessment is required to confirm both maternal *and* fetal well-being prior to discharge or transfer to another area or healthcare facility [12]. Pregnancy is a crucial part of the assessment and not merely an afterthought.

Because of the infrequency of obstetric emergencies, establishing and maintaining competencies can be difficult, especially in non-obstetric settings. There may be inadequate resources and trained personnel to care for obstetric patients. Policies and procedures may be insufficient to facilitate quick access and appropriate management of an obstetric patient [13]. Therefore a decision tree algorithm is useful for triage of the maternal–fetal dyad to determine whether the woman should remain in the emergency department or be transferred to surgery, critical care, or the obstetric unit [1,13]. Each institution should have a written guideline or triage decision tree developed jointly between the emergency and obstetric departments. This document addresses at which gestational age care is managed in an emergency department versus an obstetric setting, which conditions prompt obstetric consultations, situations in which an obstetric healthcare provider is present in the emergency department, and guidelines for discharge or transfer to another care setting [1]. Several useful references about triaging and caring for the pregnant woman in the non-obstetric setting are readily accessible for creating or updating institutional guidelines [14–17].

Patients presenting to an emergency department at 20 weeks' gestation or greater are often referred to an obstetric setting, although it is important to understand that this gestational age is not absolute. The criteria for an internal transfer from the emergency department to the obstetric setting is dependent on the patient's chief complaint, institutional policies, procedures, and resources. It is important to remember that specific diagnoses are often limited to certain gestational ages, such as preeclampsia in the second and third trimester, and should be included in the treatment algorithms when addressing the assessment of a pregnant patient in the emergency department. Women who present with complaints of well-recognized obstetric concerns (e.g., vaginal bleeding, contractions, rupture of membranes, abdominal pain, pelvic pressure, decreased fetal movement) should be transferred to the obstetric unit in an expedited manner for further assessment and management. For those women with vague symptoms, such as headache, edema, nausea, and vomiting, or "just not feeling well," the decision about where to evaluate is not always so clear unless a policy or guideline is in place. Well-meaning care in a non-obstetric setting for the woman with a complicated disorder only found in pregnancy has the potential of being detrimental to both the woman and the fetus. Discussion between the emergency department and the obstetric setting is crucial in determining whose expertise is most needed for the evaluation and care of the maternal–fetal dyad.

When a woman presents to the emergency department with cardiovascular or respiratory complaints, the maternal vital signs must be assessed and documented without delay. There are specific abnormalities or "triggers" in the patient's vital signs and condition that point to the need for immediate notification and potentially bedside evaluation by a qualified healthcare clinician resulting in the activation of diagnostic and intervention resources. Although not perfect, early warning systems are an example of how vital signs and clinical observations based on specifically designed charts and escalation protocols can positively effect maternal care in terms of improved quality of care, prevention of progressive obstetric morbidity, and better maternal health outcomes [18,19]. For example, the Modified Early Obstetric Warning System (MEOWS) can be

TABLE 8.1   Maternal Early Obstetric Warning System Color-Coded Trigger Parameters

Parameter	Trigger: Red	Trigger: Yellow
Temperature (°C)	<35 or >38	35–36
Systolic blood pressure (mm Hg)	<90 or >160	150–160 or 90–100
Diastolic blood pressure (mm Hg)	>100	90–100
Heart rate (beats per minute)	<40 or >120	100–120 or 40–50
Respiratory rate (breaths per minute)	<10 or >30	21–30
Oxygen saturation (%)	<95	—
Pain score	—	2–3
Neurologic response	Unresponsive, pain	Voice

From S. Singh, A. McGlennan, A. England, R. Simons R, A validation study of the CEMACH recommended modified early obstetric warning system (MEOWS), Anaesthesia 67 (1) (2012) 12–18.

used in emergency departments and in protocols to recognize a deteriorating healthcare situation. In the MEOWS system, a physician or other qualified clinician is called for prompt bedside evaluation when the pregnant patient exhibits any one warning sign in the red area or two warning signs in the yellow at any one time [16,20] (Table 8.1). A similar system, referred to as the Maternal Early Warning Criteria (MEWC) protocol, requires immediate action when specific abnormal maternal parameters meet preestablished criteria [21] (Table 8.2).

TABLE 8.2   Maternal Early Warning Criteria Abnormal Parameters Requiring Bedside Evaluation

Parameter	Values
Systolic blood pressure (mm Hg)	<90 or >160
Diastolic blood pressure (mm Hg)	>100
Pulse rate (beats per minute)	<50 or >120
Respiratory rate (breaths per minute)	<10 or >30
Oxygen saturation (%)	<95
Oliguria (mL/hr for 2 hours)	<35
Maternal agitation, confusion, or unresponsiveness	—
Hypertension accompanied by nonremitting headache or shortness of breath	—

From J.M. Mhyre, R. D'Oria, A. B. Hameed, et al., The maternal early warning criteria: a proposal from the national partnership for maternal safety, J. Obstet. Gynecol. Neonatal. Nurs. 43 (6) (2014) 771–779.

Federal Law and Emergency Medical Treatment and Active Labor Act

Triage incorporates a rapid assessment of the woman, identification of the concerns, determination of the acuity of the problem, and arrangement for the appropriate personnel and equipment to meet the woman's needs. Triage of pregnant patients is regulated by federal law via the Emergency Medical Treatment and Active Labor Act [12]. This act ensures public access to emergency services regardless of insurance or capacity to pay. Hospitals must triage and provide a medical screening examination (MSE) to determine whether an emergency medical condition exists, including labor. A licensed clinician performs the MSE based on the history and physical and consists of procedures and tests that will identify medical and obstetric conditions [1]. Triage and an MSE are performed in a timely manner, with appropriate treatment and stabilization based on the clinical situation. The patient may require transfer, once stabilized, when a higher level of care is necessary, there are capacity limitations in bed management at the transferring facility, or the patient requests transfer [1]. A patient's care should take place in the area best prepared to handle her needs. This supports the development of hospital policies and procedures that specifically outline triage, care, and disposition of the patient [13,15,17,22,23].

Pregnant Trauma Victim Assessment and Care

Unintentional injuries and trauma during pregnancy are the leading contributors to maternal morbidity and mortality [24–26]. Specifically in pregnancy, blunt abdominal trauma is a common type of injury, with motor vehicle accidents, falls, and assault being the most common etiologies [27,28]. More precisely, other mechanisms of injury outside the realm of motor vehicle accidents include domestic violence penetrating trauma, suicide, and homicide. Although all forms of injury are serious, trauma resulting from motor vehicle accidents are concerning in that maternal and fetal mortality may be secondary to underlying factors such as compliance with consistent seat belt practices, improper seat belt placement, and airbag deployment [29,30]. Another major cause of trauma in pregnancy is related to slips and falls because pregnancy predisposes women to these types of accidents. This is related to joint laxity and weight gain that affects postural stability, especially in the third trimester [28,31,32].

TABLE 8.3   Trauma Concerns Specific to Pregnancy

Abruption	
Result of "shearing" effect when uterus is deformed by external forces, causing separation from placenta	Can trigger diffuse intravascular coagulation because of high concentration of thromboplastin in placenta@@@Electronic fetal monitoring is most sensitive means of detecting abruption@@@Ultrasound most specific but lacks sensitivity
Vaginal bleeding poor predictor of abruption	May be a later sign; watch for increasing fundal height, increased uterine activity, increased pain
Uterine Rupture	
Blunt trauma	Use ultrasound, x-ray; palpate fetal parts outside uterus; assess pain
Maternal–Fetal Hemorrhage	
Four to five times more common in injured woman than in noninjured woman	Fetal anemia, death, or isoimmunization
Fetal Compromise	
Nonspecific complication, but most common	Late decelerations, tachycardia, loss of variability
Preterm Contractions	
Common after blunt trauma	Abruption with potential for fetal hypoxia
Fetal Injuries	
Skull fractures, intracranial hemorrhage	More common in third trimester

Regardless of the type of trauma, a minor situation can be life-threatening to the patient and fetus [25,33]. Injuries that are unique to the pregnant trauma patient include uterine rupture, placental abruption, preterm labor and birth, pelvic fracture, and intrauterine fetal demise [27,29]. Consideration of gestational age is an essential factor because a crucial decision may be required regarding performing an operative intervention on behalf of the fetus. Trauma concerns specific to pregnancy are listed in Table 8.3.

Maternal–Fetal Transport

In trauma situations, first responders provide the initial evaluation and management that is consistent with advanced trauma life support protocols with the primary focus on maternal resuscitation [34].

The foremost reason for a fetal death that occurs in the trauma setting is maternal shock [23]. Alerting the emergency department early during transport allows the staff to inform the obstetric staff of the need for collaborative care immediately on arrival. First responders must promote maternal circulation and oxygenation and consider occult hemorrhage and shock in the pregnant trauma victim. Modifications of trauma guidelines that should be provided without delay include supplementary oxygen, intravenous access, and maternal positioning to a slight left lateral position as long as there is assurance of cervical spine stability. Otherwise, elevation of the right side of a spine board will assist with preventing supine hypotension [29,34]. Vital signs are assessed at the same frequency as a nonpregnant patient, and fetal status is considered once maternal stability has been established [34,35]. Once maternal stabilization has been confirmed, obtaining a fetal heart rate (FHR) with a Doppler may be considered. If the patient is conscious, information regarding fetal activity and the presence or absence of contractions is solicited. Determination of the gestational age may be of great benefit in determining fetal age and the need for prompt obstetric intervention on arrival to an emergency department. Clinical evaluation of the fundal height allows for a rough estimation of gestational age because fetal viability is more probable if the uterine fundal height is between the umbilicus and xiphoid process [33] (Fig. 8.1). Simply noting a fundal height being above or below the maternal umbilicus may help determine whether a pregnancy is more than or less than 20 weeks' gestation. Also, marking the top of the fundus will assist the obstetric team in establishing if there is a potential concealed abruption [33].

Primary and Secondary Survey in the Emergency Department

Primary Survey

Similar to the first responders, the emergency department will complete a *primary survey* of a pregnant trauma patient on arrival, which again will encompass the immediate evaluation of the patient, not the fetus. Initial management of the pregnant patient is no different from that of the nonpregnant patient, so maternal health will take priority over fetal health unless the patient is undergoing cardiopulmonary resuscitation and surgical intervention is required. The primary

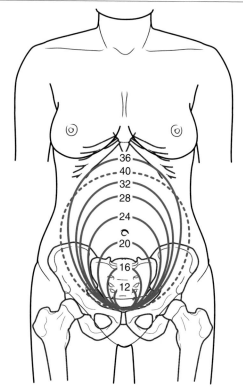

Fig. 8.1 Uterine size and gestational age. (From M.V. Muench, J.C. Canterino, Trauma in pregnancy, Obstet. Gynecol. Clin. North Am. 34 (3) (2007) 555–583.)

survey of the patient with trauma is an assessment based on the letters A-B-C-D-E. The components are [8,34]

Airway
Breathing
Circulation
Disability (neurologic: alert, voice, pain, unresponsive)
Exposure (examine)

Foremost in the primary survey is to assess the establishment of *airway* (A) stabilization. Adequate respirations (B, *breathing*) must be established, with administration of supplemental oxygen to prevent maternal hypoxia and desaturation, which in turn can lead to fetal hypoxemia [35]. Pulse oximetry and arterial blood gases will verify that the patient is adequately oxygenated when necessary. Blood pressure, pulse, and capillary refill (C, *circulation*) will typically verify how well the patient is perfusing. Uterine blood flow represents 10% to 15% of maternal cardiac output or approximately 700 to 800 mL/min. Significant blood loss, especially if a blunt or penetrating injury has occurred, may set off a cascade of maternal blood flow being shunted away from the uterus to permit maternal self-preservation at the expense of the fetus. The fetus can act as an early warning system for a patient's deteriorating hemodynamic status. An FHR is frequently considered another vital sign because adequate uterine perfusion can correlate with normal FHR characteristics, whereas abnormal FHR characteristics may reflect inadequate maternal oxygenation and circulation [23,33]. In some cases, maternal vital signs may not reflect the extent of the underlying injury [33]. Therefore FHR characteristics that reflect fetal hypoxemia secondary to maternal hypovolemia and reduced uteroplacental perfusion, including fetal tachycardia, decreasing variability, and recurrent decelerations, require the implementation of corrective measures. Compared with the nonpregnant patient, average blood volume expansion in the pregnant woman is approximately 40% to 50%, but as blood volume is lost, there is a decrease in cardiac output and arterial pressure [5]. When about 40% of total blood volume is lost, cardiac output and arterial pressures will reach critical levels and tissue hypoxia will occur [29]. Catecholamines are released as a result of volume loss, leading to vasoconstriction of blood vessels that facilitate maternal perfusion to the vital organs at the expense of uteroplacental blood flow and an intact oxygenation pathway. Thus aggressive volume resuscitation through two large-bore intravenous catheters is encouraged even when the hypovolemic woman is normotensive to maintain maternal–fetal hemodynamics [36]. As discussed previously, attention is focused on maintaining lateral positioning. This corrective measure is critical to sustaining adequate preload and cardiac output because supine positioning results in compression of the inferior vena cava in a pregnant patient after 20 weeks' gestation, which produces as much as a 30% reduction in cardiac output [25,33]. The neurologic evaluation (D, *disability assessment*) is performed by using the A-V-P-U method (alert, voice, pain, and unresponsive) of the Glasgow Coma Scale. By following steps A to D, cardiovascular or central nervous system trauma can be identified [34]. The patient can then be *exposed* (E) to examine for other obvious signs of physical trauma [33].

Secondary Survey

Once a primary survey is completed, and a patient is stabilized, the *secondary survey* is initiated. A detailed pregnancy history and head-to-toe physical examination are performed to gather pertinent pregnancy information and identify all injuries that may have been overlooked in the primary survey [33,37]. Evaluation of fetal well-being is parallel to maternal care but not at the expense of maternal resuscitation [25]. A thorough maternal–fetal assessment includes the following [11,25,33,35]:

■ Past and current pregnancy history

■ Estimated gestational age (fundal height or ultrasound)

■ Marking the top of the fundus to observe for an increasing fundal height

■ Sterile speculum examination if vaginal bleeding is present or there is evidence of ruptured membranes

■ Focused assessment sonographic trauma (FAST) ultrasound for potential intraabdominal hemorrhage; may be incorporated with obstetric ultrasound

■ Obstetric ultrasound performed by appropriately trained personnel for fetal number, cardiac activity, fetal position, biometrics, placental location, visualization of possible streaming vessels or placental hematoma indicating placental injury, amniotic fluid volume, biophysical profile, Doppler of pertinent fetal vessels such as the middle cerebral artery

■ Doppler ultrasound of middle cerebral artery identifying possible acute fetal anemia

■ Kleihauer–Betke test to evaluate for maternal–fetal hemorrhage dependent on the type of trauma

Fetomaternal hemorrhage is reported in up to 30% of obstetric trauma patients and is more common with an anterior placenta [38,39]. The Kleihauer–Betke test is performed to detect the degree of maternal–fetal hemorrhage in which fetal cells are circulating in the maternal circulation in excess of what is treated with a standard dose of Rho(D) immune globulin. This test determines the amount of Rho(D) immune globulin that is needed in the unsensitized Rh-negative pregnant trauma patient as additional fetal cells may come in contact with maternal circulation. The Kleihauer–Betke test is not used to determine the need for RhoGAM [33,35,40]. Changes in the FHR combined with a positive Kleihauer–Betke may signal hypoxemia, fetal anemia, and potential fetal compromise. If significant fetal hemorrhage has occurred, it may manifest into tachycardia or a sinusoidal pattern on the FHR tracing [40–42]. Doppler ultrasound of the middle cerebral artery may also demonstrate a compensatory response to hemorrhage.

Electronic fetal monitoring (EFM) can be a useful adjunct tool for fetal evaluation in the pregnant trauma victim with a viable fetus as long as it does not interfere with vital maternal treatment [28]. It is important to note that indeterminate and abnormal FHR tracings after trauma may not be as statistically reliable in predicting adverse perinatal outcomes with a sensitivity of 62% and specificity of 49% [23]. Continuous fetal monitoring versus intermittent auscultation is preferred, because auscultation limits the ability to detect specific FHR characteristics, such as variability and deceleration type [25,38]. Loss of variability and late or prolonged decelerations are the most sensitive findings in the detection of abruption, although other FHR characteristics such as tachycardia, bradycardia, or a sinusoidal pattern may be observed [42,43]. Regardless of monitoring mode, it is imperative to establish a baseline FHR. Similar to the laboring patient, any FHR tachycardia should be regarded with suspicion and managed, as outlined in Chapter 6. EFM should not be initiated until it is reasonable to perform an emergent cesarean birth [28].

Although there is a general consensus that EFM is an integral part of the ongoing assessment of the maternal–fetal dyad, there are no established standards for the duration of monitoring, especially after a trauma [11]. Experts advocate for a minimum of 2 to 6 hours. However, monitoring time can be extended to 24 hours or more in those patients experiencing a Category II FHR tracing, uterine activity (generally more than once per 10 minutes), vaginal bleeding, ruptured membranes, uterine or abdominal tenderness or pain, serum fibrinogen less than 200 g/L, high-risk mechanism of injury, or significant maternal injury [23,28,29,33,35]. Uterine irritability or contractions may provide clues to placental abruption. Ultrasound has limited usefulness and low sensitivity in distinguishing a placental abruption, so a negative result does not exclude the possibility [25,35,39,44,45]. Increased abruption rates are even more increased in those patients with greater than eight contractions in the first 4 hours [39]. At greater than 20 weeks' gestation, 90% of pregnant trauma patients will demonstrate some type of uterine activity in the first 4 hours. Data show that within the first hour, 64% of women will contract every 5 minutes or less, declining to 29% of women by the fourth hour. Patients without contractions or with less than one contraction every 10 minutes may be removed from the EFM and discharged as long as there is evidence of fetal movement, normal FHR characteristics, and absence of vaginal bleeding or ruptured membranes [23,46]. At discharge, labor instructions, how to perform fetal kick counts, and when to notify the healthcare clinician should be reviewed with the patient and documented in the medical record.

Emergent Cesarean Birth and Resuscitative Hysterotomy

As mentioned previously, the gravid uterus in the supine position compresses the inferior vena cava, resulting in reduced cardiac output [25,33]. Compression of the inferior vena cava is relieved once a cesarean birth is performed. This may result in restoring or improving maternal hemodynamics with a return in pulse rate and blood pressure, which in turn causes blood volume to be shunted back into the systemic system. Emergency cesarean birth in the patient with a viable gestational age is distinguished from a resuscitative hysterotomy, also known as a *perimortem cesarean birth*, which has historically been considered solely as a heroic effort for the fetus. Literature has shown that the performance of a resuscitative hysterotomy may aid in a return of spontaneous circulation [47]. This procedure is indicated in the obstetric trauma patient who is 20 weeks or greater when cardiopulmonary resuscitation has not resulted in a return of spontaneous circulation with usual measures, such as left lateral positioning and manual displacement of the uterus (Fig. 8.2) [29,47,48]. To be most effective, this surgical procedure should be initiated by 4 minutes with completion of the procedure by 5 minutes to minimize hypoxia and improve maternal and neonatal neurologic outcomes [47]. The optimal location is where the trauma patient is being resuscitated to avoid delay between cardiopulmonary resuscitation and surgery [25,29]. A decision tree for the unstable pregnant trauma patient may be a useful resource (Fig. 8.3).

Stabilization and Discharge

If the patient is unstable, transfer from the emergency department to the operating room or a critical care unit may occur. A collaborative approach among the obstetric, surgical, and critical care staff needs to be comprehensive, accurate, timely, and direct to promote an optimal environment for maternal–fetal well-being [11,49]. Once stabilized, the complex pregnant trauma patient may be transferred to an obstetric unit for continued care and monitoring. Once the patient is ready to be discharged, education regarding pregnancy warning signs, follow-up appointments, and specific instructions related to the injury are completed. For example, counseling about correct seat belt use is appropriate if the patient was involved in a motor vehicle accident. The lap belt and shoulder harness are both worn simultaneously, with the lap belt being securely placed under the abdomen and over the anterior superior iliac spine and symphysis pubis. The shoulder

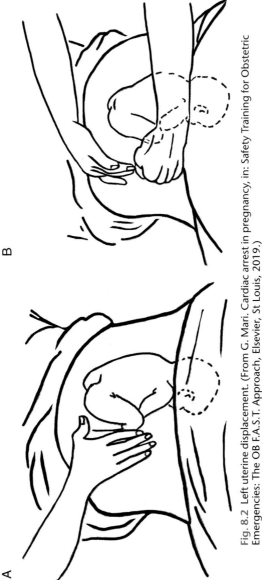

Fig. 8.2 Left uterine displacement. (From G. Mari. Cardiac arrest in pregnancy, in: Safety Training for Obstetric Emergencies: The OB F.A.S.T. Approach, Elsevier, St Louis, 2019.)

A

B

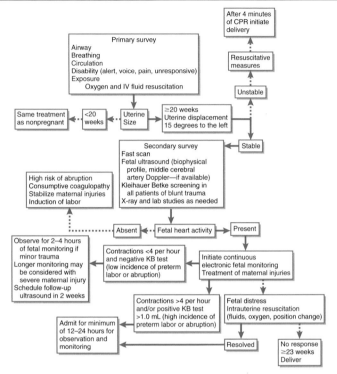

Fig. 8.3 Maternal trauma algorithm. CPR, cardiopulmonary resuscitation; IV, intravenous; KB, Kleihauer–Betke. (From M.V. Muench, J.C. Canterino, Trauma in pregnancy, Obstet. Gynecol. Clin. North Am. 34 (3) (2007) 555–583.)

harness should cross between the patient's breasts and under the neck [38,50]. Discharge instructions for a patient who has fallen might include avoiding walking on slippery or icy walkways or carrying heavy objects and using safety features such as staircase handrails.

NON-OBSTETRIC SURGICAL PROCEDURES: MATERNAL–FETAL ASSESSMENT AND CARE

Surgery during pregnancy related to non-obstetric reasons occurs in approximately 0.7% to 1.6% of women and can occur at any gestational age [51,52]. Elective surgery is best delayed until the pregnancy has ended [14,53]. If surgery is medically indicated for an urgent or emergent situation in the pregnancy patient, such as an orthopedic procedure after a motor vehicle accident, surgery should not be delayed regardless of the gestational age [14]. Major presenting conditions requiring surgical intervention can include trauma, appendicitis, biliary diseases (i.e., cholecystitis and pancreatitis), bowel obstructions, adnexal masses, and cancers [4,52,54]. Key points in coordinating surgical care for the maternal–fetal dyad include collaboration within an interdisciplinary team comprised of the obstetrician, surgical staff, anesthesia, neonatology, and nursing personnel as adjustments in management may be required during the procedure [4,49,55]. The surgeon and anesthesiologist should further collaborate with an obstetrician to determine whether an intraoperative fetal assessment is necessary.

Intraoperative Maternal–Fetal Assessment

There is a lack of standard recommendations related to the type and frequency of fetal assessment during non-obstetric surgical procedures or when to intervene. Depending on the type of surgery, intraoperative monitoring can be done with a Doppler or an EFM. These devices may need to be covered with a sterile sleeve when sterility is required. In cases in which EFM is not practical, transvaginal Doppler ultrasound may be used in selected cases [4].

Situations in which fetal surveillance is being considered is individualized based on gestational age, type of surgery, and facilities available such as a neonatal intensive care unit [14,53]. The advantage of fetal assessment for surgical procedures includes enhanced communication among disciplines related to altered maternal anatomy and physiology, patient positioning to optimize blood flow and oxygenation to the fetus, the safety of medications used during the procedure, and prompt identification of an FHR pattern requiring emergent cesarean birth [14,22]. Furthermore, fetal assessment during the surgical procedure demonstrates that the healthcare team acknowledges a second patient [53]. One approach in the decision-making process is to answer several key questions after determining fetal viability. These include whether there is a significant risk of intraoperative maternal hypotension or hypoxia and if EFM is technically feasible [14,55]. The cascading effects of an interrupted maternal–fetal oxygen transfer may be related to events that occur intraoperatively. These may include decreased uterine blood flow, hypotension, and uterine contractions [53,55]. Therefore intraoperative EFM can provide information about uteroplacental perfusion.

The following guidelines should be followed if fetal monitoring is used [14]:

- Doppler FHR pre- and postprocedure for the previable fetus.
- At a minimum, simultaneous FHR and uterine contraction monitoring in the viable fetus should be performed pre- and postprocedure to assess the fetal status and uterine quiescence.
- A qualified individual adept at both performing fetal assessment and interpreting FHR characteristics and the status of uterine activity should be readily available.
- A healthcare clinician with cesarean birth privileges should be readily available.
- Neonatal and pediatric service should be available in the institution performing the surgery.
- Intraoperative fetal monitoring may be appropriate when all of the following can be accomplished:
  - Viable fetus.
  - External application of ultrasound and tocotransducer, if feasible.
  - Informed consent for cesarean birth before surgery, if time permits.
  - Type of surgical procedure allows for safe interruption or alteration to provide access for emergency cesarean birth.
  - Appropriate equipment to perform a cesarean birth and neonatal resuscitation.

The FHR characteristically demonstrates a decreasing baseline that may remain in the lower limits of normal and decreasing variability with induction of general anesthesia (Fig. 8.4). Minimal or absent variability without decelerations is not associated with an interruption of the oxygenation pathway when an obstetric patient is receiving general anesthesia [56].This change in variability may be related to a portion of the fetal brain stem, which regulates the FHR being anesthetized [57,58]. Moderate FHR variability will return when inhalation anesthesia is discontinued [56]. Baseline FHR and variability changes caused by intraoperative medication administration must be differentiated from FHR alterations that result from fetal hypoxia such as recurrent decelerations, tachycardia, or bradycardia. Tachycardia and spontaneous decelerations are usually not found in these patients unless a woman is febrile or hemodynamically unstable [56,59,60]. Postoperative monitoring of FHR characteristics and uterine activity is continued as appropriate for gestational age, type of surgery performed, physician orders, and presence or absence of uterine contractions. Interpretation and management of intraoperative and postoperative FHR changes should be guided by the principles outlined in Chapters 2, 5, and 6.

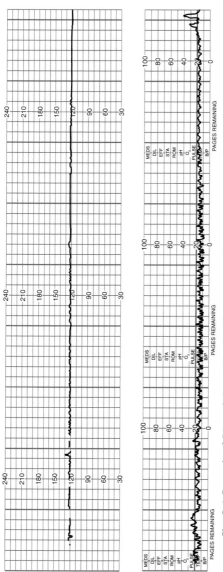

Fig. 8.4 Example of 34 weeks' gestation fetal heart rate tracing in a pregnant patient undergoing unilateral mastectomy under general anesthesia. Note the normal range baseline, minimal to absent variability, and lack of periodic and nonperiodic changes. (From Giancarlo Mari. Cardiac Arrest in Pregnancy. In: Safety Training for Obstetric Emergencies: The OB F.A.S.T. Approach. Elsevier. 2020.)

Tocolytic Agents and Antenatal Corticosteroids

The preterm birth rate in women having non-obstetric surgical procedures is higher than national vital statistics data, but this is often related to the surgical procedure, uterine manipulation, or the underlying condition requiring surgery [56]. For example, appendicitis activates the inflammatory process making it difficult to conclude if preterm birth is related to the actual surgery or the pathophysiologic pathway of infection. Routine administration of prophylactic tocolytic agents is not beneficial because these agents are not indicated for preterm labor prevention [61]. Evaluation using methods such as fetal fibronectin or transvaginal cervical length may be more useful.

A prophylactic course of antenatal corticosteroids may be considered between 23 and 24 0/7 to 36 6/7 weeks' gestation to enhance fetal lung maturity, given that there may be a potential increased risk for preterm birth. The decision to administer antenatal corticosteroids is individualized to the patient, the clinical situation, and risk factors [62]. Refer to Chapter 7 for dosing and FHR tracing interpretation after administration of this class of medication.

Fundamentals of Non-Obstetric Surgery

When surgery becomes necessary, especially in the second and third trimester, the following points should be kept in mind:

- Preoperative cervical examination
- Preoperative medications to assist with gastric emptying and neutralizing gastric contents
- Left uterine displacement after 20 weeks' gestation
- Maintaining maternal oxygen saturation greater than 95% and maternal mean arterial pressure greater than 65 mm Hg
- Neonatal equipment such as a radiant warmer, incubator, and resuscitation equipment if surgery is performed outside an obstetric unit and the fetus is considered viable

SUMMARY

A sound knowledge of maternal–fetal physiologic alterations is essential to providing appropriate care to patients presenting for emergent care or non-obstetric surgery. This allows for the implementation of a robust plan of care directed at reducing complications during these unique situations. Adequate training, exceptional interdisciplinary collaboration, clear communication, and practical institutional protocols and checklists are the foundation for optimizing care. Collaboration between the emergency department, the surgical department, and the obstetric staff ensures that evaluation and management is the same regardless of the location in the hospital.

References

[1] D.J. Angelini, E.D. Howard, Overview of obstetric triage, in: D.J. Angelini, D. LaFontaine (Eds.), Obstetric Triage and Emergency Care Protocols, 2nd edition, Springer, New York, 2017, pp. 1–10.

[2] K. O'Rourke, J. Teel, E. Nicholls, et al., Improving staff communication and transitions of care between obstetric triage and labor and delivery, J. Obstet. Gynecol. Neonatal Nurs. 47 (2) (2018) 264–272.

[3] J.A. Smith, A. Sosulski, R. Eskander, et al., Implementation of a multidisciplinary perinatal emergency response team (PERT) improves time to definitive obstetrical evaluation and fetal assessment, J. Trauma Acute Care Surg. (2020), in press.

[4] M.K. Stewart, K.P. Terhune, Management of pregnant patients undergoing general surgical procedures, Surg. Clin. North Am. 95 (2) (2015) 429–442.

[5] N.H. Troiano, Physiologic and hemodynamic changes during pregnancy, AACN Adv. Crit. Care 29 (3) (2018) 273–283.

[6] K. Torgersen, C.A. Curran, A systematic approach to the physiologic adaptations of pregnancy, Crit. Care Nurs. Q. 29 (1) (2006) 2–19.

[7] A. Mockridge, K. Maclennan, Physiology of pregnancy, Anaesthesia & Intensive Care Medicine 20 (7) (2019) 397–401.

[8] M.T. Coleman, V.A. Trianfo, D.A. Rund, Nonobstetric emergencies in pregnancy: Trauma and surgical conditions, Am. J. Obstet. Gynecol. 177 (3) (1997) 497–502.

[9] L. Uscher-Pines, J. Pines, E.Gillen A.Kellermann, A. Mehrotra, Emergency department visits for nonurgent conditions: systematic literature review, Am. J. Manag. Care 19 (1) (2013) 47–59.

[10] K.A. Kilfoyle, R. Vrees, C.A. Raker, K.A. Matteson, Nonurgent and urgent emergency department use during pregnancy: an observational study, Am. J. Obstet. Gynecol. 216 (2) (2017) 181–e1.

[11] B. MacArthur, M. Foley, K. Gray, A. Sisley, Trauma in pregnancy: A comprehensive approach to the mother and fetus, Am. J. Obstet. Gynecol. 220 (5) (2019) 465–468.

[12] Centers for Medicare and Medicaid Services, Emergency Medical Treatment and Labor Act, Available from: http://www.cms.gov/Regulations-and-Guidance/Legislation/EMTALA/index.html?redirect=/EMTALA/, 2012 (accessed 3-1-2020).

[13] Emergency Nurses Association, Emergency Care for Patients During Pregnancy and the Postpartum Period: Emergency Nurses Association and Association of Women's Health, Obstetric and Neonatal Nurses Joint Position. Available from: https://www.ena.org/docs/default-source/resource-library/practice-resources/position-statements/joint-statements/emergency-care-for-patients-during-pregnancy.pdf?sfvrsn=37506eab_4, 2020 (accessed 12-3-2020).

[14] American College of Obstetricians and Gynecologists, Nonobstetric surgery during pregnancy. ACOG Committee Opinion no. 775, Obstet. Gynecol. 133 (4) (2019) e285–e286.

[15] American College of Obstetricians and Gynecologists, Society of Maternal-Fetal Medicine, Levels of maternal care. ACOG Obstetric Care Consensus no. 9, Obstet. Gynecol. 134 (2) (2019) 342–355.

[16] American College of Obstetricians and Gynecologists, Preparing for clinical emergencies in obstetrics and gynecology. ACOG Committee Opinion no. 590, Obstet. Gynecol. 123 (2) (2014) 722–725.

[17] American College of Obstetricians and Gynecologists, Hospital-based triage of obstetric patients. ACOG Practice Bulletin, no. 211, Obstet. Gynecol. 113 (5) (2019) e303–e319.

[18] A. Umar, C.A. Ameh, F. Muriithi, M. Mathai, Early warning systems in obstetrics: A systematic literature review, PloS One 14 (5) (2019) 1–15.

[19] T. Robbins, A. Shennan, J. Sandall, Modified early obstetric warning scores: A promising tool but more evidence and standardization is required, Acta. Obstet. Gynecol. Scand. 98 (1) (2019) 7–10.

[20] S. Singh, A. McGlennan, A. England, R. Simons, A validation study of the CEMACH recommended modified early obstetric warning system (MEOWS), Anaesthesia 67 (1) (2012) 12–18.

[21] J.M. Mhyre, R. D'Oria, A.B. Hameed, et al., The maternal early warning criteria: a proposal from the national partnership for maternal safety, J. Obstet. Gynecol. Neonatal Nurs. 43 (6) (2014) 771–779.

[22] American College of Obstetricians and Gynecologists, Critical care in pregnancy. ACOG Practice Bulletin no. 211, Obstet. Gynecol. 133 (5) (2019) e303–e319.

[23] V. Jain, R. Chari, S. Maslovitz, et al., Guidelines for the management of a pregnant trauma patient, J. Obstet. Gynaecol. Can. 37 (6) (2015) 553–574.

[24] N.A. Deshpande, L.M. Kucirka, R.N. Smith, et al., Pregnant trauma victims experience nearly 2-fold higher mortality compared to their non-pregnant counterparts, Am. J. Obstet. Gynecol. 217 (5) (2017) 590.e1–e9.

[25] J. Sakamoto, C. Michels, B. Eisfelder, N. Joshi, Trauma in Pregnancy, Emerg. Med. Clin. North Am. 37 (2) (2019) 317–338.

[26] Leading Causes of Death in Females, 2014. Atlanta: CDC Office of Women's Health, 2017. Available at: https://www.cdc.gov/women/lcod/2014/all-females/index.htm. Accessed March 2, 2020.

[27] P.S. Greco, L.J. Day, M.D. Pearlman, Guidance for evaluation and management of blunt abdominal trauma in pregnancy, Obstet. Gynecol. 134 (6) (2019) 1343–1357.

[28] H. Mendez-Figueroa, J.D. Dahlke, R.A. Vrees, D.J. Rouse, Trauma in pregnancy: an updated systematic review, Am. J. Obstet. Gynecol. 209 (1) (2013) 1–10.

[29] C.K. Huls, C. Detlefs, Trauma in pregnancy, Semin. Perinatol. 42 (1) (2018) 13–20.

[30] M.B. Mulder, H.J. Quiroz, W.J. Yang, et al., The unborn fetus: The unrecognized victim of trauma during pregnancy, J. Pediatr. Surg. 2020, in press.

[31] J.L. McCrory, A.J. Chambers, A. Daftary, M.S. Redfern, Dynamic postural stability during advancing pregnancy, J. Biomech. 43 (12) (2010) 2434–2439.

[32] S.T. Blackburn, Maternal, Fetal, & Neonatal Physiology: A Clinical Perspective, fifth ed., Elsevier, St. Louis, MO, 2018.

[33] M.V. Muench, J.C. Canterino, Trauma in pregnancy, Obstet. Gynecol. Clin. North Am. 34 (3) (2007) 555–583.

[34] S.M. Galvagno, J.T. Nahmias, D.A. Young, Advanced trauma life support® Update 2019: Management and applications for adults and special populations, Anesthesiol. Clin. 37 (1) (2019) 13–32.

[35] S. Einav, H.Y. Sela, C.F. Weiniger, Management and outcomes of trauma during pregnancy, Anesthesiol. Clin. 31 (1) (2013) 141–156.

[36] Lyndon, D. Lagrew, L. Shields, E. Main, V. Cape V. Improving health care response to obstetric hemorrhage. (California Maternal Quality Care Collaborative Toolkit to Transform Maternity Care) Developed under contract #11-10006 with the California Department of Public Health; Maternal, Child and Adolescent Health Division; Published by the California Maternal Quality Care Collaborative, 2015.

[37] D.C. Ruffolo, Trauma care and managing the injured pregnant patient, J. Obstet. Gynecol. Neonatal Nurs. 38 (6) (2009) 704–714.

[38] M.C. Chames, M.D. Pearlman, Trauma during pregnancy: outcomes and clinical management, Clin. Obstet. Gynecol. 51 (2) (2008) 398–408.

[39] M.D. Pearlman, J.E. Tintinalli, R.P. Lorenz, A prospective controlled study of outcome after trauma during pregnancy, Am. J. Obstet. Gynec. 162 (6) (1990) 1502–1510.

[40] B.J. Wylie, M.E. D'Alton, Fetomaternal hemorrhage, Obstet. Gynecol. 115 (5) (2010) 1039–1051.

[41] H.D. Modanlou, R.K. Freeman, Sinusoidal fetal heart rate pattern: its definition and clinical significance, Am. J. Obstet. Gynecol. 142 (8) (1982) 1033–1038.

[42] H.D. Modanlou, Y. Murata, Sinusoidal heart rate pattern: reappraisal of its definition and clinical significance, J. Obstet. Gynaecol. Res. 30 (3) (2004) 169–180.

[43] J.K. Williams, L. McClain, A.S. Rosemurgy, et al., Evaluation of blunt abdominal trauma in the third trimester of pregnancy: maternal and fetal considerations, Obstet. Gynecol. 75 (1) (1990) 33–37.

[44] T.M. Goodwin, M.T. Breen, Pregnancy outcome and fetomaternal hemorrhage after noncatastrophic trauma Am. J. Obstet. Gynecol. 162 (3) (1990) 665–671.

[45] M.A. Dahmus, B.M. Sibai, Blunt abdominal trauma: are there any predictive factors for abruptio placentae or maternal-fetal distress? Am. J. Obstet. Gynecol. 169 (4) (1993) 1054–1059.

[46] M. Curet, C.R. Schermer, G.B. Demarest, et al., Predictors of outcome in trauma during pregnancy: Identification of patients who can be monitored for less than 6 hours, J. Trauma. 49 (1) (2000) 18–25.

[47] P.N. Soskin, J. Yu, Resuscitation of the pregnant patient, Emerg. Med. Clin. North Am. 37 (2) (2019) 351–363.

[48] C.H. Rose, A. Faksh, K.D. Traynor, Challenging the 4- to 5-minute rule: from perimortem cesarean to resuscitative hysterotomy, Am. J. Obstet. Gynecol. 213 (5) (2015) 653–656.

[49] K.L. Torgersen, Communication to facilitate care of the obstetric surgical patient in a postanesthesia care setting, J. Perianesth. Nurs. 20 (3) (2005) 177–184.

[50] M.D. Pearlman, M.E. Phillips, Safety belt use during pregnancy, Obstet. Gynecol. 88 (6) (1996) 1026–1029.

[51] V. Balinskaite, A. Bottle, V. Sodhi, et al., The risk of adverse pregnancy outcomes following nonobstetric surgery during pregnancy: estimates from a retrospective cohort study of 6.5 million pregnancies, Ann. Surg. 266 (2) (2017) 260–266.

[52] A.S. Rasmussen, C.F. Christiansen, N. Uldbjerg, M. Nørgaard, Obstetric and non-obstetric surgery during pregnancy: A 20-year Danish population-based prevalence study, BMJ Open 9 (5) (2019) e028136.

[53] M.F. Higgins, L. Pollard, S.K. Mcguinness, J.C. Kingdom, Fetal monitoring in non-obstetric surgery: systematic review of the evidence, Am. J. Obstet. Gynecol. 1 (4) (2019) 1–14.

[54] J. Vujic, K. Marsoner, A.H. Lipp-Pump, et al., Non-obstetric surgery during pregnancy–an eleven-year retrospective analysis, BMC Pregnancy Childbirth 19 (1) (2019) 382–386.

[55] M.C. Tolcher, W.E. Fisher, S.L. Clark, Nonobstetric surgery during pregnancy, Obstet. Gynecol. 132 (2) (2018) 395–403.

[56] G. Po, R. McCurdy, C.H. Rose, et al., Intraoperative fetal heart monitoring for non-obstetric surgery: a systematic review, Eur. J. Obstet. Gynecol. Reprod. Biol. 238 (2019) 12–19.

[57] P.L. Liu, T.M. Warren, G.W. Ostheimer, J.B. Weiss, L.M. Liu, Fetal monitoring in parturients undergoing surgery unrelated to pregnancy, Obstet. Anesth. Digest. 6 (1) (1986) 185.

[58] M. Van De Velde, F. De Buck, Anesthesia for non-obstetric surgery in the pregnant patient, Minerva Anesthesiol. 73 (4) (2007) 235–240.

[59] M.A. Rosen, Management of anesthesia for the pregnant surgical patient, Anesthesiology 91 (4) (1999) 1159–1163.

[60] M. Balki, P.H. Manninen, Craniotomy for suprasellar meningioma in a 28-week pregnant woman without fetal heart rate monitoring, Can. J. Anaesth. 51 (6) (2004) 573–576.

[61] American College of Obstetricians and Gynecologists, Prediction and prevention of preterm birth. ACOG Practice Bulletin no. 130, Obstet. Gynecol. 120 (4) (2012) 964–973.

[62] American College of Obstetricians and Gynecologists, Antenatal corticosteroid therapy for fetal maturation. ACOG Committee Opinion no. 713, Obstet. Gynecol. 130 (2) (2017) e102–e109.

CHAPTER 9

Antepartum Fetal Assessment

Electronic fetal heart rate (FHR) monitoring originally relied on electrical signals derived from transducers that were applied directly to the fetus. The requirement for membrane rupture limited the technology to the intrapartum period. Later, the development of Doppler ultrasound technology made it possible to monitor the FHR externally, expanding the application of fetal monitoring to the antepartum period. Observations and experience gained from early intrapartum monitoring were applied to the antepartum period, leading to the development of antepartum testing.

The goals of antepartum testing are to identify

1. Fetuses at risk for injury caused by interrupted oxygenation so that permanent injury or death might be prevented
2. Appropriately oxygenated fetuses so that unnecessary intervention can be avoided

COMPARING ANTEPARTUM TESTING METHODS

The *false-negative rate* is the key measure of effectiveness of any antepartum test. It is most often defined in the literature as the *incidence of fetal death within 1 week of a normal antepartum test* (Box 9.1). Reported false-negative rates range from 0.4 to greater than 6 per 1000 with current testing methods. The *false-positive rate* is another important feature in antepartum testing. A false-positive test usually is defined as an *abnormal test that prompts delivery but that is not associated with evidence of acute interruption of fetal oxygenation* (meconium-stained amniotic fluid, intrapartum FHR abnormalities, abnormal umbilical artery blood gas results, low Apgar scores), *or chronic interruption of fetal oxygenation* (fetal growth restriction under the 10th percentile for gestational age). False-positive rates range from 30% to 90% with current testing methods.

In August 2007, the Eunice Kennedy Shriver National Institute of Child Health and Human Development (NICHD), the National Institutes of Health Office of Rare Diseases, the American College of Obstetricians and Gynecologists (ACOG), and the American Academy of Pediatrics jointly sponsored a 2-day workshop to

---

BOX 9.1   Key Measures of the Effectiveness of Antepartum Testing

---

False negative: fetal death within 1 week of a normal antepartum test
　False positive: abnormal test that prompts delivery but is not associated with acute or chronic interruption of fetal oxygenation

---

evaluate and summarize the scientific evidence supporting the use of antepartum assessment of fetal condition [1].

Antepartum testing is used primarily in patients who are considered to be at *increased risk for interruption of fetal oxygenation* by any of the mechanisms described in Chapter 2. The participants of the 2007 NICHD workshop reviewed the evidence regarding indications for antepartum testing, the reported gestational ages at which to initiate testing for various conditions, and the recommended options for testing mode and schedule. They published their findings in 2009 [1]. Table 9.1 provides a summary of the available evidence regarding testing indication, initiation, and mode and schedule of testing from the 2009 report.

The panel concluded that data were insufficient to support recommendations for the following conditions:

- Advanced maternal age (≥35 years)
- Advanced maternal age (≥40 years)
- Black race
- Maternal age <20 years
- Nulliparity
- Parity >10
- Assisted reproductive technology
- Abnormal serum markers
- Obesity (body mass index ≥25)
- Less than 12 years of education
- Smoking >10 cigarettes per day
- Thrombophilia
- Thyroid disorders

If testing is to be used in these conditions, it should be initiated in general no earlier than 32 to 34 weeks [2]. Possible exceptions include conditions such as poorly controlled chronic hypertension with fetal growth restriction, poorly controlled diabetes, or collagen vascular disease [2]. Earlier initiation is likely to result in false-positive tests, possible unnecessary interventions, and potential iatrogenic prematurity. The relative capabilities and limitations of various methods of antepartum testing, including test indications, timing

TABLE 9.1   Recommendations for Initiation of Antepartum Testing

Maternal and Fetal Indications	Reported Gestational Age at Initiation	Reported Options for Testing Mode and Schedule
Diabetes: diet controlled	Not indicated	Not applicable
Diabetes: insulin controlled Class A2, B, C, D without hypertension, renal disease, or fetal growth restriction	32 weeks	Weekly CST with midweek NST
Diabetes: insulin controlled Class A2, B, C, D without hypertension, renal disease, or fetal growth restriction	32 weeks	Twice-weekly NST or Twice-weekly BPP
Diabetes: insulin controlled Class A2, B, C, D without hypertension, renal disease, or fetal growth restriction	34 weeks	Twice-weekly NST with weekly AFI
Diabetes: insulin controlled Class R or F	26 weeks	Weekly CST with midweek NST
Diabetes: insulin controlled Any class with hypertension, renal disease, or fetal growth restriction	26 weeks	Weekly CST with midweek NST
Diabetes: insulin controlled Any class with hypertension, renal disease, or fetal growth restriction	28 weeks	Twice-weekly NST or Twice-weekly BPP
Chronic hypertension	26 weeks	Twice-weekly NST plus AFI
Chronic hypertension	33 weeks	Twice-weekly MBPP
Chronic hypertension with SLE, fetal growth restriction, diabetes, or pregnancy-induced hypertension	26 weeks	Twice-weekly NST with AFI
Mild pregnancy-induced hypertension	At diagnosis	Twice-weekly MBPP
Severe pregnancy-induced hypertension	At diagnosis	Daily NST with BPP if nonreactive and AFI twice weekly
Suspected fetal growth restriction	At diagnosis	Weekly NST plus AFI
Suspected fetal growth restriction	At diagnosis	UAD 1–2 times weekly

Continued

TABLE 9.1 Recommendations for Initiation of Antepartum Testing—cont'd

Maternal and Fetal Indications	Reported Gestational Age at Initiation	Reported Options for Testing Mode and Schedule
Confirmed fetal growth restriction	At diagnosis	Twice-weekly MBPP
Confirmed fetal growth restriction	At diagnosis	UAD 1–2 times weekly
Concordant twins	32 weeks	Weekly NST plus AFI
Discordant twins	At diagnosis	Twice-weekly MBPP
Triplets	28 weeks	Twice-weekly BPP
Oligohydramnios	At diagnosis	Twice-weekly NST plus AFI
Preterm premature rupture of membranes	At diagnosis	Daily NST or daily BPP
Gestational age 41 weeks	41 weeks	Twice-weekly BPP or weekly MBPP
Gestational age ≥42 weeks	42 weeks	Twice-weekly MBPP
Previous stillbirth	32 weeks	Twice-weekly MBPP or weekly BPP or weekly CST
Previous stillbirth	34 weeks or 1 week before previous stillbirth	Weekly MBPP
Decreased fetal movement	At diagnosis	MBPP
SLE	26 weeks	Weekly CST, BPP, or NST
Renal disease	30–32 weeks	Twice-weekly BPP
Cholestasis of pregnancy	34 weeks	Weekly MBPP

AFI, amniotic fluid index; *BPP,* biophysical profile; *CST,* contraction stress test; *MBPP,* modified biophysical profile; *NST,* nonstress test; *SLE,* systemic lupus erythematosus; *UAD,* umbilical artery Doppler.

From C. Signore, R.K. Freeman, C.Y. Spong, Antenatal testing—a reevaluation: executive summary of a Eunice Kennedy Shriver National Institute of Child Health and Human Development workshop, Obstet. Gynecol. 113 (3) (2009) 687–701. Available at www.ncbi.nlm.nih.gov/pmc/articles/PMC2771454/.

of initiation, and frequency of testing are summarized in ACOG Practice Bulletin Number 145 [2]. Examples of indications for antepartum testing identified by ACOG are listed as follows.

Maternal conditions:

- Pregestational diabetes
- Hypertension
- Systemic lupus erythematosus
- Chronic renal disease

- Antiphospholipid syndrome
- Hyperthyroidism (poorly controlled)
- Hemoglobinopathies (sickle cell, sickle cell–hemoglobin C, or sickle cell–thalassemia disease)
- Cyanotic heart disease
  Pregnancy-related conditions:
- Gestational hypertension
- Preeclampsia
- Decreased fetal movement
- Gestational diabetes mellitus (poorly controlled or medically treated)
- Oligohydramnios
- Fetal growth restriction
- Late-term or postterm pregnancy
- Isoimmunization
- Previous fetal demise (unexplained or recurrent risk)
- Monochorionic multiple gestation (with significant growth discrepancy)

METHODS OF TESTING

Contraction Stress Test and Oxytocin Challenge Test

The first antepartum testing technique, the contraction stress test or oxytocin challenge test, arose from intrapartum observations linking late decelerations with poor perinatal outcome. The test sought to identify transient fetal hypoxemia by demonstrating late decelerations in fetuses exposed to the stress of spontaneous (contraction stress test) or induced (oxytocin challenge test) uterine contractions. Kubli and associates reported that late decelerations occurring during spontaneous uterine contractions were associated with increased rates of fetal death, growth restriction, and neonatal depression [3]. Similar observations were made by other investigators using oxytocin or nipple stimulation to provoke uterine contractions.

Interpretation and Management

The contraction stress test is considered *negative* if there are at least three uterine contractions in a 10-minute period with no late decelerations on the tracing. In this case the routine weekly testing schedule usually is resumed. Failure to produce three contractions within a 10-minute window, or inability to trace the FHR, results in an *unsatisfactory* test. Prolonged decelerations, variable decelerations, or late decelerations occurring with less than 50% of the contractions constitute a *suspicious* or *equivocal* test. Decelerations that occur in the presence of contractions more frequent than every 2 minutes or lasting longer than 90 seconds constitute an equivocal test. Unsatisfactory, suspicious, or equivocal tests usually are managed by further evaluation in the form of prolonged monitoring or repeat testing after a reasonable interval, often the next day.

The contraction stress test or oxytocin challenge test is considered *positive* when at least half of the contractions during a 10-minute window are associated with late decelerations. Usually, a positive contraction stress test or oxytocin challenge test warrants hospitalization for further evaluation and/or delivery. Freeman and colleagues tested more than 4600 women with the contraction stress test and reported a false-negative rate of 0.4/1000 [4]. When the last test before delivery was a negative contraction stress test, the perinatal mortality rate was 2.3/1000, compared with a mortality rate of 176.5/1000 when the last test was a positive contraction stress test. Reported false-positive rates for the contraction stress test range from 8% to 57%, with an average of approximately 30% [5].

Interpretation summary of the contraction stress test is as follows:

- *Negative:* no late or significant variable decelerations
- *Positive:* late decelerations with 50% or more of contractions (even if there are fewer than three contractions in 10 minutes)
- *Equivocal-suspicious:* intermittent late decelerations or significant variable decelerations
- *Equivocal:* FHR decelerations that occur in the presence of contractions more frequently than every 2 minutes or lasting longer than 90 seconds
- *Unsatisfactory:* fewer than three contractions in 10 minutes or an uninterpretable tracing

Advantages and Limitations

Principal advantages of the contraction stress test include excellent sensitivity and a weekly testing interval. Limitations include a high rate of equivocal results requiring repeat testing, increased expense and inconvenience (particularly if oxytocin is required), and increased time requirement compared with the nonstress test (NST).

Procedures for Contraction Stress Testing

The contraction stress test can be performed by breast or nipple stimulation or by administering an intravenous infusion with oxytocin. Note that the contraction stress test is contraindicated in several clinical situations, including preterm labor, placenta previa, vasa previa, cervical incompetence, multiple gestation, and previous classical cesarean delivery. The procedure for performing the contraction stress test follows.

Procedure for Nipple-Stimulated Contraction Stress Test

1. Assist the woman into a semi-Fowler's position with a lateral tilt.
2. Position the tocodynamometer above the uterine fundus.
3. Place the ultrasound transducer on the maternal abdomen where the clearest fetal signal can be obtained.
4. Monitor baseline FHR and uterine activity until 10 minutes of interpretable data are obtained (defer nipple stimulation if three spontaneous contractions of more than 40 seconds' duration occur within a 10-minute period).
5. Instruct the woman to brush the surface of the fingers over the nipple of one breast through her clothes; continue four cycles of 2 minutes on and 2 to 5 minutes off; stop when contraction begins and restimulate when contraction ends (if a 2-minute period has elapsed).
   a. If unsuccessful after four cycles, restimulate the breasts for 10 minutes, stopping when contraction begins and resuming when contraction ends.
   b. If unsuccessful, begin bilateral continuous stimulation for 10 minutes, stopping when contraction begins and resuming when contraction ends.
6. Discontinue nipple stimulation when three or more spontaneous contractions lasting longer than 40 seconds occur in a 10-minute period and are palpable to the examiner.
7. Interpret results and continue monitoring until uterine activity has returned to the prestimulation state.

If nipple stimulation does not produce the desired uterine activity, an oxytocin-stimulated contraction stress test may be necessary.

Procedure for Oxytocin Challenge Test

The oxytocin challenge test is performed in the inpatient setting because labor may be stimulated in some sensitive women.

1. Assist the woman into a semi-Fowler's position with a lateral tilt.
2. Place the tocodynamometer above the uterine fundus.
3. Place the ultrasound transducer on the maternal abdomen where the clearest fetal signal can be obtained.
4. Monitor baseline FHR and uterine activity until 10 minutes of interpretable data are obtained.
5. Check the woman's blood pressure and pulse.

6. If fewer than three spontaneous contractions occur within a 10-minute period and if late decelerations do not occur with spontaneous contractions, oxytocin can be initiated.

7. Piggyback oxytocin into the primary intravenous line in the port nearest the intravenous insertion site.

8. Administer oxytocin, beginning with 0.5 to 2.0 mU/min, with a constant infusion pump per facility protocol.

9. Increase the dosage of oxytocin infusion by 0.5 to 1.0 mU/min at 15-minute intervals until the contraction frequency is three in 10 minutes of 40 seconds' or more duration and contractions are palpable to the examiner.

10. Discontinue the oxytocin when three contractions have occurred within a 10-minute period of interpretable data.

11. Discontinue the oxytocin any time there is evidence of excessive uterine activity, prolonged deceleration, or recurrent late decelerations; be prepared to administer terbutaline for tocolysis.

12. Continue to monitor until uterine activity and FHR return to baseline status.

The Nonstress Test

FHR accelerations that occur in association with fetal movements form the basis of the NST. Although many criteria have been reported, a normal or "reactive" NST usually is defined by two or more accelerations in a 20-minute period, each lasting at least 15 seconds and peaking at least 15 bpm above the baseline. Before 32 weeks, an acceleration is defined as a rise of at least 10 bpm with a duration of at least 10 seconds from the beginning of the acceleration until return to baseline.

The NST is considered "nonreactive" if, *after 40 minutes of continuous monitoring,* the FHR tracing does not demonstrate at least two qualifying accelerations within a 20-minute window [2,6]. In most institutions, the test is repeated once or twice weekly. Boehm and colleagues reported that twice-weekly testing yielded a threefold reduction in the incidence of fetal death [7].

Alternately, fetal acoustic stimulation testing (FAST) can be used. As discussed in Chapter 6, an FHR acceleration in response to fetal vibroacoustic stimulation is highly predictive of the absence of fetal metabolic acidemia and ongoing hypoxic injury [8–16]. Using an artificial larynx placed on the maternal abdomen near the fetal head, vibroacoustic stimulation is applied for 1 to 2 seconds. The test is considered *reactive* if stimulation results in an FHR acceleration.

(NOTE: The gestational age–related criteria for acceleration peak and duration are the same for FAST as they are for the NST). Clinicians should note that with FAST, only one application of vibroacoustic stimulation is performed; if the fetus does not respond with an acceleration, the FAST is considered *nonreactive.*

Among 1542 women tested weekly with the NST, Freeman reported a corrected fetal false-negative rate of 1.9/1000 [4]. Assessment of FHR characteristics other than accelerations (baseline rate, variability, decelerations) may improve the sensitivity of the test. Decelerations may be observed in 33% to 50% of patients undergoing weekly NSTs [17–19]. In one study, reactive tests accompanied by variable decelerations were associated with rates of meconium passage and cesarean delivery for fetal indications that were similar to those encountered with nonreactive tests [18]. Manning and colleagues concluded that FHR decelerations during the NST, regardless of reactivity, warrant consideration of delivery [20]. Reported false-positive rates of the NST vary widely, with an average rate of approximately 50%.

Interpretation and Management

The NST is interpreted as reactive or nonreactive (see Figs. 9.1 and 9.2).

- A reactive NST is defined as two accelerations in a 20-minute period, each lasting at least 15 seconds and peaking at least 15 bpm above the baseline. (Before 32 weeks an acceleration is defined as a rise of at least 10 bpm lasting at least 10 seconds from onset to offset.)

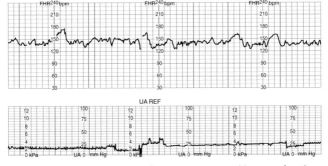

Fig. 9.1 Reactive nonstress test in term pregnancy. Note accelerations meet minimum criteria of 15 bpm or greater and last a minimum of 15 seconds or longer duration (onset to offset). *FHR,* fetal heart rate; *REF,* Reference; *UA,* uterine activity.

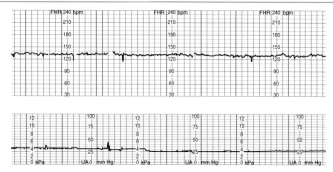

Fig. 9.2 Segment of nonreactive nonstress test in term pregnancy. The lack of accelerations meeting minimum criteria continued for 40 minutes. *FHR,* fetal heart rate; *UA,* uterine activity.

- A nonreactive NST is a test that does not demonstrate at least two qualifying accelerations within a 20-minute window.

A reactive NST with no significant decelerations is considered normal, and the routine testing schedule is resumed (usually once or twice weekly). A nonreactive NST requires further evaluation. In most cases, a backup test is performed (a contraction stress test or a biophysical profile [BPP]) [2]. Management is guided by the results of the backup test. When performed twice weekly and interpreted in the context of associated FHR patterns, the NST alone appears to be an acceptable, although not optimal, method of antepartum testing.

Advantages and Disadvantages

Advantages of the NST include ease of use and interpretation, low cost, and minimal time requirement. The chief disadvantages include a twice-weekly testing interval, a high false-positive rate, and a higher false-negative rate than achieved with other methods. Management of the NST is illustrated in Fig. 9.3.

The Biophysical Profile

The BPP, as described by Manning and colleagues [20], assesses five biophysical variables. FHR reactivity, fetal movement, tone, and breathing reflect acute central nervous system function, whereas amniotic fluid volume serves as a marker of the longer term adequacy of placental function. Two points are assigned for each normal

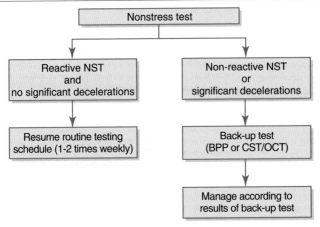

Fig. 9.3 Management of the nonstress test (NST). *BPP,* biophysical profile; *CST,* contraction stress test: *OCT,* oxytocin challenge test.

variable and zero points for each abnormal variable, for a maximum score of 10.

Interpretation and Management

Scoring the BPP is outlined in Table 9.2. A BPP score of 8 to 10, with normal amniotic fluid volume, is considered normal, and the routine testing schedule is resumed. A score of 6 is considered suspicious, and testing is usually repeated the next day. Scores less than 6 are associated with increased perinatal morbidity and mortality and usually warrant hospitalization for further evaluation or delivery.

The BPP is a reliable indicator of fetal well-being. The false-negative rate is superior to that of the NST alone and compares favorably with the false-negative rate of the contraction stress test. One study reported a false-negative rate of 0.6/1000 among 12,620 women tested weekly with the BPP [21]. Another study reported significantly lower rates of cesarean delivery for fetal distress (3% vs. 22%), low 5-minute Apgar scores (1.6% and 3.2% vs. 12.5%), and meconium aspiration syndrome when the last BPP before delivery was normal versus when it was abnormal [22]. Among 19,221 referred high-risk pregnancies, Manning and colleagues [23] reported a false-negative rate of 0.7/1000. The false-positive rate of the BPP varies with the score of the last test before delivery, ranging from 0% if the last BPP

TABLE 9.2   Scoring the Biophysical Profile

Biophysical Variable	Score 2	Score 0
Fetal breathing movements	At least one episode of fetal breathing movements of at least 30-second duration in a 30-minute observation	Absent fetal breathing movements or less than 30 seconds of sustained fetal breathing movements in 30 minutes
Fetal movements	At least three trunk/limb movements in 30 minutes	Fewer than three episodes of trunk/limb movements in 30 minutes
Fetal tone	At least one episode of active extension with return to flexion of fetal limb or trunk; opening and closing of hand considered normal tone	Absence of movement or slow extension/flexion
Amniotic fluid	Deepest vertical pocket >2 cm	Deepest vertical pocket ≤2 cm
Nonstress test	Reactive	Nonreactive

score before delivery was 0, to more than 40% if the last BPP score was 6.

Advantages and Limitations

Advantages of the BPP include excellent sensitivity, a weekly testing interval, a low false-negative rate, and improved detection of structural fetal anomalies. The primary limitation is the requirement for personnel trained in sonographic visualization of the fetus. Additionally, although the duration of ultrasound observation is less than 10 minutes in the majority of cases, the complete BPP is more time-consuming than other noninvasive tests. However, when all ultrasound variables are normal, addition of the NST does not appear to alter the discriminative accuracy of the test.

The Modified Biophysical Profile

The modified BPP (MBPP) combines the strengths of the NST (ease of use, low cost) and the complete BPP (improved sensitivity, low false-negative rate), while minimizing the requirement for additional training in sonographic visualization of the fetus. The test is performed once or twice weekly and uses the NST as a short-term marker of fetal status and the amniotic fluid volume as a marker of longer term placental function. In 2014 ACOG changed the requirement for evaluation of amniotic fluid volume in an MBPP from the traditional four-quadrant amniotic fluid index to a single deepest vertical pocket of greater than 2 cm [2].

Interpretation and Management

Interpretation of the NST incorporates assessment of reactivity, baseline rate, variability, and FHR decelerations. Late, prolonged, or significant variable decelerations, particularly in the setting of low-normal amniotic fluid volume (single deepest vertical pocket 2 cm or less), are considered abnormal. The MBPP is considered normal if the NST is reactive and the amniotic fluid volume measurement is a single deepest vertical pocket of greater than 2 cm [2]. Regardless of reactivity of the NST, oligohydramnios constitutes an abnormal test.

If the MBPP is normal, the routine testing schedule is resumed. If the MBPP is abnormal, a backup test is warranted. The BPP and the contraction stress test are the most common backup tests and perform similarly with respect to perinatal morbidity and mortality [2]. Further management is guided by the results of the backup test. Management of the MBPP is summarized in Fig. 9.1.

Nageotte and coworkers [24] evaluated 2774 high-risk pregnancies with twice-weekly MBPPs and reported one unexplained fetal death within 1 week of a normal test result, for a false-negative rate of 0.36/1000. Another study, by Miller and colleagues [25], reported 54,617 MBPPs in 15,482 high-risk pregnancies. Antepartum testing in high-risk pregnancies yielded a fetal death rate that was nearly sevenfold lower than that in the untested, "low-risk" population. The overall false-negative rate of the MBPP was 0.8/1000, and the false-positive rate was 60%. Abnormal test results prompted intervention in 15.5% of the tested population; however, iatrogenic prematurity occurred in only 1.5% of women tested before 37 weeks. Large studies reveal the false-negative rate of the MBPP to be similar to that of the contraction stress test and the complete BPP. When using the MBPP, amniotic fluid evaluation may be done weekly or twice weekly, depending on gestational age and initial and ongoing evaluation of amniotic fluid volume [26,27].

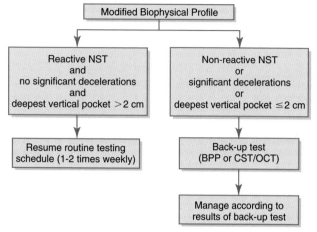

Fig. 9.4 Management of the modified biophysical profile. *BPP,* bio-physical profile; *CST,* contraction stress test; *OCT,* oxytocin challenge test.

Advantages and Limitations

Advantages of the MBPP are that it is easier to perform and less time-consuming than the contraction stress test or the complete BPP. The sensitivity of the MBPP is superior to that of the NST alone. Limitations include the need for backup testing in 10% to 50% of patients, a high false-positive rate, and a twice-weekly testing interval. Fig. 9.4 depicts a schematic for management of the MBPP.

Fetal Movement Counts

Maternal perception of normal fetal movement has long been recognized as a reliable indicator of fetal well-being. Conversely, prolonged absence of fetal movement may signal fetal death. Cessation of fetal movement in response to hypoxia has been demonstrated in animal studies; however, controlled data in human fetuses are lacking. Nevertheless, any acute change in the number or strength of fetal movements should prompt further evaluation. Many clinicians recommend routine fetal movement counting, particularly in women who are considered high risk [28–30].

Interpretation and Management

A common approach is to recommend the pregnant woman count fetal movements for 1 hour each day.

- Ten fetal movements in a 1-hour period are considered reassuring.
- If fewer than 10 movements are perceived, counting is continued for another hour.
- Fewer than 10 movements in a 2-hour period should alert the patient to contact her physician for further evaluation.

Another approach calls for the pregnant woman to count movements for 1 hour three times per week. Yet another calls for movement counting two to three times daily for 30 minutes. With this latter approach, further evaluation is recommended if there are fewer than four strong movements in a 30-minute period.

Evidence from one study using nonconcurrent controls demonstrated a lower rate of fetal death and a higher incidence of intervention for fetal distress in patients using a formalized protocol of fetal movement counting [29]. Although there is insufficient evidence to recommend routine fetal movement counting in all pregnancies, fetal movement counting is an inexpensive method of involving the patient in her own care and carries few if any risks [1].

Doppler Velocimetry of Maternal and Fetal Blood Vessels

Doppler velocimetry of fetal, umbilical, and uterine vessels has been the focus of intensive study in the last years. This technology uses systolic/diastolic flow ratios, such as resistance and pulsatility indices, to estimate blood flow in various arteries. In pregnancies complicated by fetal growth restriction, addition of Doppler velocimetry has been shown to improve perinatal outcome [1,31,32]. Although severe restriction of umbilical artery blood flow—as evidenced by absent or reversed flow during diastole—has been correlated with fetal growth restriction, acidosis, and adverse perinatal outcome, the predictive values of less extreme deviations from normal remain undefined. In conditions other than fetal growth restriction resulting from placental dysfunction, Doppler velocimetry does not appear to be a useful screening test for the detection of fetal compromise. Umbilical artery Doppler velocimetry it is not recommended for use as a screening test in the general obstetric population.

Doppler velocimetry of the fetal middle cerebral artery (MCA) demonstrates increased diastolic flow velocity in the setting of reduced fetal oxygenation, reflecting decreased resistance to flow. This autoregulatory reflex is known as the *brain-sparing effect* of hypoxemia [33]. The peak systolic velocity in the MCA has been shown to increase significantly in the setting of fetal anemia, and it can predict moderate to severe anemia with sensitivity and negative predictive values that equal or exceed those of the traditional method of amniocentesis for delta OD 450 determination [22,34–38].

The cerebroplacental ratio (CPR) is the ratio of the pulsatility indices of the MCA and the umbilical artery. The pulsatility index is an indicator of resistance to blood flow; high pulsatility indices reflect increased resistance to blood flow, low pulsatility indices reflect low resistance. In the setting of suboptimal fetal oxygenation caused by placental dysfunction, the numerator of the ratio (MCA pulsatility index) will decrease, reflecting decreased resistance to forward flow in the MCA. At the same time, the denominator of the ratio (the umbilical artery pulsatility index) will increase, reflecting increased resistance to forward flow in the umbilical arteries. The combination of a decreasing numerator and a rising denominator results in a greater change in the CPR than that observed individually in either the MCA or umbilical artery pulsatility indices. This has led some to suggest that the CPR is more accurate than either of its individual components. A 2018 systematic review and meta-analysis included 128 studies of CPR, umbilical artery Doppler, and MCA Doppler [39]. The CPR performed better than umbilical artery Doppler alone in identifying the need for emergency delivery for fetal distress and in composite adverse neonatal outcomes in singleton pregnancies. CPR and umbilical artery Doppler performed similarly for all other outcomes. The authors could not demonstrate a benefit of the CPR over umbilical artery Doppler alone in the setting of late fetal growth restriction.

A number of studies have evaluated the utility of uterine artery Doppler waveform analysis in the prediction of fetal growth restriction [40]. In the setting of an abnormal uterine artery Doppler waveform, the pooled likelihood ratio was 3.67 for the development of fetal growth restriction. When Doppler velocimetry measurements are used in antepartum fetal surveillance, they should be interpreted in the context of the clinical setting and the results of other tests of fetal status. In the setting of fetal growth restriction, Doppler velocimetry used in conjunction with standard fetal surveillance, such as NST or BPP, is associated with improved outcomes [2].

Biochemical Assessment

Amniocentesis for Fetal Lung Maturity

Amniocentesis is an invasive procedure in which a needle is introduced into the amniotic cavity to remove amniotic fluid for analysis. It is performed under ultrasound guidance using a 20- to 22-gauge spinal-type needle placed transabdominally to withdraw 5 to 20 mL of amniotic fluid (Fig. 9.5). In the second trimester, amniocentesis is used frequently to detect a number of abnormalities, including aneuploidy. In the third trimester, it is used primarily to assess fetal lung maturity (FLM). Risks in the third trimester are relatively few and include bleeding, infection, membrane rupture, preterm labor,

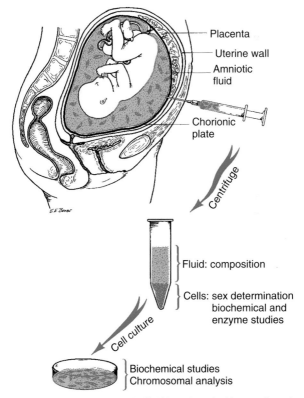

Fig. 9.5 Amniocentesis. Amniotic fluid is aspirated with a sterile syringe. The sample is centrifuged to separate cells and fluid.

preterm delivery, and alloimmunization in the setting of blood type incompatibility. Amniotic fluid can be used to assess FLM by a number of methods.

Lecithin-to-Sphingomyelin Ratio

Pulmonary surfactant contains primarily phospholipids. Surfactant acts as a surface detergent at the air–liquid interface of the alveoli, preventing collapse at the end of expiration. The lecithin-to-sphingomyelin (L/S) ratio compares the concentrations of two phospholipids, lecithin and sphingomyelin, which are major components of surfactant. In the third trimester, an increase in lecithin causes a rise in the L/S ratio. A ratio of 2.0 or greater is associated with a low risk of neonatal surfactant-deficient respiratory distress syndrome (RDS).

The following interpretation is generally accepted:

L/S Ratio	Fetal Lung	Risk for RDS
>2.0	Mature	Minimal
1.5–2.0	Transitional	Moderate
<1.5	Immature	High

L/S, lecithin-to-sphingomyelin; *RDS,* respiratory distress syndrome.

Note that the presence of blood or meconium can interfere with the results of the L/S ratio.

Foam Stability Test

This test is based on the ability of surfactant to generate stable foam when ethanol is added to the amniotic fluid specimen. Ethanol, isotonic saline, and amniotic fluid at varying dilutions are shaken together for 15 seconds. At the proper dilution, a ring of bubbles at the air–liquid interface after 15 minutes indicates probable FLM (Fig. 9.6).

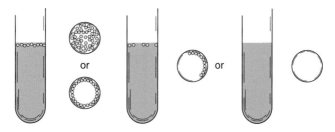

Positive foam test   Negative foam test

Fig. 9.6 Foam stability test (shake test). For the test to be positive, bubbles must be seen around the entire circumference of the tube.

Phosphatidylglycerol

The presence of phosphatidylglycerol can be ascertained quickly and is not affected by blood or meconium. The presence of phosphatidylglycerol indicates a low risk for RDS. Whenever possible, FLM assessment should be based on phosphatidylglycerol in combination with the L/S ratio.

Fluorescence Polarization (Fetal Lung Maturity-II Assay)

The FLM-II assay uses fluorescence polarization to determine lipid membrane fluidity in amniotic fluid.

Interpretation of the FLM-II assay is summarized as follows:
Mature >55 mg/g
Transitional 40 to 54 mg/g
Immature <39 mg/g

Lamellar Body Count

Lamellar body counting measures the number of surfactant-containing particles in amniotic fluid directly by using the platelet channel of a standard hematology cell counter. The size and number of lamellar bodies in the amniotic fluid are predictive of FLM [41]. Interpretation is summarized as follows:

Mature ≥50,000/μL
Transitional >15,000 to <50,000/μL
Immature ≤15,000/μL

SUMMARY

Our ability to assess the condition of the fetus has improved dramatically since fetal monitoring was introduced into clinical practice. Although diagnostic precision is enhanced by electronic FHR monitoring and ultrasound technology, room for improvement remains. Electronic FHR monitoring is a very sensitive tool for the detection of interrupted fetal oxygenation; truly compromised fetuses rarely fail to exhibit abnormal FHR patterns. The converse, however, is not true. FHR patterns such as decelerations, tachycardia, and intermittent reduction in variability and/or accelerations are frequently observed in the absence of fetal compromise. The limited positive predictive value is the principal shortcoming of FHR monitoring. Accuracy may be improved by combining FHR analysis with assessment of biophysical variables, such as amniotic fluid volume, fetal movement, breathing, tone, and blood flow characteristics. The most effective combination of variables has not been defined, and no one approach to fetal surveillance has demonstrated clear superiority over the others. Despite the limitations, antepartum testing in high-risk pregnancies has been reported to yield a fetal death rate lower than that observed in untested, low-risk pregnancies [25]. If this observation is substantiated, future investigation will be needed to address the role of antepartum fetal surveillance in uncomplicated, low-risk pregnancies.

References

[1] C. Signore, R.K. Freeman, C.Y. Spong, Antenatal testing-a reevaluation: executive summary of a Eunice Kennedy Shriver National Institute of Child Health and Human Development workshop, Obstet. Gynecol. 113 (3) (2009) 687–701.

[2] American College of Obstetricians and Gynecologists, Antepartum fetal surveillance. ACOG Practice Bulletin No. 145, Obstet. Gynecol. 124 (2014) 182–192.

[3] F.W. Kubli, E.H. Hon, A.F. Khazin, et al., Observations on heart rate and pH in the human fetus during labor, Am. J. Obstet. Gynecol. 104 (8) (1969) 1190–1206.

[4] R.K. Freeman, G. Anderson, W. Dorchester, A prospective multi-institutional study of antepartum fetal heart rate monitoring. II. Contraction stress versus nonstress test for primary surveillance, Am. J. Obstet. Gynecol. 143 (7) (1982) 778–781.

[5] D.C. Lagrew Jr, The contraction stress test, Clin. Obstet. Gynecol. 38 (1) (1995) 1–25.

[6] National Institute of Child Health and Human Development Research Planning Workshop, Electronic fetal heart rate monitoring: research guidelines for interpretation, Am. J. Obstet. Gynecol. 177 (6) (1997) 1385–1390.

[7] F.H. Boehm, S. Salyer, D.M. Shah, et al., Improved outcome of twice weekly nonstress testing, Obstet. Gynecol. 67 (4) (1986) 566–568.

[8] S.L. Clark, M.L. Gimovsky, F.C. Miller, Fetal heart rate response to scalp blood sampling, Am. J. Obstet. Gynecol. 144 (6) (1982) 706–708.

[9] S.L. Clark, M.L. Gimovsky, F.C. Miller, The scalp stimulation test: a clinical alternative to fetal scalp blood sampling, Am. J. Obstet. Gynecol. 148 (3) (1984) 274–277.

[10] T.G. Edersheim, J.M. Hutson, M.L. Druzin, et al., Fetal heart rate response to vibratory acoustic stimulation predicts fetal pH in labor, Am. J. Obstet. Gynecol. 157 (6) (1987) 1557–1560.

[11] A. Elimian, R. Figueroa, N. Tejani, Intrapartum assessment of fetal well-being: a comparison of scalp stimulation with scalp blood pH sampling, Obstet. Gynecol. 89 (3) (1987) 373–376.

[12] I. Ingemarsson, S. Arulkumaran, Reactive fetal heart rate response to VAS in fetuses with low scalp blood pH, Br, J. Obstet. Gynaecol. 96 (5) (1989) 562–565.

[13] G.B. Polzin, K.J. Blakemore, R.H. Petrie, et al., Fetal vibro-acoustic stimulation: magnitude and duration of fetal heart rate accelerations as a marker of fetal health, Obstet. Gynecol. 72 (4) (1988) 621–626.

[14] D.W. Skupski, C.R. Rosenberg, G.S. Eglington, Intrapartum fetal stimulation tests: a meta-analysis, Obstet. Gynecol. 99 (1) (2002) 129–134.

[15] C.V. Smith, H.N. Nguyen, J.P. Phelan, et al., Intrapartum assessment of fetal well-being: a comparison of fetal acoustic stimulation with acid-base determinations, Am. J. Obstet. Gynecol. 155 (4) (1986) 726–728.

[16] J.A. Spencer, Predictive value of a fetal heart rate acceleration at the time of fetal blood sampling in labour, J. Perinat. Med. 19 (3) (1991) 207–215.

[17] P.J. Meis, J.R. Ureda, M. Swain, et al., Variable decelerations during nonstress tests are not a sign of fetal compromise, Am. J. Obstet. Gynecol. 154 (3) (1986) 586–590.

[18] J.P. Phelan, P.E. Lewis Jr, Fetal heart rate decelerations during a nonstress test, Obstet. Gynecol. 57 (2) (1981) 228–232.

[19] J.P. Phelan, L.D. Platt, S.Y. Yseh, et al., Continuing role of the nonstress test in the management of post-dates pregnancy, Obstet. Gynecol. 64 (5) (1984) 624–628.

[20] F.A. Manning, L.D. Platt, L. Sipos, Antepartum fetal evaluation: development of a fetal biophysical profile, Am. J. Obstet. Gynecol. 136 (6) (1980) 787–795.

[21] F.A. Manning, I. Morrison, I.R. Lange, et al., Fetal assessment based upon fetal BPP scoring: experience in 12,620 referred high risk pregnancies. I. Perinatal mortality by frequency and etiology, Am. J. Obstet. Gynecol. 151 (3) (1985) 343–350.

[22] J.M. Johnson, C.R. Harman, I.R. Lange, et al., Biophysical profile scoring in the management of postterm pregnancy: an analysis of 307 patients, Am. J. Obstet. Gynecol. 154 (2) (1986) 269–273.

[23] F.A. Manning, I. Morrison, C.R. Harman, et al., Fetal assessment based on fetal biophysical profile scoring: experience in 19,221 referred high-risk pregnancies. II. An analysis of false-negative fetal deaths, Am. J. Obstet. Gynecol. 157 (4 Pt 1) (1987) 880–884.

[24] J.P. Nageotte, C.V. Towers, T. Asrat, et al., Perinatal outcome with the MBPP, Am. J. Obstet. Gynecol. 170 (6) (1994) 1672–1676.

[25] D.A. Miller, Y.A. Rabello, R.H. Paul, The modified biophysical profile: antepartum testing in the 1990s, Am. J. Obstet. Gynecol. 174 (3) (1996) 812–817.

[26] D.C. Lagrew, R.A. Pircon, M. Nageotte, et al., How frequently should the amniotic fluid index be repeated?, Am. J. Obstet. Gynecol. 167 (4 Pt 1) (1992) 1129–1133.

[27] D.A. Wing, A. Fishman, C. Gonzalez, et al., How frequently should the amniotic fluid index be performed during the course of antepartum testing?, Am. J. Obstet. Gynecol. 174 (1 Pt 1) (1996) 33–36.

[28] A. Grant, D. Elbourne, L. Valentin, et al., Routine formal fetal movement counting and risk of antepartum late death in normally formed singletons, Lancet 2 (8659) (1989) 345–349.

[29] T.R. Moore, K. Piacquadio, A prospective evaluation of fetal movement screening to reduce the incidence of antepartum fetal death, Am. J. Obstet. Gynecol. 60 (5 Pt 1) (1989) 1075–1080.

[30] S. Neldam, Fetal movements as an indicator of fetal well-being, Dan. Med. Bull 30 (4) (1983) 274–278.

[31] Z. Alfirevic, J.P. Neilson, Doppler ultrasonography in high-risk pregnancies: systematic review with meta-analysis, Am. J. Obstet. Gynecol. 172 (5) (1995) 1379–1387.

[32] G. Mari, R.L. Deter, R.L. Carpenter, et al., Noninvasive diagnosis by Doppler ultrasonography of fetal anemia due to maternal red cell alloimmunization. Collaborative Group for Doppler Assessment of the Blood Velocity in Anemic Fetuses, N. Engl. J. Med. 342 (1) (2000) 9–14.

[33] R.O. Bahado-Singh, E. Kovanci, A. Jeffres, U. Oz, et al., The Doppler cerebroplacental ratio and perinatal outcome in intrauterine growth restriction, Am. J. Obstet. Gynecol. 180 (3 Pt 1) (1999) 750–756.

[34] D. Dukler, D. Oepkes, G. Seaward, et al., Noninvasive tests to predict fetal anemia: a study comparing Doppler and ultrasound parameters, Am. J. Obstet. Gynecol. 188 (5) (2003) 1310–1314.

[35] G. Mari, A. Adrignolo, A.Z. Abuhamad, et al., Diagnosis of fetal anemia with Doppler ultrasound in the pregnancy complicated by maternal blood group immunization, Ultrasound Obstet. Gynecol. 5 (6) (1995) 400–405.

[36] G. Mari, L. Detti, U. Oz, R. Zimmerman, et al., Accurate prediction of fetal hemoglobin by Doppler ultrasonography, Obstet. Gynecol. 99 (4) (2002) 589–593.

[37] G. Mari, F. Hanif, M. Kruger, et al., Middle cerebral artery peak systolic velocity: a new Doppler parameter in the assessment of growth-restricted fetuses, Ultrasound Obstet. Gynecol. 29 (3) (2007) 310–316.

[38] G. Mari, F. Rahman, P. Olofsson, et al., Increase of fetal hematocrit decreases the middle cerebral artery peak systolic velocity in pregnancies complicated by rhesus alloimmunization, J. Matern. Fetal Med. 6 (4) (1997) 206–208.

[39] C.A. Vollgraff Heidweiller-Schreurs, M.A. De Boer, M.W. Heymans, et al., Prognostic accuracy of cerebroplacental ratio and middle cerebral artery Doppler for adverse perinatal outcome:systematic review and meta-analysis, Ultrasound Obstet. Gynecol. 51 (2018) 313–322.

[40] A.T. Papageorghiou, C.K. Yu, K.H. Nicolaides, The role of uterine artery Doppler in predicting adverse pregnancy outcome, Best Pract. Res. Clin. Obstet. Gynaecol. 18 (3) (2004) 383–396.

[41] M.G. Neerhof, J.C. Dohnal, E.R. Ashwood, et al., Lamellar body counts: a consensus on protocol, Obstet. Gynecol. 97 (2) (2001) 318–320.

CHAPTER 10

Patient Safety, Risk Management, and Documentation

Knowledge of the basic principles of law and the effect on the obstetric clinicians who provide patient care is an essential aspect of professional practice. In today's healthcare climate, there is a reasonable expectation for clinicians to stay abreast of key aspects of obstetric care and electronic fetal monitoring (EFM) including clinical reasoning and information to determine a diagnosis, terminology, and evidence-based interventions and processes to uphold patient safety's basic tenets [1]. This chapter provides an overview of the relevant litigation issues and documentation principles that clinicians practicing in the obstetric specialty are challenged with understanding and practicing in daily clinical practice.

RISK MANAGEMENT

Risk management related to healthcare organizations is a continual process of identifying and mitigating, and when necessary controlling liability risks to a healthcare organization [2]. Two critical elements of risk management include risk reduction and risk mitigation. Risk reduction seeks to avoid preventable adverse outcomes, decreasing the risk of litigation. Risk mitigation is overseeing liability exposure after a preventable or unpreventable adverse outcome [3]. In obstetrics, safety initiatives such as quality improvement efforts have gradually transitioned from being local programs from a single hospital to statewide efforts through state-based perinatal quality collaboratives [4]. Presently, national initiatives are being incorporated into these perinatal collaboratives across the United States to improve the quality of care of women and newborns. Multiple studies have been published regarding the use of patient safety bundles, evidence-based guidelines, and interdisciplinary education to improve processes of care and patient outcomes. This includes literature that supports the use of interdisciplinary teamwork in EFM interpretation and data that consistently demonstrated significant decreases in perinatal morbidity and mortality related to intrapartum asphyxia, low Apgar scores, hypoxic-ischemic encephalopathy, and suboptimal obstetric care [5–11]. In all healthcare specialties, initiatives in patient safety share several general themes, including a human factor approach to error, standardization of clinical practice, and emphasis on a team approach that places high value on communication.

THE DECISION-MAKING PROCESS IN ELECTRONIC FETAL MONITORING AND INTERMITTENT AUSCULTATION

In daily clinical practice, clinicians often engage patients in healthcare discussions in one-way conversations that are based on best practices and available evidence [12]. These dialogues often include benefits, risks, and alternatives that are parallel to what a reasonably prudent individual of similar training and background would do under the same circumstances. This is referred to as *informed consent* because a patient will either agree or refuse a proposed option in regard to invasive treatments and procedures [13]. Although written informed consent is not a legal requirement for either intermittent auscultation (IA) or EFM, a discussion regarding mode of monitoring is the responsibility of the midwife or physician with the nurse having an independent duty to act as a patient advocate. For example, a woman may not understand why a physician has planned to start oxytocin for labor augmentation and placement of an internal monitor. A nurse may provide basic patient education regarding EFM, but he or she is obligated to notify the primary provider if the patient continues to have questions regarding the intent of the procedure. This allows the provider to have further discussion and clarification before instituting the procedure.

In the current healthcare climate, there is a movement to change these one-way informed consent conversations into two-way discussions in which a partnership is formed with a patient during the decision-making process. This exchange of information, commonly referred to as *shared decision-making* (SDM), incorporates an individual's values, goals, and preference before giving informed consent [12]. There are three fundamental components of the SDM model

[12,14]. First, accurate, impartial, and comprehensible information, including the right to refuse the proposed plan of care is relayed to the patient. Second, the SDM process requires a clinician be present and proficient in communication to that the data presented are individualized to a particular situation. Last, the woman's individual's values, goals, informed preferences, and concerns are incorporated into this conversation.

In obstetric practice, there is a plethora of information that needs to be conveyed to the pregnant patient. Depending on the clinical scenario, this information can be overwhelming and a patient may feel compelled to agree to a plan of care without fully understanding the associated risks, benefits, and alternatives. Therefore institutions that provide labor and birth services may consider creating patient decision aids regarding fetal surveillance options and other antepartum and intrapartum topics. These tools allow patients to be better participants in the decision-making process and contain information on the risks, benefits, and alternatives, and burdens of options [14]. Additionally, these fact sheets help patients clarify and communicate personal values on different aspects of the options being presented. Basically, decision aids help educate patients in an unbiased format. Box 10.1 provides a list of discussion points that an interdisciplinary team may incorporate into these fact sheets during the development phase of a fetal surveillance tool. These instruments can be particularly important when discussing IA as the guidance from several professional organizations can be incorporated into the document. More specifically, the American College of Obstetricians and Gynecologists (ACOG) has stated that there

---

BOX 10.1   Discussion Points for Electronic Fetal Monitoring and Intermittent Auscultation Decision Aid

1. Clinical indications for IA or EFM (e.g., risk factors).
2. Description of the procedure that will be used for fetal surveillance, which could include the technique (Doppler vs. fetoscope, abdominal fetal electrocardiogram or telemetry) and the frequencies of assessment based on risk factors and the stage of labor.
3. Review of risks and benefits with discussion concerning the lack of quality evidence and the grading quality of evidence and strength of recommendations made in the literature.
4. Alternatives to an absolute use of either IA or EFM as there are clinical situations that may warrant some combination of intermittent EFM with IA.

EFM, electronic fetal monitoring; *IA,* intermittent auscultation.

is no clear benefit for EFM over IA in women not experiencing complications [15]. The Association of Women's Health, Obstetric and Neonatal Nurses (AWHONN) asserts a woman's preferences and clinical presentation should guide selection of FHM techniques and that the least invasive method of monitoring is preferred to promote physiologic labor and birth [16]. The American College of Nurse-Midwives (ACNM) affirms that IA is the preferred method for intrapartum fetal surveillance for women who are considered to be low risk at labor onset for developing fetal acidemia and are at a term gestational age [17]. Nevertheless, both EFM and IA may be the basis of a malpractice allegation in the event of an unexpected adverse outcome. Providing evidence that the patient received informed consent using an SDM model is both ethically correct and sound risk management.

CENTRAL CONCEPTS IN LIABILITY CLAIMS

Failure to do something that a reasonable and prudent clinician would do in the same circumstances is known as *malpractice* or *professional negligence*. Clinicians are held to national standards of care and practice within the "same or similar circumstances" and "reasonably expected" parameters. Standards of care come from a variety of sources as shown in Fig. 10.1 *Negligence* is the failure to act in the required manner, causing harm to an individual. *Malpractice* is an unintentional act performed by a professional acting in a professional capacity that causes harm to an individual. Under the rule *respondeat superior,* "let the master answer," an employer is held liable for acts of malpractice committed by an employee while performing duties for which he or she was hired. Clinicians are encouraged to have a rudimentary understanding of the law and the medical malpractice claim process, which has predictable steps and elements that must be proven [1]. Tort is a form of civil law addressing an act or omission that causes injury or harm to a person and is divided into three categories: intentional, strict, and negligence. To establish negligence in a medical liability claim, four criteria must be satisfied: duty, breach of duty, causation, and harm or injuries [1,18].

- *Duty:* a professional relationship that is established between a patient and a clinician or a legal obligation to an individual who may be affected by specific actions.
  - For example, the primary nurse who cares for the laboring patient throughout the duration of the shift fulfills this criteria.

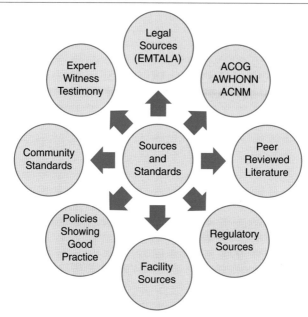

Fig. 10.1 Standard of care sources. *ACNM,* American College of Nurse-Midwives; *ACOG,* American Congress of Obstetricians and Gynecologists; *AWHONN,* Association of Women's Health, Obstetric and Neonatal Nurses; *EMTALA,* Emergency Medical Treatment and Active Labor Act. (Courtesy Rebecca L. Cypher, MSN, PNNP.)

- *Breach of duty:* a clinician's practice has neglected to meet an appropriate standard of care in which a reasonably prudent person of similar experience and training would do under the same circumstances.
  - For example, failure to perform corrective interventions for a Category III tracing is a breach of duty.
- *Causation:* a causal connection between harm and a clinician's actions or lack of actions (breach of duty) caused by a failure to meet a standard of care.
  - For example, causation can be established between 100 mcg of vaginal misoprostol, tachysystole, and uterine rupture when administered for cervical ripening in a postterm labor induction.
- *Harm or injury:* actual harm or injury occurred to the woman, fetus, or neonate as a result of the breach of duty.

- This takes the form of punitive, economic, or noneconomic damages such as payment for healthcare expenses; loss of past, present, and future wages; or loss of a chance of survival.

COMPONENTS OF CARE: ASSESSMENT, COMMUNICATION, AND DOCUMENTATION

There are three critical components to providing adequate patient care: assessment, communication, and documentation (Fig. 10.2). At times, hospital policies and protocols, especially those related to documentation, fail to appreciate that there are distinct differences between these elements. This results in clinician's being unable to remain in compliance with policies that have been set forth while spending excessive amounts of time "nursing the chart" and "monitoring the computer" instead of providing direct patient care. A brief review of these components is necessary.

Assessment is the evaluation of a patient's status and is constant, ongoing, and detailed. Healthcare professionals observe and perform tasks that are clinically relevant but do not warrant communication or documentation in a medical record. Examples include introducing the healthcare team at the beginning of a work shift, changing a disposable underpad after amniotic membrane rupture, or simply offering words

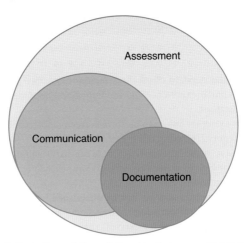

Fig. 10.2 Illustration of the relationship between assessment, communication, and documentation in daily clinical practice. (Courtesy Lisa A. Miller, CNM, JD.)

of encouragement to a woman experiencing painful uterine contractions. Realistically, there is absolutely no rationale and nor is it physically possible to either communicate or document all the assessments and activities of any clinician. *Thus the frequently quoted adage "if it wasn't charted, it wasn't done" has never been and will never be true because it has no legal basis* [19]. Yet many clinicians readily agree with this statement because a plaintiff attorney will have only the medical record and the patient or support system's story to rely on when determining whether an allegation of malpractice has any merit [19]; except, the defense team has a number of options for providing proof at deposition or trial outside the medical record. Testimony on the basis of what a defendant clinician can recall or remember from caring for the patient can be used. A clinician's usual or routine practice also can be used at the time of testimony.

Communication is slightly less broad than assessment but also encompasses more than any clinician can or should document in the medical record. Oftentimes, communication in the obstetric setting is routine, consisting of sharing information or giving instructions to patients and their support systems. For example, notification of the senior obstetric resident by an intern or a discussion between a staff nurse and the charge nurse in relationship to a patient's ongoing Category I tracing may not require documentation in the medical record depending on the clinical scenario. Conversely, notification of the midwife regarding labor progress and fetal status may be quite detailed in communication but could be documented simply as "Provider updated as to patient status." as the actual data are reflected in ongoing documentation. There is no legal requirement to document verbatim each and every conversation that occurs over the course of labor and birth. In addition, this is not an effective use of a clinician's time.

Documentation is the least broad of the three categories. Yet a clinician's documentation is the most singularly important piece of evidence in litigation because the primary exhibit in a malpractice case is the medical record. Accordingly, a complete, accurate, and contemporaneous record is the foundation of a plaintiff or defense attorney's ability to demonstrate the merits of a liability claim. The best evidentiary friend of a plaintiff attorney is either absent, inaccurate, or inconsistent documentation of the care provided. Inaccurate documentation can stem from a competency issue, for example, if the fetal heart rate (FHR) or uterine activity (UA) is not appropriately interpreted or when inappropriate terminology is used to describe what is present on the tracing. One illustration of unacceptable documentation is found in Fig. 10.3. Both physician and nursing summary

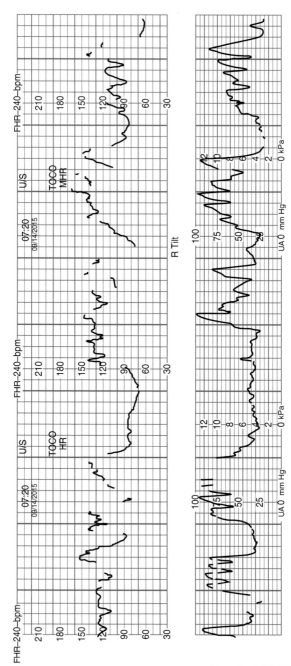

Fig. 10.3 Tracing described as "sketchy" by the healthcare team. *FHR*, fetal heart rate; *U/A*, uterine activity. (Courtesy Rebecca L. Cypher, MSN, PNNP.)

documentation described the tracing as *sketchy* in relationship to a noncontiguous tracing that had transitioned to a Category II tracing. In situations similar to this example, immediate impressions are often formed when clinical notes such as these are reviewed from a medicolegal perspective [20].

LIABILITY IN FETAL MONITORING

Litigation related to healthcare is a relatively prevalent occurrence in the United States. Traditionally, obstetrics has had one of the highest rates of paid malpractice claims to include higher average indemnity payments and higher paid-to-closed ratios than most medical specialties [21]. One of the most commonly cited motives to pursue litigation in the obstetric environment is from the EFM perspective because ongoing tracing interpretation and management is the most common task clinicians perform during the intrapartum period. Common allegations that are frequently cited in malpractice claims related to EFM include:

- Failure to recognize Category II or III FHR tracings and appropriately manage indeterminate and abnormal patterns
- Failure to maintain an adequate FHR and UA signal source for interpretation
- Failure to recognize signal ambiguity in a timely manner
- Failure to complete ongoing EFM education as an individual clinician or in a collaborative setting
- Failure to adhere to policies and procedures
- Failure to communicate because of lack of knowledge or fear of conflict
- Failure to maintain an organizational culture
- Failure to use the chain of command when required
- Failure to maintain situational awareness
- Failure to provide adequate documentation in the medical record
    Table 10.1 outlines potential ways to decrease the risk of liability related to fetal monitoring.

FETAL MONITORING DOCUMENTATION

Obstetric safety is a high priority in today's healthcare environment with contemporaneous, complete, and objective documentation being the foundation for continuity of care and communication between clinicians [21]. Documentation promotes improved quality of care by encouraging assessment and reevaluation of progress and clinical management plans while meeting professional and legal standards. The American Reinvestment and Recovery Act introduced language that paper medical records would be replaced with electronic health records (EHRs) to

TABLE 10.1   Limiting Liability Mistakes in Electronic Fetal Monitoring

1. Establish a patient relationship from admission to discharge that allows for open communication that is timely, straightforward, and transparent.
2. Keep current with evidence-based practice related to maternal–fetal physiology, fetal heart rate interpretation, and interventions.
3. Know and use applicable published standards and guidelines for electronic fetal monitoring.
4. Follow unit policies, to include electronic fetal monitoring and documentation.
5. Maintain adequate interpretable fetal heart rate and uterine activity tracing.
6. Recognize indeterminate and abnormal fetal heart characteristics.
7. Attend interdisciplinary fetal monitoring education to include formal in-person lectures, case reviews, and debriefs after unanticipated outcomes.
8. Membership in professional organizations.
9. Maintain professional licensure and certification, including electronic fetal monitoring.

Adapted from: R. L. Cypher, Electronic fetal monitoring documentation, J. Obstet. Gynecol. Neonatal Nurs. 32 (1) (2018) 24–33.

allow for greater interoperability. This would allow for health information exchange as an initiative to improve the quality of healthcare [22]. Today's EHRs have reached a higher level of precision incorporating technology that incorporates a variety of features. These records are a vital attribute of a clinician's responsibility to document certain aspects of healthcare, communication with the clinical team, and patient education, thus promoting patient safety [23]. Regardless of the healthcare specialty, adherence to fundamental documentation strategies is crucial because thorough and complete documentation reflects a healthcare professional's character, competency, and care delivery [24]. In contrast, incomplete and insufficient charting can affect healthcare delivery, bedside care, professional accountability, and increase an individual's or hospital's risk for a liability claim. Three leading professional organizations in the United States, including the ACOG, AWHONN, and ACNM, endorse the National Institute of Child Health and Human Development (NICHD) standardized approach to terminology and nomenclature to describe FHR tracings and UA and use of a three-tier categorization system [15–17,25]. Unfortunately, selected healthcare clinicians remain slow in accepting the use of these standardized terms or decline to use approved nomenclature despite publications from recognized organizations and up-to-date EFM education. Similar to other obstetric situations, this creates an increased risk for patient safety errors and liability claims caused by inaccurate communication between healthcare clinicians and inconsistencies in medical records related to the absence of critical thinking in interpretation, continuity of care, clinical decisions, and interventions [20,26].

DOCUMENTATION COMPONENTS OF THE ELECTRONIC FETAL MONITORING EVALUATION

Six components form the basis of EFM interpretation and management. These characteristics should be included in all FHR and UA documentation when data are able to be interpreted:

1. Baseline rate
2. Baseline variability
3. Presence of accelerations
4. Presence of periodic or episodic decelerations
5. UA: frequency, duration, intensity, and resting tone
6. Changes or trends over time

The last component, changes or trends over time, is apparent by reviewing previous FHR and UA documentation or examining several hours of the FHR tracing. However, when clinicians use narrative charting, as is the case for physicians and midwives, changes or trends over time may need to be specifically acknowledged. Regardless of the method of charting or clinical context, clinicians can remember the important aspects of documentation by use of the simple acronym CLEAR [19,20]:

- *Contemporaneous:* charted near the time of the assessment, procedure, or occurrence (i.e., 30–60 minutes).
- *Logical:* easily understood and clear.
  - Consider SOAP (subjective, objective, assessment, plan) for progress notes.
- *Explicit:* use standardized FHR and UA terminology.
  - Avoid vague or ambiguous terms.
- *Accurate:* Reflects correct times and sequence of events.
  - Record must be truthful.
- *Readable:* Entries must be legible if paper charting is used.

Integrating these key concepts with EFM documentation can result in the development of sound, clinically realistic documentation policies that reflect interdisciplinary collaboration. In addition, clinicians and organizational leadership must be able to articulate and endorse the six key principles that are essential to effective documentation and communication [27]. These principles are outlined in Table 10.2 and include specific recommendations that are applicable to EFM.

TABLE 10.2   Principles of Effective Obstetric Documentation and Communication

Documentation quality	■ Permanently accessible, retrievable, and available for audits ■ Thorough, accurate, relevant, and consistent ■ Clear, concise, timely, and complete ■ Legible regardless if paper or electronic format ■ Entered contemporaneously and sequentially ■ Reflective of nursing process and critical thinking ■ Apply standardized EFM nomenclature to entries ■ Avoidance of nonspecific terms such as *reassuring* and *nonreassuring* ■ Provide evidence of patient handoffs
Interdisciplinary education and training to include physicians, midwives, and nurses	■ Comprehensive EFM education and training plan for new employees incorporating technical elements of charting with organization or unit documentation policies ■ Ongoing follow-up education for all employees to reinforce information and documentation trend updates ■ Conduct team training
Documentation and communication policies	■ Familiarization with organization and work location documentation and communication policies that include chain of command, consultation and on-call policies, transfer policies, and conflict resolution ■ Consider annual review of key policy by bedside clinicians and leadership
Medical record security	■ Integrated into documentation systems that abide by recommended industry standards, governmental mandates, accrediting agencies, and organizational policies ■ Includes: data security, protection of patient identification, confidentiality of patient information, clinical professionals' information, and organizational information
Documentation entries	Medical record entries must be: ■ Accurate, valid, and complete ■ Authenticated demonstrating entries are truthful, the clinician is readily identified, and information has not been added or inserted ■ Dated and time-stamped by the clinician ■ Legible/readable ■ Completed using standardized terminology and abbreviations

TABLE 10.2   Principles of Effective Obstetric Documentation and Communication—cont'd

Standardized nomenclature	Standardized terminologies and The Joint Commission–approved abbreviations that are used to describe plan, deliver, and evaluate nursing care based on professional organizational guidelines and position statements

EFM, electronic fetal monitoring.
From: R. L. Cypher, Electronic fetal monitoring documentation, J. Obstet. Gynecol. Neonatal Nurs. 32 (1) (2018) 24–33.

COMMON DOCUMENTATION DILEMMAS

A number of EFM documentation issues come into question in clinical practice that can create difficulties in litigation if not addressed in policies or handled before an adverse event occurs in the obstetric setting. Several common documentation questions center around what should be included in a complete and thorough notation and what should be avoided in medical record entries. Are summary terms, such as FHR categories, required in all entries? Is quantification of FHR deceleration, specifically depth and duration, necessary? How frequently are FHR and UA assessments documented? In addition, concerns may arise when clinicians use conflicting or contradictory statements or nomenclature that can confuse the clinical picture. Each hospital must address these issues and provide guidance for staff members that is reasonable and based on evidence-based guidelines when possible. There are few absolutes for any of these issues, and institutional approaches will naturally vary, but some general principles will provide a starting point for team discussion.

Use of Fetal Heart Rate Categories

Prior to 2008, poorly defined summary terms, specifically *reassuring* and *nonreassuring,* were used to classify FHR tracings. Although both terms are frequently found in the literature, there are no standardized definitions based on the NICHD recommendations and these terms should be abandoned in both communication and documentation. Instead, a three-tiered system for the categorization of FHR patterns is used in the United States [25]. For purposes of documentation, assessment and interpretation of the individual components of the FHR tracing are charted at specific intervals rather than the category. Although some hospitals have mandated categories be documented in addition to the six components of adequate FHR and UA documentation, there are no published recommendations from professional organizations requiring categories should be charted in a medical record [20]. Several issues should be considered when policies require categories to be charted with all FHR entries. Documenting redundant information is time-consuming because FHR characteristics are already documented. This also is counterproductive, considering the already burdensome paperwork responsibilities of the bedside nurse [19]. In the event an allegation of harm is claimed, FHR and UA characteristics, and corrective measures and presence of communication between healthcare providers, are reviewed, not which category was identified in the medical record. Additionally, if the wrong category is charted, this may be viewed as an example of a clinician who has insufficient education and competency related to FHR interpretation. Fig. 10.4

	05:30
Vital Signs	
HR	
SpO2 (%)	
Uterine Activity	
Monitor Mode	Palpation
Frequency (min)	5
Duration (sec)	60-80
Quality	Moderate
Pattern	Normal: ≤ 5 Contractions in 10 Minutes
Resting Tone Toco	Relaxed
Fetal Assessment A	
Monitor Mode	External US
FHR Baseline Rate	150
Variability	Moderate 6-25 bpm
Decelerations	Early; Late
Actions for Fetal Decelerations	Side to Side
Category	Category I
Interventions	
IV/Blood Work	
Patient Care Comments	
Communication	

Fig. 10.4 Incorrect documentation of fetal heart rate (FHR) category. *HR,* heart rate; *IV,* intravenous; *US,* ultrasound.

is an example of the misuse of category terminology. When using EFM, a record is created and is archived permanently in a paper format or electronically. Both formats have the potential to be compromised either because the paper tracing is lost or for the electronic archival system fails to store data. Clinicians who document the FHR components always can determine what the corresponding category was at the time in question, but the reverse is not true [28]. The clinician who simply documents a category will not be able to later articulate the FHR components if the tracing is unavailable. Clearly stated, although FHR categories can be helpful in writing policies and procedures, these terms are limited in usefulness during deposition or trial, during which clinicians are expected to be able to provide specific answers regarding patient assessment. *FHR categories are summary terms that clinicians should know and be able to apply and articulate if queried; they are not required documentation components.*

Documentation of Uterine Activity

Patients may be placed at an increased risk for harm, which is an entryway to liability when healthcare providers are not adept at understanding uterine physiology and using appropriate terminology when documenting UA [29]. Therefore clinicians are responsible for recognizing that the terms *normal* and *tachysystole* are summary terms used to describe UA based on frequency of contractions in 10 minutes averaged over a 30-minute time frame [25]. Terms such as *hyperstimulation, hypercontractility, hypertonic, hypotonic, polysystole, skewed contractions,* and *paired contractions* are ill defined in the literature and not supported by the NICHD document or professional organizations. These terms should be abandoned and not used in communication, documentation, or published literature as this serves as a vehicle for further errors. Comprehensive documentation includes a clear picture of all the UA components of assessment as a whole, including frequency, duration, strength, and resting tone (see Chapter 4). Documentation related to UA also should reflect the mode of assessment (external or internal), resting tone and intensity to palpation when using a tocodynamometer, and resting tone and intensity to palpation when intrauterine pressures need to be confirmed. Similar to FHR categories, *there is no justification for adding a summary term, such as tachysystole, to each UA entry where documentation already includes the individual components assessed.*

Quantification of Decelerations

Historically, clinicians were instructed to document the presence of periodic and episodic patterns by name (e.g., accelerations and early, late, variable, and prolonged decelerations) and extensive details about the FHR pattern, especially decelerations (e.g., variable decelerations with pushing lasting 60 to 90 seconds down to 50 to 65 bpm at nadir lasting 10 to 15 seconds with quick return to baseline). This practice is no longer encouraged or recommended in routine practice. On occasion, variable, late, and prolonged deceleration patterns may need to be further quantified based on data showing a relationship between deceleration area and the risk for fetal acidemia to guide clinical management [30–32]. This is accomplished with a summary note documenting the components of the FHR pattern, whether the decelerations are recurrent, and the duration (onset to offset) and depth of nadir to show trends over time.

Frequency of Electronic Fetal Monitoring Assessment and Documentation

Although assessment and documentation are often used interchangeably with EFM, these are two separate tasks. Assessment is a systematic and dynamic way to collect and analyze data [33]. Documentation is simply a tool to record this information in one place as a mechanism to communicate these findings. There is a paucity of literature detailing the optimal frequency of FHR assessment and documentation [20]. There are no published peer-reviewed data demonstrating a positive effect on perinatal outcomes when current EFM assessment guidelines are applied at the beside and used for charting frequencies [20]. Frequency of assessment of a FHR tracing varies depending on the stage of labor, the risk status of the patient in labor, and other clinical factors such as previous FHR characteristics or interventions that have been performed. For physicians and midwives, there are specific time and date requirements to complete a medical record that are dictated by regulatory and insurance agencies related to the history and physical, surgical procedure. and postoperative notes, and discharge summaries. Writing notes at regular intervals related to individual encounters between a physician or midwife with a patient is common sense. This demonstrates continuity of care, especially if different healthcare professionals are involved in treating a patient. Additionally, ongoing documentation can ensure appropriate information is accessible to relevant clinicians and will assist in management of the patient throughout the labor course. In regard to nursing documentation, Table 10.3 illustrates

TABLE 10.3 Electronic Fetal Monitoring Assessment

	Labor Stage: Latent Phase (<4 cm)	Labor Stage: Latent Phase (<4–5 cm)	Labor Stage Active Phase (≥6 cm)	Labor Stage: Second Passive Fetal Descent	Labor Stage: Second Active Pushing
Low-risk without oxytocin	Insufficient evidence for recommendation	Every 30 minutes	Every 30 minutes	Every 30 minutes	Every 15 minutes
With oxytocin or risk factors	Every 15 minutes with oxytocin; every 30 minutes without	Every 15 minutes	Every 15 minutes	Every 15 minutes	Every 5 minutes

Note: Assessment frequency should always be determined based on the status of the mother and fetus and will need to occur more frequently often based on a patient's clinical needs, e.g., in response to a temporary or ongoing change. Summary documentation is acceptable, and individual hospital policy should be followed.

Adapted from Association of Women's Health, Obstetric and Neonatal Nurses, Fetal heart monitoring: position statement, J. Obstet. Gynecol. Neonatal Nurs. 47 (6) (2018) 874–877.

the recommended *assessment* intervals, not documentation intervals, for FHR and UA patterns. *More clearly, this table does not make recommendations for documentation intervals because each institutional protocol should delineate both the frequency of FHR tracing and frequency of documentation findings. The concept of simultaneous assessment and documentation, especially in high-risk and second-stage labor, is unrealistic and unnecessary.*

Appropriate Use of Fetal Heart Rate and Uterine Activity Terminology

The incorrect use of nomenclature often creates difficulties for clinicians in both the screening and testimonial phases of malpractice litigation. When a medical record is initially reviewed by the plaintiff's counsel to determine whether there is merit to a medical malpractice claim, the record provides the only documentation available at that point in time. Flow sheet and narrative entries will be read against subsequent clinician's notes and an EFM tracing. Accurate recognition and description of FHR and UA assessments in the patient's chart demonstrate attentive and competent care. Inaccurate or incorrect terminology in a medical record when read and compared with the objective fetal heart tracing increases the likelihood of litigation. Statements such as "doing well" or "no change" are vague and do not describe the clinical scenario. Another example is that of a nursing summary note in regard to a laboring patient on oxytocin.

Patient with complaints of leaking fluid. Significant amount of bleeding noted. Dr. Jones called to come to bedside—currently en route. Verbal order to check patient. Writer unable to reach cervix, but one golf ball–sized clot came out with exam. FHR tracing reactive.

In this scenario, there are several criticisms, but the highlighted issue related to documentation is the use of the word *reactive*. This term is reserved for patients that are receiving antepartum fetal surveillance and not for intrapartum care.

Compounding the matter further, *inconsistent and inaccurate terminology or an inability to define FHR and UA terms* according to recognized standard terminology also creates difficult obstacles later, such as during the testimonial phase of litigation. When a clinician uses modified or nonstandardized terminology, other healthcare clinicians and potentially expert witnesses will not understand the full extent of what is meant. For example, terms such as "spikes," "nitnoids," "ditzels," "little variables," "variables with late components," "beat-to-beat variability," and "short-term and long-term variability" have no place in communication between clinicians caring for an obstetric patient. This creates unclear communication, which can result in medical errors or the appearance of errors within a medical record. Use of these terms also can send the wrong message to not only a plaintiff attorney's team during deposition but also to the jury at the time of trial. Another example is exemplified by the following deposition excerpt that occurred after the NICHD consensus statement was published.

Deposition Excerpt

A certified nurse midwife (CNM) was questioned in deposition by the plaintiff's attorney (PA) to define the categories of variability that have been identified in the portion of the FHR tracing that was under scrutiny.

> PA: I see that you have circled the sections in this 10-minute period of the FHR tracing that you believe to be minimal variability. By the way, can you define what minimal variability is?
>
> CNM: I can't remember the exact beats per minute off the top of my head. But in general, I look at minimal variability as being more of a flat tracing. It's when you aren't able to observe as many jiggles or grass marks in the FHR tracing.
>
> PA: That being said, can you define moderate variability?
>
> CNM: If you were to look at a tracing in between the 10-second blocks, you'll have an increase within 6 to 15 bpm. Anything greater than that is considered marked variability.

Clinicians should use standardized terminology that can support the defense of a medical malpractice action; more importantly, it allows the obstetric team to communicate clearly and make certain they are accurately discussing the findings and placing the same significance on each term.

Location of Nursing Assessment and Documentation

Intrapartum care is often delivered in an environment that is centered primarily on technology such as EFM and vital sign equipment, intravenous pumps, and computer documentation stations surrounding a patient's bedside. This atmosphere and a clinician's ability to be receptive to each patient's individual needs can interfere with effective patient care, especially from the nursing perspective [20]. Group interactions on an inpatient unit for social and nonsocial reasons are also a frequent occurrence. Priority should be placed on assessment and documentation taking place at the bedside [20]. By charting at the bedside, clinicians are less likely to be faced with interruptions from other individuals or asked to perform non–nursing-related tasks that have been shown to have a negative effect on individualized care and patient safety [34,35]. On occasion, assessment and documentation may need to occur from a remote location, such as an outpatient clinic, triage, the operating room, or when staffing requires a nurse to care for more than one patient. In general, the practice from charting at the desk or other alternative location should not be exercised on a routine basis.

Late Entry

Late entry notes are generally considered to be those entries that are not made in a reasonable time period in conjunction with assessments or after an event has occurred. Delays in documentation can potentially affect a clinician's memory, leading to uncertainty about vital details or sequence and timing of actions and interventions [20]. Contemporaneous data entry is not always possible because clinicians are required to dedicate full attention to changes in maternal–fetal condition, such as an emergent cesarean birth for an umbilical cord prolapse, and not on documentation. Late entries should follow a format established by each healthcare facility, if available, and are completed as soon as possible after an event [20]. Documentation policies should dictate the maximum time period an entry on patient care can be made before becoming late. There are no legal or professional organization time frame recommendations for what constitutes a noncontemporaneous note, but using the phrase "Late Entry" in charting that is greater than 1 to 2 hours seems practical [20,28]. After an event or other clinical situation has been resolved, patient care needs or obstetric unit responsibilities can affect a healthcare provider's ability to complete a contemporaneous note. In these cases, clinicians have a professional responsibility to ensure late entries are written prior to the end of a scheduled shift. Completing a late entry on another shift or several days later is not acceptable and may be interpreted as being self-serving or defensive, making the clinician appear unreliable and less credible [28]. Regardless of whether paper or electronic documentation is used, notes are labeled as late with the date and time charting took place if electronic charting is not available. Other requirements include stating why a note was delayed, the events in the sequence of order as it occurred with times recorded whenever possible, and a complete EFM assessment if applicable to the clinical situation. Here is one example of late entry: Late entry because of urgency of patient care situation. Patient presented to triage at 0425 via ambulance with painful contractions, bright red vaginal bleeding and ping pong ball–sized clots at 38 2/7 weeks' gestation. Monitoring showed FHR baseline 180, absent variability, recurrent late decelerations that quickly deteriorated to a bradycardic rate to the 50 to 60s. Contractions every 1 to 2 minutes lasting 70 to 90 seconds. IV fluids, oxygen, and lateral positioning initiated. Patient quickly moved to OR per Dr. Buck for emergent cesarean at approximately 0450. Pediatrics paged with arrival in OR at approximately 0455. FHR 50s via doptone in OR. Time of birth 0506. Apgars 1, 2, and 5. Refer to delivery summary and neonatal resuscitation flow sheet for further details. Some clinicians, specifically nurses, think short-interval EFM documentation (e.g., every 15 minutes) as outlined in organizational policies is a time-consuming nuisance that can be left until the end of a shift or several hours after a birth is complete. This results in rushed entries that lack depth, detail, and do not represent the general context of late entry documentation. This places an increased risk of critical data being lost, potentially leading to adverse outcomes [36]. Also, hours of "catch-up" charting, especially in nonemergent scenarios or when the nurse to patient ratio cannot be achieved, can potentially influence how a case is defended as the jury may find this practice unacceptable. An audit trail will verify who entered data, location of entry (bedside or remote location), and the date and time of all entries. Some documentation systems also reflect the time the entry was actually made. In situations where clinicians back chart for several hours of data, the entry time is recorded wherever a clinician desires the entry to be placed, and an actual time documentation also is recorded. Fig. 10.5 represents an example of a reasonably timed entry. Fig. 10.6 characterizes an entry that was made on the next shift after an adverse neonatal outcome. These entries will be scrutinized closely as being reflective of a patient not being monitored closely, poor time management skills, or that care was negligent.

ELECTRONIC FETAL MONITORING DOCUMENTATION POLICIES

Hospital policies are designed to [37]
- Facilitate adherence with recognized professional practices
- Promote compliance with regulations, statutes, and accreditation requirements
- Reduce practice variation between clinicians
- Standardize processes and practices across multiple entities within a hospital or a health system

Ent:05/15/12 23:33:58 * Note:05/15/12 23:32 -   FHR Eval: Baseline 140 bpm / Variability
                                                 Moderate / Accelerations Present / Decelerations
                                                 Absent

Fig. 10.5 Example of contemporaneous documentation entry verified by system logs entry program. *FHR,*
fetal heart rate.

Ent:05/16/12 19:11:03 * Note:05/16/12 00:52 -   Comment : US shows the HR in the 90's to 110's.
                                                 Holding the US in place to monitor FHT, MD feels
                                                 this may still be moms HR which is picking up at
                                                 91

Fig. 10.6 Example of documentation demonstrating an entry made over 18 hours after an event that resulted
in an intrapartum fetal death. *FHT,* fetal heart tone; *HR,* heart rate; *US,* ultrasound.

- Serve as a resource for all staff
- Reduce reliance on memory, which increases the risk of error

Unfortunately, hospitals often can have policies that can create inconsistent or conflicting standards. On occasion, policies are outdated or have not been reviewed or revised to reflect more contemporary recommendations and literature [20]. Documentation policies will vary depending on the type of medical record (paper or computerized), style of charting (flow sheet or narrative), clinical context (labor evaluation or nonlabor complaint), and other factors. Nevertheless, fetal monitoring policies must be reasonable and rational regarding all three areas, *assessment, communication,* and *documentation,* as previously discussed. One example of an unreasonable documentation policy written by a director who lacked an obstetric background who misinterpreted a professional organization's position statement stated:

- When FHR is outside normal range, the FHR should be assessed and documented
    - Every 15 minutes in latent phase
    - Every 5 minutes during the active and transition phases
    - Every 2 to 3 minutes during the second stage

This policy is useless from the standpoint of a clinician who cannot meet this hospital's documentation expectations. Lack of documentation or inadequate documentation policies can have significant legal consequences [20]. This can lead to a plaintiff expert or attorney's accusations that a clinician is not meeting the standard of care as set forth by the hospital. A more logical and practical policy that is achievable by clinicians may state the following:

- Recommended documentation intervals in the high-risk patient include a summary note of FHR and UA activity every 15 to 30 minutes or more frequently based on the clinical scenario. Documentation policies related to EFM should address the following:
    - Recognition of the difference between assessment and documentation
    - Components of FHR evaluation to include baseline rate, baseline variability, presence of accelerations, and periodic/episodic decelerations with each FHR entry when data are interpretable
    - Components of UA evaluation, including frequency, duration, strength, and resting tone with FHR entry when data are interpretable

- Frequency of FHR and UA evaluation/assessment
- Minimum frequency of documentation of FHR and UA findings

SUMMARY

Fetal monitoring is a screening tool that can potentially prevent adverse outcomes only when used by competent clinicians who have been adequately trained to use a standardized approach for EFM interpretation and management. Progressive high-reliability obstetric units can use an SDM model in conjunction with patient safety bundles, evidence-based guidelines, and interdisciplinary education to improve healthcare processes of care as a mechanism to improve patient outcomes. Clinicians that have the context for understanding the basics principles of the law and the effect on a legal claim will be able to respond appropriately. Furthermore, healthcare professionals will know what to expect during the investigation and potential discovery and deposition process that may lead to trial or settlement. Prompt recognition of frequently encountered EFM challenges may reduce potential liability as long as there is evidence that interpretation and clinical management is conducted in a collaborative environment. The obstetric liability environment will continue to generate much discussion in the future. Therefore incorporating patient safety programs and other initiatives into healthcare reform is an important aspect of reducing adverse events that result in medical malpractice.

References

[1] R.L. Cypher, Demystifying the 4 elements of negligence, J. Perinat. Neonatal Nurs. 34 (2) (2020) 108–109.

[2] V.R. Klein, Risk management in obstetrics and gynecology, Clin. Obstet. Gynecol. 62 (3) (2019) 550–559.

[3] K.R. Simpson, G.E. Knox, Risk management and EFM: decreasing risk of adverse outcomes and liability exposure, J. Perinat. Neonatal Nurs. 14 (3) (2000) 40–52.

[4] P.D. Schneider, B.A Sabol, P.A. King, A.B. Caughey, A.E. Borders, The hard work of improving outcomes for mothers and babies: Obstetric and perinatal quality improvement initiatives make a difference at the hospital, state, and national levels, Clin. Perinatol. 44 (3) (2017) 511–528.

[5] R. von Benzon Hollesen, R.L. Johansen, C. Rørbye, et al., Successfully reducing newborn asphyxia in the labour unit in a large academic medical centre: A quality improvement project using statistical process control, BMJ Qual. Saf. 27 (8) (2018) 633–642.

[6] P. Amin, S. Zaher, R. Penketh, et al., Falling caesarean section rate and improving intra-partum outcomes: a prospective cohort study, J. Matern Fetal Neonatal. Med. 32 (15) (2019) 2475–2480.

[7] C.A. Ameh, M. Mdegela, S. White, N. van den Broek, The effectiveness of training in emergency obstetric care: a systematic literature review, Health Policy Plan 34 (4) (2019) 257–270.

[8] M. Battin, L, Sadler, Neonatal encephalopathy: How can we improve clinical outcomes? J. Paediatr. Child Health 54 (11) (2018) 1180–1183.

[9] K. M., Mehlhaff, C.M. Pettker, H. Hosier, et al., Putting teamwork to the test: A randomized trial of collaboration in electronic fetal monitoring (EFM), Am. J. Obstet. Gynecol. 222 (1) (2020) S351.

[10] C.M. Pettker, S.F. Thung, H.S. Lipkind, et al., A comprehensive obstetric patient safety program reduces liability claims and payments, Am. J. Obstet. Gynecol. 211 (4) (2014) 319–325.

[11] J. Antony, W. Zarin, V. Nincic, et al., Patient safety initiatives in obstetrics: a rapid review, BMJ Open 8 (7) (2018) e020170.

[12] R.L. Cypher, Shared decision-making: A model for effective communication and patient satisfaction, J. Perinat. Neonatal Nurs. 33 (4) (2019) 285–287.

[13] J.S. Kingman, B.W. Moulton, Rethinking informed consent: the case for shared medical decision-making, Am. J. Law Med. 32 (4) (2006) 429–501.

[14] National Quality Forum, National quality partners playbook: Shared decision making in healthcare, Washington, DC: National Quality Forum, 2018.

[15] American College of Obstetricians and Gynecologists, Intrapartum fetal heart rate monitoring: nomenclature, interpretation, and general management principles, ACOG Practice Bulletin No. 106, Obstet. Gynecol. 114 (1) (2009) 192–202.

[16] Association of Women's Health, Obstetric and Neonatal Nurses, Fetal heart monitoring: position statement, J. Obstet. Gynecol. Neonatal Nurs. 47 (6) (2018) 874–877.

[17] American College of Nurse–Midwives, Intermittent auscultation for intrapartum fetal heart rate surveillance, J. Midwifery Womens Health 60 (5) (2015) 626–632.

[18] S.B. Bal, An introduction to medical malpractice in the United States, Clin. Orthop. Relat. Res. 467 (2) (2009) 339–347.

[19] L.A. Miller, Intrapartum fetal monitoring: liability and documentation, Clin. Obstet. Gynecol. 54 (2011) 50–55.

[20] R.L. Cypher, Electronic fetal monitoring documentation, J. Perinat. Neonatal Nurs. 32 (1) (2018) 24–33.

[21] L.M. Glaser, F.A. Alvi, M.P. Milad, Trends in malpractice claims for obstetric and gynecologic procedures, 2005 through 2014, Am. J. Obstet. Gynecol. 217 (3) (2017) 340-e1-e6.

[22] Centers for Disease Control and Prevention, Meaningful Use Introduction CDC. Available from: https://www.cdc.gov/ehrmeaningfuluse/introduction.html, 2019 (accessed 5-15-2020).

[23] E.A. Malane, C. Richardson, K.G. Burke, A novel approach to electronic nursing documentation dducation: Ambassador of learning program, J. Nurses Prof. Dev. 35 (6) (2019) 324–329.

[24] S. Feutz-Harter, Documentation principles and pitfalls, J. Nurs. Adm. 19 (12) (1989) 7–9.

[25] G.A. Macones, G.D. Hankins, C.Y. Spong, et al., The 2008 National Institute of Child Health and Human Development workshop report on electronic fetal monitoring: update on definitions, interpretation, and research guidelines, Obstet. Gynecol. 112 (3) (2008) 661–666.

[26] S.L. Clark, M.A. Belfort, G.A. Dildy, J.A. Meyers, Reducing obstetric litigation through alterations in practice patterns, Obstet. Gynecol. 112 (6) (2008) 1279–1283.

[27] American Nurses Association, Principles of nursing documentation: Guidance for registered nurses. Silver Spring, MD: American Nurses Association; 2010.

[28] L.A. Miller, Common questions on documentation, J. Perinat. Neonatal. Nurs. 30 (1) (2016) 9–10.

[29] L.A. Miller, Uterine activity: What you don't know can hurt you, MCN Am. J. Matern Child Nurs. 43 (3) (2018) 180.

[30] A.G. Cahill, K.A. Roehl, A.O Odibo, G.A. Macones, Association and prediction of neonatal acidemia, Am. J. Obstet. Gynecol. 207 (3) (2012) e201–e208.

[31] S. Martí Gamboa, M. Lapresta Moros, J Pascual Mancho, et al., Deceleration area and fetal acidemia, J. Matern Fetal Neonatal. Med. 30 (21) (2016) 2578–2584.

[32] A.G. Cahill, M.G. Tuuli, M.J. Stout, J.D. Lopez, G.A. Macones, A prospective cohort study of fetal heart rate monitoring: Deceleration area is predictive of fetal acidemia, Am. J. Obstet. Gynecol. 218 (5) (2018) 523e1–523e12.

[33] American Nurses Association, The nursing process. Available from: https://www.nursingworld.org/practice-policy/workforce/what-is-nursing/the-nursing-process/, no date (accessed 5-15-2020).

[34] L.M. McGillis Hall, M. Ferguson-Paré, E. Peter, et al., Going blank: factors contributing to interruptions to nurses' work and related outcomes, J. Nurs. Manag. 18 (8) (2010) 1040–1047.

[35] L.M. McGillis-Hall, C. Pedersen, P. Hubley, et al., Interruptions and pediatric patient safety, J. Pediatr. Nurs. 25 (3) (2010) 167–175.

[36] W. Blair, B. Smith, Nursing documentation: frameworks and barriers, Contemp. Nurse 41 (2) (2012) 160–168.

[37] A. V. Irving, Policies and procedures for healthcare organizations: A risk management perspective. Perinatal Safety & Quality Healthcare. Available from: https://www.psqh.com/analysis/policies-and-procedures-for-healthcare-organizations-a-risk-management-perspective/, 2014 (accessed 5-15-2020).

Obstetric Models of Care and Electronic Fetal Monitoring Outside the United States

Similar to the United States, continuous electronic fetal monitoring (EFM) in the obstetric setting is prevalent in many high-income countries [1–3]. However, there are variations in models of antepartum and intrapartum care, scenarios in which EFM is implemented, terminology to interpret fetal heart rate (FHR) characteristics, and adjuncts to fetal surveillance compared with the United States. This chapter provides a brief overview of these differences.

OBSTETRIC MODELS OF CARE

Globally, physician-led, midwifery-led, or shared models of inter- and intradisciplinary healthcare provides continuity care for pregnant women in the antepartum, intrapartum, and postpartum settings [4–6]. In some countries, physicians undertake complete responsibility for obstetric patients. In other nations, midwifery-led care is a core part of universal healthcare coverage and is representative of the primary source of obstetric care, with patients only being transferred or referred to a physician when a complication is suspected or diagnosed [4,7]. Last, the responsibility may be collectively shared among midwives, nurse practitioners, and physicians throughout the pregnancy course.

Regardless of the model of care, there is no decisive consensus on the optimal birth setting. For example, guidelines in the United Kingdom state that low-risk obstetric patients have several birth setting options including physician-led hospital units, midwifery-supervised hospital-based or free-standing community-based birth centers, or at home [8,9]. In 2018 the World Health Organization published a comprehensive, evidence-based, and consolidated guideline on key recommendations in intrapartum care regardless of the setting or level of care [10] (Table 11.1). One fundamental concept is that birth will occur in

TABLE 11.1 Care Throughout Labor and Birth

WHO Recommendation	Description
Respectful maternity care	Healthcare that maintains dignity, privacy, and confidentiality ensures freedom from harm and mistreatment, and enables informed choice and continuous support throughout labor and birth
Effective communication	Effective communication between clinicians and patients in labor, using simple and culturally acceptable methods
Companionship during labor and birth	Support person of choice throughout labor and birth
Continuity of care	Midwifery-led care model to support patients throughout the antepartum, intrapartum, and postpartum continuum in settings in which trained midwives are available

From World Health Organization (WHO), Intrapartum care for a positive child-birth experience. Available from: https://www.who.int/reproductivehealth/publications/intrapartum-care-guidelines/en/, 2018. (accessed 03-04-20).

a clinically and psychologically safe environment with a technically competent staff [10]. The physician-led model of care is a separate service from other healthcare disciplines [11]. In many countries, this type of care can have an effective and powerful influence on women's care decisions [12]. For example, physicians may take a more medicalized approach by treating pregnancy as a pathologic condition using a "high-tech" approach. This type of care may subsequently escalate into unnecessary interventions and procedures that potentially cause an increased risk to the maternal–fetal dyad [11,12].

Midwifery-led care is differentiated from other models of care based on variations in philosophy about pregnancy and birth, the goals and objectives of care, type of patient seeking midwifery-led care, provider–client relationships, use of interventions during labor, and the care setting [4,11,13,14]. Midwifery-led care is also distinctive from other healthcare models because it unites public health with clinical health, while combining access to all women and newborns across the care continuum in both community and clinical facilities [15]. In many countries outside the United States, midwives are the primary obstetric care providers [4]. Women who receive midwifery-led care experience fewer intrapartum interventions, a reduction in the use of analgesia and regional anesthesia, more spontaneous vaginal births, fewer episiotomies, and less operative vaginal births [4,16,17].

Interprofessional models of care, or shared models of care, are those in which groups or individuals that represent the same or similar field of work come together to provide specific patient care services [18]. The focal point in this healthcare framework is the role this methodology plays in delivering high-quality patient-oriented services. Shared models of care can decrease cost, allow for increased access to obstetric care, and are able to provide more effective healthcare, which in turn improves quality and optimizes perinatal and neonatal outcomes [11,18,19]. This care model is essential because certain experiences and skills can only be found in a broad range of healthcare professionals and disciplines [6]. For example, a pregnancy that is complicated by an underlying fetal cardiac anomaly may be comanaged by a maternal–fetal medicine physician, pediatric cardiologists, women's health nurse practitioner, and obstetric clinical nurse specialist. Interprofessional models of care also have a similar goal: providing safe, effective, patient-centered care for women and their families guided by shared rules and structures that govern a mutually beneficial relationship [18]. In fact, studies evaluating shared models of care between midwives and physicians have demonstrated decreased rates of labor induction, oxytocin augmentation, and cesarean birth rates and in some cases similar neonatal outcomes compared with physician-led management of labor [13,19].

ELECTRONIC FETAL MONITORING: CARDIOTOCOGRAPHY

International literature frequently refers to EFM as *cardiotocography* (CTG). These terms are used interchangeably in this chapter. Additionally, publications from countries outside the United States sometimes refer to FHR tracings or monitor strips as *obstetric registrations, registers,* or simply *"traces."* Of note, when interpreting traces in other countries, international paper speeds are often 1 or 2 cm/min versus the typical 3 cm/min seen in the United States. Figs. 11.1 through 11.5 are examples of FHR tracings at 1- and 2-cm paper speeds. These tracing examples are provided to familiarize the reader with the appearance of tracings at different paper speeds. Consistent with the state of current practice, the figure legends reflect the terminology in use at the center in which the tracing

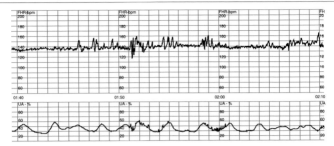

Fig. 11.1 Normal cardiotocography with accelerations, paper speed 1 cm/min. *FHR*, fetal heart rate; *UA*, uterine activity. (Courtesy Neoventa Medical, Mölndal, Sweden.)

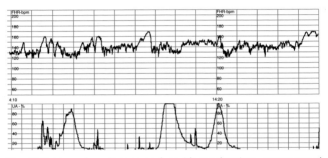

Fig. 11.2 Normal cardiotocography with accelerations, paper speed 2 cm/min. *FHR*, fetal heart rate; *UA*, uterine activity. (Courtesy Neoventa Medical, Mölndal, Sweden.)

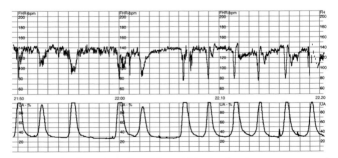

Fig. 11.3 Cardiotocography with variable decelerations, paper speed 1 cm/min. *FHR*, fetal heart rate; *UA*, uterine activity. (Courtesy Neoventa Medical, Mölndal, Sweden.)

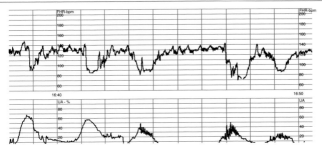

Fig. 11.4 Cardiotocography with variable decelerations, paper speed 2 cm/min. *FHR*, fetal heart rate; *UA*, uterine activity. (Courtesy Neoventa Medical, Mölndal, Sweden.)

was obtained and do not necessarily coincide with guidelines from the International Federation of Gynecology and Obstetrics (FIGO), the Royal Australian and New Zealand College of Obstetricians and Gynaecologists (RANZCOG), the National Institute for Health and Care Excellence (NICE), or the Society of Obstetricians and Gynaecologists of Canada (SOGC). Regardless of the country providing the obstetric care or the birth setting (home, birth center, hospital), one of three types of fetal surveillance can be used throughout the course of labor: intermittent auscultation (IA), CTG, or a combination of both methods. IA is discussed in greater detail in Chapter 3. Data regarding the exact percentage of intrapartum patients monitored with IA compared with EFM are scarce. For example, by 2004, the United States ceased to report EFM utilization rates in annual birth-related vital statistics because of the high and stable rate of 89% of all births [20]. The introduction of EFM in high-income countries has resulted in decreased IA rates as a primary fetal surveillance option during the intrapartum period [21,22].

INTERNATIONAL INTERMITTENT AUSCULTATION AND CARDIOTOCOGRAPHY GUIDELINES

In 1987 a consensus development group presented a fetal monitoring document to FIGO, which was subsequently adopted. The guidelines promulgated by FIGO were an important landmark in CTG history, and they still represent the sole international consensus document on the topic [23]. Subsequently, multiple international professional organizations have published guidelines and recommendations regarding IA and intrapartum fetal surveillance [9,10,23–29]. For example,

NICE, which is supported by the Royal College of Obstetricians and Gynaecologists (RCOG), is responsible for producing evidence-based guidelines and quality standards for the United Kingdom. These intra-partum guidelines recommend IA be offered to low-risk patients in the first stage of labor regardless of the birth setting. Routine CTG is

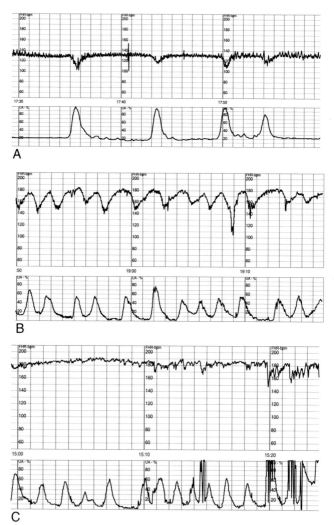

Fig. 11.5 Examples of various cardiotocography traces at 1 cm/min. (A) Early decelerations. (B) Late decelerations. (C) Tachycardia.

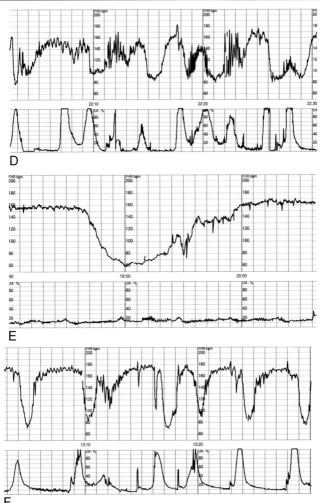

Fig. 11.5—cont'd (D) Prolonged decelerations. (E) Bradycardia. (F) "Complicated" or "atypical" variable decelerations. *FHR,* fetal heart rate; *UA,* uterine activity. (Courtesy Neoventa Medical, Mölndal, Sweden.)

not performed on every patient. The NICE intrapartum guidelines also have an inclusive list of risk factors that indicate the need for CTG. For instance, continuous CTG is recommended if any of the following risk factors occur: suspected chorioamnionitis, sepsis, or maternal temperature of 38 °C or higher; severe hypertension (160/110 mm Hg or greater); oxytocin use; "significant" meconium; or vaginal bleeding that occurs in labor. Continuous CTG is also advised if two or more of the following are present: prolonged rupture of membranes (≥24 hours), moderate hypertension (150/100–159/109 mm Hg), delay in first- or second-stage labor; or the presence of "nonsignificant" meconium [9].The RANZCOG has a comparable guideline on intrapartum fetal surveillance. This document lists IA as an appropriate method of fetal monitoring in patients without preexisting risk factors. Similar to the NICE guideline, continuous CTG is recommended when specific antepartum risk factors are identified and include but are not limited to abnormal Doppler flow studies, amniotic fluid abnormalities, hypertension, or diabetes. Intrapartum risk factors requiring CTG also are similar to the NICE guideline and include risk factors such as abnormal IA characteristics, labor induction, tachysystole, regional anesthesia, or prolonged first- or second-stage labor and other conditions [26]. Similarly, IA is the SOGC's recommended method of fetal surveillance in low-risk pregnancies [27].

Guidelines for Terminology and Interpretation

Standardization of the visual interpretation of FHR characteristics was developed to overcome intra- and interobserver variability during fetal surveillance [30]. A single universal standardized system of EFM terminology, interpretation, and management remains elusive. When there is a lack of standardization regarding fetal surveillance definitions, classification, and management, there is a risk for conflict and error, especially when healthcare providers travel abroad for employment or when volunteering professional services to other organizations or humanitarian efforts. For example, the RANZCOG defines a prolonged deceleration as a decrease in the FHR baseline for more than 90 seconds and up to 5 minutes as opposed to the NICE guidelines, which define a prolonged deceleration as a decrease in the FHR baseline by greater than 15 bpm lasting longer than 3 minutes [9,26,31]. Also, like the recommendations in the United States, other international professional organizations have created three-tier classification systems for CTG patterns, although each organization uses different terminology. For example, the NICE guidance uses normal, suspicious, and pathologic [9]. The SOGC use normal, atypical, and abnormal [27]. A separate classification system for antepartum versus intrapartum tracings is found in the FIGO document [23]. Therefore being familiar with each country's IA and CTG guidelines is encouraged to optimize patient safety (Table 11.2).

FIGO (Intrapartum)	RCOG/NICE	SOGC	RANZCOG
Normal ■ FHR BL 110–150 bpm ■ FHR variability 5–25 bpm	**Normal** (must meet all four features) ■ FHR BL 110–160 bpm ■ FHR variability ≥5 bpm ■ No decelerations ■ No accelerations	**Normal** ■ FHR BL 110–160 bpm ■ FHR variability 6–25 bpm or ≤5 bpm for <40 seconds	**Normal** ■ FHR BL 110–160 bpm ■ Variability 6–26 bpm ■ Accelerations ■ No decelerations
Suspicious ■ FHR BL 150–170 bpm ■ Variability 5–10 bpm for >40 minutes ■ Variability >25 bpm ■ Variable decelerations	**Suspicious** (one of the following is present in conjunction with a normal tracing) ■ FHR BL 100–109 bpm or 161–180 bpm ■ FHR variability <5 bpm for 40–90 minutes ■ Typical variable decelerations >50% of contractions for >90 minutes ■ Single prolonged deceleration up to 3 minutes ■ No accelerations with normal features ■ Is of uncertain significance	**Atypical** ■ FHR 100–110 bpm or >160 bpm for 30–80 minutes ■ Rising baseline ■ Arrhythmia ■ Variability ≤5 bpm for 40–80 minutes ■ Absent acceleration with scalp stimulation ■ Repetitive uncomplicated variable decelerations ■ Nonrepetitive complicated variables ■ Intermittent late decelerations ■ Single prolonged deceleration ≥2 minutes but <3 minutes	**Abnormal: unlikely to be associated with fetal compromise if isolated** ■ FHR BL 100–109 bpm ■ FHR variability reducing or reduced 3–5 bpm ■ Absent accelerations ■ Early decelerations ■ Variable decelerations without complicating features
Pathologic ■ FHR BL <100 or >170 bpm ■ Persistent FHR variability <5 bpm for >40 minutes	**Pathologic** ■ FHR BL 100 bpm or >160 bpm ■ Persistent FHR variability <5 bpm for >40 minutes ■ Severe variable decelerations ■ Severe early decelerations	**Abnormal** ■ FHR BL <100 bpm or >160 bpm for >80 minutes or erratic baseline ■ FHR variability ≤5 bpm for >80 minutes or ≥25 bpm for >10 minutes ■ Sinusoidal pattern	**Abnormal: associated with fetal compromise and requires further action** ■ FHR BL >160 bpm or rising where rate remains in normal range

Continued

TABLE 11.2 Comparison of International Category Classification Criteria—cont'd

FIGO (Intrapartum)	RCOG/NICE	SOGC	RANZCOG
■ Severe variable decelerations ■ Severe early repetitive decelerations ■ Late decelerations ■ Sinusoidal pattern	■ Prolonged decelerations ■ Late decelerations ■ Sinusoidal pattern	■ Absent accelerations ■ Repetitive complicated variable decelerations ■ Recurrent late decelerations ■ Single prolonged Deceleration ≥3 minutes but <10 minutes	■ Complicated variable decelerations ■ Late decelerations ■ Prolonged decelerations **Abnormal: associated with fetal compromise and requires immediate management to include an expedited birth** ■ Bradycardia ■ FHR variability absent ■ Complicated variable decelerations with reduced or absent FHR variability ■ Late decelerations with reduced or absent FHR variability

Note: The categories listed in the table are for international use only. Refer to Chapter 6 for categories and definitions in the United States.

BL, baseline; *FHR,* fetal heart rate; *FIGO,* International Federation of Gynecology and Obstetrics; *NICE,* National Institute for Health and Care Excellence; *RANZCOG,* Royal Australian and New Zealand College of Obstetricians and Gynaecologists; *RCOG,* Royal College of Obstetricians and Gynaecologists; *SOGC,* Society of Obstetricians and Gynaecologists of Canada.

From National Institute of Health and Care Excellence, Intrapartum care of healthy women and their babies during childbirth. NICE Clinical Guideline 190. Available from: https://www.nice.org.uk/guidance/cg190, 2014 (accessed 03-04-20); D. Lewis, S. Downe, FIGO Intrapartum Fetal Monitoring Expert Consensus Panel, FIGO consensus guidelines on intrapartum fetal monitoring: Intermittent auscultation, Int. J. Gynecol. Obstet. 131 (1) (2015) 9–12; Royal Australian and New Zealand College of Obstetricians and Gynaecologists, Intrapartum Fetal Surveillance Clinical Guidelines, fourth ed. Available from https://ranzcog.edu.au/RANZCOG_SITE/media/RANZCOG-MEDIA/Women%27s%20Health/Statement%20and%20guidelines/Clinical-Obstetrics/IFS-Guideline-4thEdition-2019,pdf?ext=.pdf, 2019 (accessed 03-04-20); S. Dore, W. Ehman, Fetal health surveillance: intrapartum consensus guideline, No. 396, J. Obstet.

METHODS OF DETERMINING FETAL ACID–BASE STATUS

EFM is an indirect method of measuring fetal oxygenation. This technology seeks to identify FHR changes that represent an interruption in the oxygenation pathway allowing for timely corrective measures and intervention to reduce the risk of hypoxic injury or death. Umbilical cord blood gas evaluation is considered the most objective method of assessing the metabolic state of the newborn at the time of birth [32]. Alternatively, obtaining an umbilical artery lactate level also may be used to predict acidemia at the time of birth. Both methods are unable to measure real-time fetal acid–base status during the intrapartum period. Umbilical cord blood gas and umbilical artery lactate level measurements are discussed more thoroughly in Chapter 6. Therefore in countries outside the United States, adjunct methods to fetal surveillance are used in an attempt to reduce the false-positive rate of CTG and identify the presence or absence of fetal acidosis during labor [33].

Fetal Blood Sampling

Fetal blood sampling (FBS) is used outside the United States as a direct approach to assessing fetal acid–base status during labor. This intrapartum procedure involves collecting blood from the fetal scalp to measure pH or to calculate lactate levels [32,34]. Specific criteria that should be met when FBS is being considered include [26,27,35,36]:

- Cephalic presentation
- Gestational age 34 weeks' gestation or greater
- Membranes are ruptured
- Minimal cervical dilation of at least 2–3 cm
- Adequate equipment and expertise to promptly perform the blood analysis
- Review of records for potential contraindications: HIV, hepatitis B or C, or fetal coagulation disorders such as suspected hemophilia

In addition, the FHR pattern should be correctly interpreted using a standardized approach to identify the indication for FBS, which is used in conjunction with CTG. It can provide additional information on fetal metabolic status at a specific moment before critical decisions are made concerning the need for and timing of birth and the type of anesthesia that will be used for either an operative vaginal or cesarean birth [27,34,37,38].

Fetal Blood Sampling for pH

FBS is considered an invasive procedure. Once the criteria mentioned previously have been met, the fetal scalp surface is punctured through an amnioscope with a small scalpel-like device. A fetal capillary blood sample is collected with a heparinized glass tube. In some facilities, two or three specimens are obtained from the same puncture site to verify results [39]. A sample size of approximately 15 to 50 μL of blood is sufficient to obtain a fetal blood pH value [35,39,40]. The procedure must be repeated on a regular basis to guide FHR management [36,40]. There are considerable clinical, facility, and equipment requirements, and precise technical skills for performing FBS, which in turn potentially increases the inaccuracy rate of pH results [32,35,36]. For instance, estimating capillary blood pH may be inaccurate as the collection site is not representative of the actual acid–base balance [34]. The presence of caput succedaneum or maternal sepsis and any samples that are contaminated with amniotic fluid or meconium can lead to erroneous values [9,33,34]. Consequently, this may result in unnecessary interventions such as cesarean birth in a fetus that is not hypoxic.

Another pitfall is the reported draw-to-result median time of 18 minutes with ranges of 12 to more than 30 minutes, which may result in a delay in delivering a compromised fetus [41]. FBS does not differentiate between metabolic and respiratory acidemia, because only the pH value is measured [34]. A pH value ≥ 7.25 is normal and represents adequate fetal oxygenation. Values between 7.21 and 7.24 are regarded as borderline and require corrective measures to improve fetal oxygenation; sampling is repeated within 20 to 30 minutes. Values of pH ≤ 7.20 (or <7.15 in the second stage of labor) are abnormal and require intervention [9,34,36,38,39]. Results should be interpreted in the entire clinical context, which includes previous FBS results, stage of labor, progress in labor, and clinical characteristics of the FHR [35,41]. Available evidence to support FBS is mixed and obstetric experts have questioned the continued use of fetal pH measurement to reduce rates of cesarean birth and neonatal seizures [9,27,33,34,42]. Nevertheless, professional organizations outside the United States continue to reference the use of FBS for fetal pH assessment in labor and a basis for clinical experience and research.

Fetal Scalp Blood Sampling for Lactate

Fetal lactate measurement has been proposed as an alternative to fetal pH. Lactate is a marker or by-product of fetal dependence on anaerobic metabolism related to periods of hypoxia [34]. Lactate measurement during the intrapartum period appears to be more specific than pH in predicting fetal acidemia. Therefore it is reasonable to assume that fetal lactate levels represent the metabolic stage of the acid–base balance, which is thought to be more closely related to the condition of the fetus compared with a pH value [37,43,44]. The procedure for lactate sampling is analogous to pH sampling but requires a smaller volume of blood (approximately 5 μL in a heparinized glass tube) [34,43,45]. Lactate test strips and a lactate analyzer are used rather than blood gas analysis equipment [41,44,46]. The test strips and lactate analyzer are similar to glucometers. Available data indicate normal lactate levels are greater than 4.2 mmol/L. Values between 4.2 and 4.8 mmol/L are considered intermediate or preacidemic. Repeat lactate testing in 20 to 30 minutes is recommended when lactate levels are within this range. Results greater than 4.8 mmol/L are abnormal and require intervention [37,38,47]. FBS for lactate levels has been shown to provide more precise information on fetal acid–base status than do the pH and base deficits, has quicker turnaround for sample results, and is quicker and easier to perform [37,46].

ST Analysis of the Fetal Electrocardiogram

In countries independent of the United States, such as Sweden and Norway, ST analysis of the fetal electrocardiogram (FECG) also may be encountered as an adjunct to CTG to identify fetal hypoxia during the intrapartum period. Unlike the other methods used to measure fetal acid–base status, ST analysis does not require blood sampling. This device assesses the fetal myocardial response to hypoxia based on fetal ECG changes [48–51]. ST analysis of the fetal ECG is used in combination with stringent FHR interpretation and published management guidelines. ST analysis automatically analyzes the ratio of the T and QRS amplitudes known as the *T/QRS ratio* and the *ST interval* [50–53]. Elevation or depression of the ST segment has been shown to represent periods of fetal hypoxia [30,53–55]. The system consists of a freestanding electronic fetal monitor with an exclusive ST analysis software feature that records data via a specialized fetal spiral electrode (FSE) (STAN; Neoventa Medical, Göteborg, Sweden). Use of the adjunctive ST analysis option requires the following patient characteristics to be met [53]:

- Planned vaginal delivery
- >36 completed weeks' gestation
- Singleton fetus

- Vertex presentation
- Ruptured amniotic membranes
  - Record review for potential contraindications: maternal infections with the risk of vertical transmission and fetal coagulation disorders such as suspected hemophilia

Multiple research studies have been published about the role of ST analysis in clinical practice. For example, several authors have suggested that ST analysis can be used as an adjunct to CTG for detecting fetal acidemia and improving perinatal and neonatal outcomes [52,56–58]. Conversely, several systematic reviews and meta-analyses propose that ST analysis does not demonstrate a significant improvement in decreasing cesarean birth rates or adverse outcomes compared with CTG alone [59–61]. The future of ST analysis remains uncertain as experts have pointed out differences in study protocols, inclusion criteria, enrollment rates, clinical guidelines, FBS use, and definitions of outcome parameters. Also, discrepancies in data management and statistical methodology have been described [52].

SUMMARY

Unfortunately, there continues to be a lack of consensus for the type of fetal surveillance in the intrapartum period and standardized definitions related to FHR characteristics. Although IA is a recommended and accepted practice for low-risk laboring patients in countries outside the United States, EFM and other adjunct methods of assessing fetal well-being remain widespread in obstetric practice. The institutional culture and other influences such as perceived legal consequences or opinions that continuous monitoring offers more authoritative information than IA may result in overreliance on EFM [62–65]. Like the United States, CTG utilization in other countries is fraught with challenges related to patient selection, standardization of terminology, interpretation, labor management, and appropriate application of adjunct tools. Regardless of the country in which healthcare is provided, clinicians will need to work together with the entire healthcare team to identify reasonable approaches to obstetric care that make the best use of information provided by technology, keeping in mind the importance of the relationship among patients and their support systems. In the case of IA and CTG, standardization of guidelines and the simplification of management algorithms should be a priority regardless of the geographic location.

References

[1] Pregnancy Outcome Unit, SA Health, Pregnancy outcome in south Australia 2016. Available from: https://www.sahealth.sa.gov.au/wps/wcm/connect/4ccbba85-14c6-4b39-a19e4e8cd54e9ea1/Pregnancy+Outcome+in+South+Australia+2016+V2.pdf?MOD=AJPEESCACHEID=ROOTWORKSPACE-4ccbba85-14c6-4b39-a19e-4e8cd54e9ea1-mXe8zjD, 2018 (accessed 20.04.18).

[2] C.E. East, S.C. Kane, M.A. Davey, C.O. Kamlin, S.P. Brennecke, Protocol for a randomised controlled trial of fetal scalp blood lactate measurement to reduce caesarean sections during labour: The Flamingo trial, BMC Pregnancy Childbirth 15 (1) (2015) 285.

[3] S. Kuah, G. Matthews, Role of computerized CTG, in: E. Chandraharan (Ed.), Handbook of CTG Interpretation, Cambridge University Press, Cambridge, UK, 2017, pp. 142–146.

[4] J. Sandall, H. Soltani, S. Gates, A. Shennan, D. Devane, Midwife-led continuity models versus other models of care for childbearing women, Cochrane Database Syst. Rev. (2016) CD004667.

[5] D.C. Smith, Interprofessional collaboration in perinatal care, J. Perinat. Neonatal Nurs. 30 (3) (2016) 167–173.

[6] J. Shamian, Interprofessional Collaboration, The only way to save every woman and every child, Lancet 384 (9948) (2014) e41–e42.

[7] R. Horton, O. Astudillo, The power of midwifery, Lancet 384 (9948) (2014) 1075–1076.

[8] B.R. Fletcher, R. Rowe, J. Hollowell, et al., Exploring women's preferences for birth settings in England: A discrete choice experiment, PLoS ONE 14 (4) (2019) 1–17.

[9] National Institute of Health and Care Excellence, Intrapartum care of healthy women and their babies during childbirth. NICE Clinical Guideline 190. Available from: https://www.nice.org.uk/guidance/cg190, 2014 (accessed 03-04-20).

[10] World Health Organization, Intrapartum care for a positive childbirth experience, Available from: https://www.who.int/reproductivehealth/publications/intrapartum-care-guidelines/en/, 2018 (accessed 03-04-20).

[11] A.B. Caughey, Midwife and obstetrician collaborative care: The whole is better than the parts, J. Midwifery Womens Health 60 (2) (2015) 120–121.

[12] E. Hadjigeorgiou, C. Kouta, E. Papastavrou, I. Papadopoulos, L.B. Mårtensson, Women's perceptions of their right to choose the place of childbirth: An integrative review, Midwifery 28 (3) (2012) 380–390.

[13] N.S. Carlson, N.K. Lowe, A concept analysis of watchful waiting among providers caring for women in labour, J. Adv. Nurs. 70 (3) (2014) 511–522.

[14] J.P. Rooks, The midwifery model of care, J. Nurse Midwifery 44 (4) (1999) 370–374.

[15] F. McConville, New global midwifery initiatives and why 2014 should be a good year for women and newborns, Midwifery 30 (5) (2014) 489–490.

[16] S.E. Lobst, C.L. Storr, D. Bingham, S. Zhu, M. Johantgen, Variation of intrapartum care and cesarean rates among practitioners attending births of low-risk, nulliparous women, Birth 47 (2) (2020) 227–236.

[17] N.S. Carlson, E.J. Corwin, T.L. Hernandez, et al., Association between provider type and cesarean birth in healthy nulliparous laboring women: A retrospective cohort study, Birth 45 (2) (2018) 159–168.

[18] D.C. Smith. Midwife–Physician collaboration, A conceptual framework for interprofessional collaborative practice, J. Midwifery Womens Health 60 (2) (2015) 128–139.

[19] I.C. Boesveld, P.P Valentijn, M. Hitzert, et al., An approach to measuring integrated care within a maternity care system: Experiences from the maternity care network study and the Dutch birth centre study, Int. J. Integr. Care 17 (2) (2017) 1–13.

[20] H.Y. Chen, S.P. Chauhan, C.V. Anath, et al., EFM and its relationship to neonatal and infant mortality in the United States, Am. J. Obstet. Gynecol. 204 (6) (2011) 491e1–49e10.

[21] C.V. Ananth, S.P. Chauhan, H.Y. Chen, M.E. D'Alton, A.M. Vintzileos, Electronic fetal monitoring in the United States: Temporal trends and adverse perinatal outcomes, Obstet. Gynecol. 121 (5) (2013) 927–933.

[22] P.R. McCartney, Intrapartum fetal monitoring: A historical perspective, in: A. Lyndon, L.U. Ali (Eds.), Fetal Heart Monitoring Principles and Practices5th Ed., Kendall Hunt, Dubuque, IA, 2015, pp. 3–47.

[23] D. Ayres-de-Campos, C.Y. Spong, E. ChandraharanFIGO Intrapartum Fetal Monitoring Expert Consensus Panel, FIGO consensus guidelines on intrapartum fetal monitoring: Cardiotocography, Int. J. Gynecol. Obstet. 131 (1) (2015) 13–24.

[24] K. Wisner, C. Holschuh, Fetal Heart Rate Auscultation, Nurs Womens Health 22 (6) (2018) e1–e32.

[25] D. Lewis, S. DowneFIGO Intrapartum Fetal Monitoring Expert Consensus Panel, FIGO consensus guidelines on intrapartum fetal monitoring: Intermittent auscultation, Int. J. Gynecol. Obstet. 131 (1) (2015) 9–12.

[26] Royal Australian and New Zealand College of Obstetricians and Gynaecologists. Intrapartum Fetal Surveillance Clinical Guidelines, fourth ed. Available from https://ranzcog.edu.au/RANZCOG_SITE/media/RANZCOG-MEDIA/Women%27s%20Health/Statement%20and%20guidelines/Clinical-Obstetrics/IFS-Guideline-4thEdition-2019.pdf?ext=.pdf., 2019 (accessed 03-04-20).

[27] S. Dore, W. Ehman, Fetal health surveillance: Intrapartum consensus guideline, No. 396, J. Obstet. Gynaecol. Can. 42 (3) (2020) 316–348.

[28] American College of Nurse-Midwives, Intermittent auscultation for intrapartum fetal heart rate surveillance, J. Midwifery Womens Health 60 (5) (2015) 626–632.

[29] G.A. Macones, G.D. Hankins, C.Y. Spong, et al., The 2008 National Institute of Child Health and Human Development workshop report on electronic fetal monitoring: update on definitions, interpretation, and research guidelines, Obstet. Gynecol. 112 (2008) 661–666.

[30] R.J. Knupp, W.W. Andrews, A.T. Tita, The future of electronic metal Monitoring, Best Pract. Res. Clin. Obstet. Gynaecol. (2020), in press.

[31] A. Garcia-Perez-Bonfils, E. Chandraharan, Physiology of fetal heart rate control and types of intrapartum hypoxia, in: E. Chandraharan (Ed.), Handbook of CTG Interpretation, Cambridge University Press, Cambridge, UK, 2017, pp. 13–25.

[32] R. Cypher, Assessment of fetal oxygenation and acid–base status, in: A. Lyndon, K. Wisner (Eds.), Fetal Heart Monitoring: Principles and Practices (6th ed.), Dubuque, IA: Kendall Hunt Publishing.

[33] E. Chandraharan, Fetal scalp blood sampling during labour: Is it a useful diagnostic test or a historical test that no longer has a place in modern clinical obstetrics? BJOG 121 (9) (2014) 1056–1062.

[34] B. Mills, E. Chandraharan, Peripheral tests of fetal well-being, in: E. Chandraharan (Ed.), Handbook of CTG Interpretation, Cambridge University Press, Cambridge, UK, 2017, pp. 147–150.

[35] M.K. Whitworth, L. Bricker, How to perform intrapartum fetal blood sampling, Br. J. Hosp. Med. 67 (9) (2006) 162–164.

[36] B. Carbonne, K. Pons, E. Maisonneuve, Foetal scalp blood sampling during labour for pH and lactate measurements, Best Pract. Res. Clin. Obstet. Gynaecol. 30 (2016) 62–67.

[37] Royal College of Obstetricians and Gynaecologists, Is It Time for UK Obstetricians to Accept Fetal Scalp Lactate as an Alternative to Scalp pH, Scientific Impact Paper, No. 47, RCOG Press, London, 2015.

[38] J.S. Jørgensen, T. Weber, Fetal scalp blood sampling in labor—a review, Acta Obstet. Gynecol. Scand. 93 (6) (2014) 548–555.

[39] Z. Henderson, J.L. Ecker, Fetal scalp blood sampling—limited role in contemporary obstetric practice: part II, Lab. Med. 34 (8) (2003) 594–600.

[40] X. Carbonell, E.F. Gonzalez, Recommendations and Guidelines for Perinatal Medicine, Matres Mundi, Barcelona, Spain, 2007 JM Carrera, Ed.

[41] C. Tuffnell, W. Haw, K. Wilkinson, How long does a fetal scalp blood sample take? BJOG 113 (3) (2006) 332–334.

[42] Z. Alfirevic, G.M. Gyte, A. Cuthbert, D. Devane, Continuous cardiotocography (CTG) as a form of electronic fetal monitoring (EFM) for fetal assessment during labour, Cochrane Database Syst. Rev. (2017) CD006066.

[43] M. Westgren, K. Kruger, S. Ek, et al., Lactate compared with pH analysis at fetal scalp blood sampling: a prospective randomised study, BJOG 105 (1) (1998) 29–33.

[44] L. Nordström, S. Achanna, K. Naka, S. Arulkumaran, Fetal and maternal lactate increase during active second stage, BJOG 108 (3) (2001) 263–268.

[45] C. Young, A. Ryce, Fetal scalp lactate testing during intrapartum pregnancy with abnormal fetal heart rate: A review of clinical effectiveness, cost-effectiveness, and guidelines. Available from: https://www.ncbi.nlm.nih.gov/books/NBK532205/pdf/Bookshelf_NBK532205.pdf, 2018 (accessed 03-04-20).

[46] A.M. Heinis, M.E. Spaanderman, J.M.K. Gunnewiek, F.K. Lotgering, Scalp blood lactate for intrapartum assessment of fetal metabolic acidosis, Acta Obstet. Gynecol. Scand. 90 (10) (2011) 1107–1114.

[47] K. Kruger, B. Hallberg, M. Blennow, M. Kublickas, M. Westgren, Predictive value of fetal scalp blood lactate concentration and pH as markers of neurologic disability, Am. J. Obstet. Gynecol. 181 (5) (1999) 1072–1078.

[48] Amer-Wåhlin, L.A. Miller, ST analysis as an adjunct to electronic fetal monitoring: an overview, J. Perinat. Neonatal Nurs. 24 (3) (2010) 231–237.

[49] K.G. Rosen, K. Lindencrantz, STAN—the Gothenburg model for fetal surveillance during labour by ST analysis of the fetal electrocardiogram, Clin. Phys. Physiol. Meas. 10 (Suppl. B) (1989) 51–56.

[50] M.A. Belfort, G.R. Saade, ST segment analysis as an adjunct to electronic fetal monitoring, part I: background, physiology, interpretation, Clin. Perinatol. 38 (2011) 143–157.

[51] M.A. Belfort, G.R. Saade, ST segment analysis (STAN) as an adjunct to electronic fetal monitoring, part II: clinical studies and future directions, Clin. Perinatol 38 (2011) 143–157.

[52] I. Amer-Wåhlin, A. Ugwumadu, B.M. Yli, Fetal electrocardiography ST-segment analysis for intrapartum monitoring: a critical appraisal of conflicting evidence and a way forward, Am. J. Obstet. Gynecol. 221 (6) (2019) 577–601.

[53] A.P. Carrillo, E. Chandraharan, ST-analyzer: Case examples and pitfalls, in: E. Chandraharan (Ed.), Handbook of CTG Interpretation, Cambridge University Press, Cambridge, UK, 2017, p. 135.

[54] P.J. Steer, L.E. Hvidman, Scientific and clinical evidence for the use of fetal ECG ST segment analysis (STAN), Acta Obstet. Gynecol. Scand. 93 (6) (2014) 533–538.

[55] K.G. Rosén, I. Amer-Wåhlin, R. Luzietti, et al., Fetal ECG waveform analysis, Best Pract. Res. Clin. Obstet. Gynaecol. 18 (3) (2004) 485–514.

[56] R.Z. Mansano, M.H. Beall, M.G. Ross, Fetal ST segment heart rate analysis in labor: improvement of intervention criteria using interpolated base deficit, J. Matern Fetal Neonatal Med. 20 (1) (2007) 47–52.

[57] C. Vayssiere, R. Haberstich, V. Sebahoun, et al., Fetal electrocardiogram ST-segment analysis and prediction of neonatal acidosis, Int. J. Gynecol. Obstet. 97 (2) (2007) 110–114.

[58] H. Norén, A.K. Luttkus, J.H. Stupin, et al., Fetal scalp pH and ST analysis of the fetal ECG as an adjunct to cardiotocography to predict fetal acidosis in labor/A multi-center, case controlled study, J. Perinat. Med. 35 (5) (2007) 408–414.

[59] G. Saccone, E. Schuit, I. Amer-Wåhlin, S. Xodo, V. Berghella, Electrocardiogram ST analysis during labor: a systematic review and meta-analysis of randomized controlled trials, Obstet. Gynecol. 127 (1) (2016) 127–135.

[60] E. Blix, K.G. Brurberg, E. Reierth, L.M. Reinar, P. Øian, ST wave-form analysis versus cardiotocography alone for intrapartum fetal monitoring: a systematic review and meta-analysis of randomized tri-als, Acta Obstet. Gynecol. Scand. 95 (1) (2016) 16–27.

[61] J.P. Neilson, Fetal electrocardiogram (ECG) for fetal monitoring during labour, Cochrane Database Syst. Rev. (2015) CD000116.

[62] M.E. Foley, M. Alarab, L. Daly, et al., The continuing effectiveness of active management of first labor, despite a doubling in overall nulliparous cesarean delivery, Am. J. Obstet. Gynecol. 191 (3) (2004) 891–895.

[63] A.M. Patey, J.A. Curran, A.E. Sprague, et al., Intermittent auscultation versus continuous fetal monitoring: Exploring factors that influence birthing unit nurses' fetal surveillance practice using theoretical domains framework, BMC Pregnancy Childbirth 17 (1) (2017) 320–338.

[64] V. Smith, C.M. Begley, M. Clarke, D. Devane, Professionals' views of fetal monitoring during labour: A systematic review and thematic analy-sis, BMC Pregnancy Childbirth 12 (1) (2012) 166–174.

[65] J.L. Neal, N.S. Carlson, J.C. Phillippi, et al., Midwifery presence in United States medical centers and labor care and birth outcomes among low-risk nulliparous women: A Consortium on Safe Labor study, Birth 46 (3) (2019) 475–486.

Amnioinfusion

Amnioinfusion is the administration of room temperature isotonic solution such as normal saline or Ringer's lactate via a double-lumen intrauterine pressure catheter (IUPC) by either a gravity flow or an infusion pump to restore amniotic fluid volume. The procedure is intended to relieve intermittent umbilical cord compression, which results in variable fetal heart rate decelerations and transient fetal hypoxemia. This procedure has no known effect on late decelerations and is no longer recommended for dilution of meconium.

An amnioinfusion generally begins by administering a bolus of fluid (250–500 mL) over 20 to 30 minutes. The maintenance dose is infused at a rate of 2 to 3 mL/min (maximum of 180 mL/hr), during which time it is imperative that the amount of fluid returning is approximated and documented to avoid overdistention of the uterus. Assessment of the output can be accomplished by weighing the absorbent pads underneath the woman (1 mL = 1 g) and counting the number of pads changed.

Assessment of uterine resting tone is also an important aspect of surveillance during the procedure, and it should not exceed 40 mm Hg. It is unlikely that more than 1000 mL of fluid will need to be administered, and if variable decelerations persist even after this amount of fluid has been instilled into the uterus, other therapies should be used as treatment. Amnioinfusion is not without risks, and iatrogenic hydramnios from amnioinfusion may cause a placental abruption or pressure on the maternal diaphragm, causing shortness of breath, tachycardia, and a change in maternal blood pressure. A rapid release, or "gush," of fluid predisposes the woman to a prolapsed umbilical cord. The preterm fetus may benefit from a warmed solution, avoiding bradycardia. A blood warmer is the safest method for administering warmed fluid. *The fluid should not be heated in a microwave or blanket warmer.* Warmed fluid also is suggested if the rate of the amnioinfusion exceeds 15 mL/min.

There are a variety of ways to perform an amnioinfusion. It is important that the institution has a policy and procedure in place and these are followed.

INDICATIONS FOR AMNIOINFUSION

1. Laboring preterm women with premature rupture of the membranes (prophylactic)
2. Variable decelerations uncorrectable with conventional interventions
3. Significant oligohydramnios at term when labor is being induced

EQUIPMENT AND SUPPLIES

- Normal saline or Ringer's lactate solution, 1000 mL at room temperature
- Intrauterine catheter equipment, preferably with a double lumen and amnioport (if using single-lumen water-filled IUPC, intravenous [IV] extension tubing with twin sites or arterial line [12 inches] and a three-way stopcock are needed)
- Volumetric infusion pump and tubing or IV pole for gravity flow
- Blood warmer or blood/fluid warming set (optional)

Procedure

Amnioinfusion should be initiated after insertion of the intrauterine catheter. Before the procedure, the intrauterine resting tone should be noted with the woman in the right and left lateral and supine positions for later comparison. Various procedures have been discussed in the literature, and each institution determines its own obstetric policies and procedures. A sample procedure follows:

1. Connect the 1000-mL bottle of amnioinfusion solution to the IV tubing.
2. Flush the tubing with the solution.
3. Connect the tubing to the woman's IUPC via the amnioport or double-lumen IUPC or via a three-way stopcock, depending on the type of IUPC used.
4. Initiate the flow of amnioinfusion and instill the initial bolus, usually 250 to 500 mL over a 20- to 30-minute period (10–15 mL/min) using either an infusion pump or gravity flow. If gravity flow is used, the solution must be hung about 3 to 4 feet above the level of the tip of the IUPC. If fluid will not run by gravity, check the position/placement of the IUPC.
5. When variable decelerations resolve, continue the infusion at a slower rate, usually about 2 to 3 mL/min (120–180 mL/hr), as ordered by the care provider. If variable decelerations are not

relieved after infusing 800 to 1000 mL of solution, discontinue the procedure and perform an alternative intervention.

6. Observe and evaluate for amount and character of vaginal drainage. Vaginal output is assessed and documented to demonstrate that the volume infused is also coming back out and not causing overdistention of the uterus. Be vigilant for sudden gushes of fluid and assess for cord prolapse.

NOTE: Intrauterine resting tone will appear higher than normal, from 25 to 40 mm Hg, because of resistance to outflow through the tiny holes in the tip of the catheter. The true resting tone can be checked by temporarily discontinuing the flow of infusion.

Patient Care

Care of the woman undergoing amnioinfusion includes the following:

1. Stop the infusion periodically, approximately every 30 to 60 minutes, to note the baseline uterine pressure. If the resting tone of the uterus exceeds 40 mm Hg, discontinue the infusion and notify the physician.

2. Change the underpads frequently to ensure the woman's comfort.

3. Note the color and amount of fluid on the underpads. The underpads may be weighed. Amounts of fluid returned should be determined (1 mL = 1 g).

4. Monitor for signs and symptoms of infection.

5. Monitor for signs and symptoms of cardiac or respiratory compromise secondary to an overdistended uterus (maternal shortness of breath, hypotension, or tachycardia).

6. Monitor fetal heart rate patterns on the electronic fetal monitoring strip.

Fetal Heart Rate Tracings Review

Appendix B consists of 40 fetal heart rate (FHR) tracings clinicians can review for the purpose of improving competency in the application of both the National Institute for Child Health and Human Development terminology and the two central principles of FHR interpretation presented in Chapter 5. Clinicians should assume that all tracings are from term pregnancies unless otherwise noted. For purposes of identifying tachysystole and the issue of recurrence with decelerations, clinicians should assume the tracings have been present for 30 minutes.

Clinicians should review the tracings provided and determine the following:

1. The components of FHR (baseline rate, baseline variability, accelerations, decelerations)
2. The category (1, 2, 3) of each tracing
3. Whether uterine contraction frequency would be summarized as normal or tachysystole, and identify any possible excessive uterine activity, such as inadequate relaxation time (see Chapter 4)
4. Whether there is evidence of interruption of the oxygen pathway
5. Whether the possibility of evolving fetal metabolic acidemia/ongoing hypoxic injury can be ruled out

A key with the answers for each tracing is provided immediately after each tracing. Please note that because FHR tracing evaluation is a visual exercise, there may be valid differences of opinion among clinicians reviewing these tracings. Whenever possible, the authors have anticipated such differences and included them in the answer key for purposes of discussion.

Finally, specific management approaches are not included in the key that follows the tracings, primarily because application of the standardized management model presented in Chapter 6 would vary widely based on the patient's clinical context.

KEY FOR APPENDIX B FETAL HEART RATE TRACINGS

Monitoring modes are identified as follows:

US: external Doppler
TOCO: external tocotransducer
IFE: internal fetal electrode
IUPC: intrauterine pressure catheter

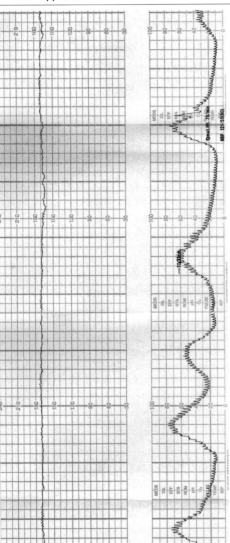

Fig. B-1

1. **Monitoring Mode:** US/TOCO
   Baseline FHR: 170 bpm. **Baseline variability:** Minimal. **Accelerations:** Absent. **Decelerations:** Depending on where the clinician would consider the onset, there is a possibility of a late deceleration at minute 7, but opinions could differ. **Uterine activity:** Tachysystole as evidenced by 5-plus contractions in the 10-minute window. **Category:** This is a Category 2 tracing.
   Interpretation
   If the FHR decrease at minute 7 is seen as a late deceleration, then there is interruption of the oxygen pathway at one or more points; the lack of either acceleration(s) or moderate variability means clinicians are unable to rule out the possibility of evolving fetal metabolic acidemia/ongoing hypoxic injury. Clinicians also should be sure to consider all causes of tachycardia when evaluating this tracing. Note that the standardized management model would require assessment of the oxygen pathway because of the Category 2 status, regardless of whether clinicians see a late deceleration or not. This provides an added level of safety in dealing with Category 2 tracings.

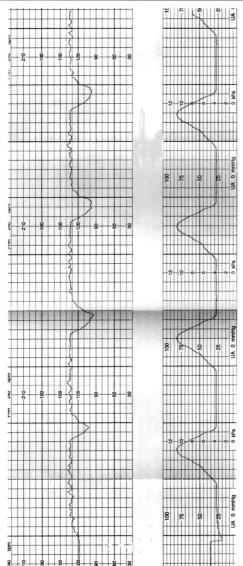

Fig. B-2

2. **Monitoring Mode:** IFE/IUPC
Baseline FHR: 135 bpm. **Baseline variability:** Moderate. **Accelerations:** Absent. **Decelerations:** Variable decelerations. Note that although some clinicians may want to label the decelerations as lates, the abrupt onset to nadir (less than 30 seconds) makes all of these variable decels, regardless of their relationship to contractions. **Uterine activity:** Normal. **Category:** This is a Category 2 tracing.
Interpretation
The variable decelerations reflect interruption of the oxygen pathway at one or more points; the moderate variability means clinicians are able to rule out the possibility of evolving fetal metabolic acidemia/ongoing hypoxic injury.

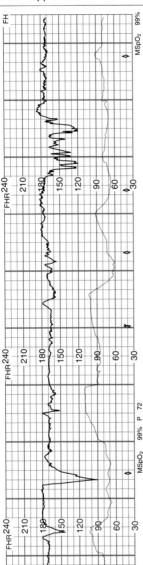

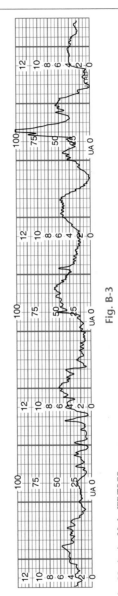

Fig. B-3

3. **Monitoring Mode:** IFE/TOCO
Baseline FHR: 170 bpm. **Baseline variability:** Minimal for the majority of the baseline. **Accelerations:** Minimal for at one or more points; the lack of either acceleration(s) or moderate variability means clini- Absent. **Decelerations:** Variable decelerations. **Uterine activity:** Tachysystole, toco needs to be adjusted to provide a clearer picture. **Category:** This is a Category 2 tracing.
Interpretation
The variable decelerations reflect interruption of the oxygen pathway at one or more points; the lack of either acceleration(s) or moderate variability means clinicians are unable to rule out the possibility of evolving fetal metabolic acidemia/ongoing hypoxic injury. Clinicians should consider all causes of tachycardia when evaluating this tracing. Note the swings in maternal heart rate (MHR) during and between contractions.

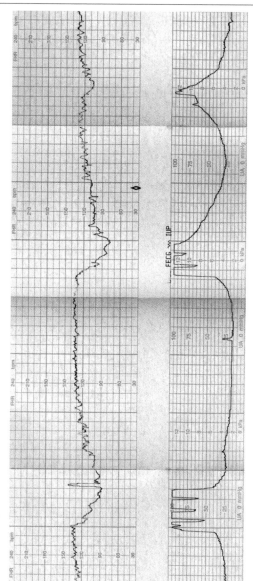

Fig. B-4

4. **Monitoring Mode:** IFE/IUPC
    Baseline FHR: 130 bpm. **Baseline variability:** Moderate, but there is very limited baseline to assess. **Accelerations:** Absent. **Decelerations:** Two prolonged decelerations followed by a late or variable deceleration (depending on how the clinician views deceleration onset). **Uterine activity:** Normal, however, it appears the patient is performing coached, long-Valsalva pushing and this should be corrected. **Category:** This is a Category 2 tracing.
    Interpretation
    The decelerations reflect interruption of the oxygen pathway at one or more points; the moderate variability means clinicians are able to rule out the possibility of evolving fetal metabolic acidemia/ongoing hypoxic injury.

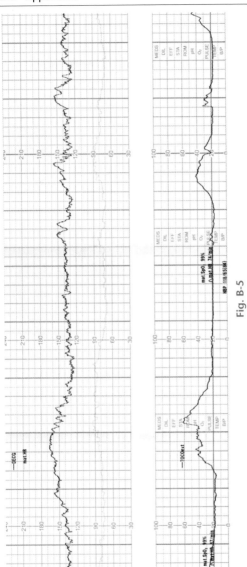

Fig. B-5

5   Monitoring Mode: IFE/TOCO
Baseline FHR: 135 bpm. **Baseline variability:** Moderate. **Accelerations:** Multiple accelerations, including a prolonged acceleration. **Decelerations:** None.
Uterine activity: Normal. **Category:** This is a Category 1 tracing.
Interpretation
There are no decelerations reflecting interruption of the oxygen pathway at one or more points; the accelerations and the moderate variability means clinicians are able to rule out the possibility of evolving fetal metabolic acidemia/ongoing hypoxic injury.

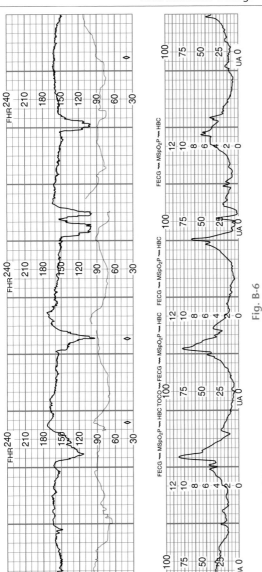

Fig. B-6

6. **Monitoring Mode:** IFE/TOCO
Baseline FHR: 160 bpm. **Baseline variability:** Minimal. **Accelerations:** None. **Decelerations:** Variable decelerations. **Uterine activity:** If you include what appears to be a contraction in minute 1, there is tachysystole. **Category:** This is a Category 2 tracing.
Interpretation
The variable decelerations reflect interruption of the oxygen pathway at one or more points; the absences of either accelerations or moderate variability means clinicians are unable to rule out the possibility of evolving fetal metabolic acidemia/ongoing hypoxic injury.

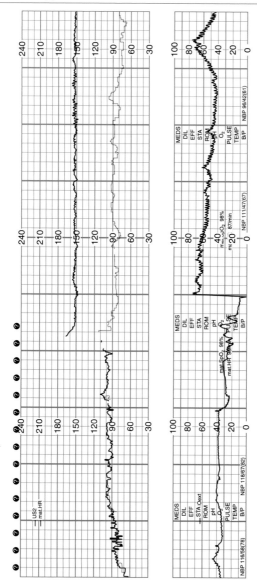

Fig. B-7

7. **Monitoring Mode:** US/TOCO
Baseline FHR: 155 bpm. Note the monitor is picking up MHR in the first 4 minutes of the tracing. **Baseline variability:** Minimal. **Accelerations:** None. **Decelerations:** None. **Uterine activity:** Likely normal, but unable to be certain, clinician would need to palpate and adjust toco. **Category:** This is a Category 2 tracing.
Interpretation
Although there are no decelerations reflecting interruption of the oxygen pathway at one or more points, the lack of accelerations or moderate variability means clinicians are able to rule out the possibility of evolving fetal metabolic acidemia/ongoing hypoxic injury.

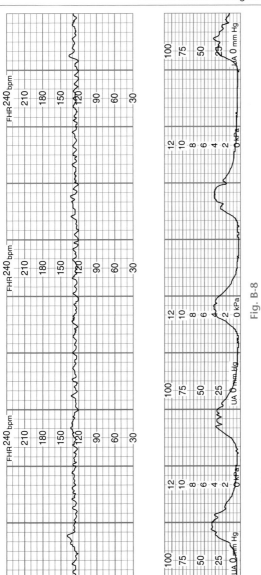

Fig. B-8

8. **Monitoring Mode:** US/TOCO
Baseline FHR: 125 bpm. **Baseline variability:** Moderate. **Accelerations:** None. **Decelerations:** None. **Uterine activity:** None. **Category:** This is a Category 1 tracing.
Interpretation
There are no decelerations reflecting interruption of the oxygen pathway at one or more points; the moderate variability means clinicians are able to rule out the possibility of evolving fetal metabolic acidemia/ongoing hypoxic injury.

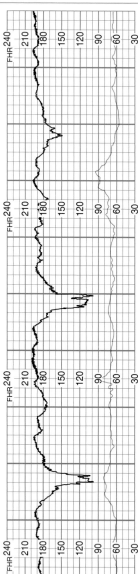
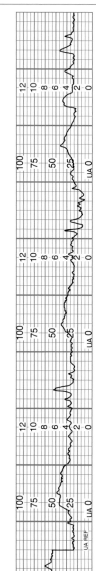

Fig. B-9

9. **Monitoring Mode:** IFE/TOCO
Baseline FHR: Difficult to assess because of the limited amount and questionable undulating pattern in areas, likely near 190 bpm. **Baseline variability:** Unclear, although some clinicians may assess the variability as moderate, the undulations at time appear regular, which is consistent with a sinusoidal baseline. **Accelerations:** None. **Decelerations:** There are three obvious variable decelerations and a questionable deceleration between minutes 3 and 4. **Uterine activity:** Unable to gauge because of the quality of the tracing. **Category:** This is a Category 2 tracing.

Interpretation

The variable decelerations reflecting interruption of the oxygen pathway at one or more points; and while some clinicians may think they can visualize moderate variability, the safest approach to interpretation in this tracing, given the entire picture (tachycardia, decelerations, possible undulating baseline characteristics) would be to proceed as unable to rule out the possibility of evolving fetal metabolic acidemia/ongoing hypoxic injury. Clinicians must remember that EFM has no diagnostic value. Its only value is as a screening tool, which requires clinicians err on the side of caution when interpreting questionable tracings.

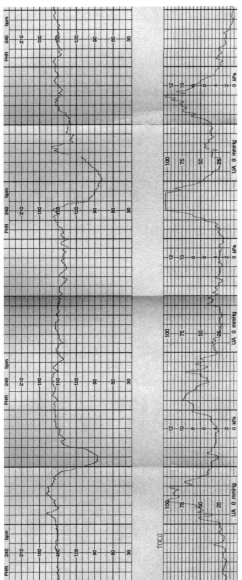

Fig. B-10

10. **Monitoring Mode:** US/TOCO

Baseline FHR: 150 bpm. **Baseline variability:** Moderate. **Accelerations:** None. **Decelerations:** Variable decelerations. Note that some clinicians may be tempted to label these decelerations as late decelerations because of their relationship to the contractions, but the onset to nadir in both decelerations is abrupt (less than 30 seconds) not gradual (30 seconds or more) making the correct assessment variable decelerations. **Uterine activity:** Normal, note that the toco may benefit from an adjustment.

Category: This is a Category 2 tracing.

Interpretation

The variable decelerations reflect interruption of the oxygen pathway at one or more points; the moderate variability means clinicians are able to rule out the possibility of evolving fetal metabolic acidemia/ongoing hypoxic injury.

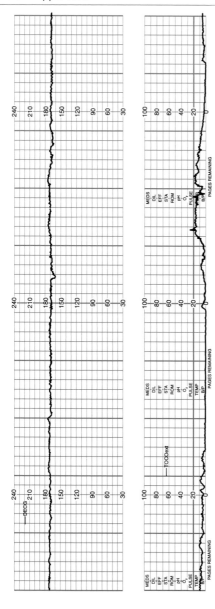

Fig. B-11

11. **Monitoring Mode:** IFE/TOCO

Baseline FHR: 170 bpm. **Baseline variability:** Minimal. **Accelerations:** Absent. **Decelerations:** Absent. **Uterine activity:** Normal (vs. tachysystole), but it appears toco may need to be adjusted, and it is possible that palpation would reveal contraction duration that is excessive. **Category:** This is a Category 2 tracing.

Interpretation

Although there are no decelerations reflecting interruption of the oxygen pathway at one or more points; the lack of either acceleration(s) or moderate variability means clinicians are unable to rule out the possibility of evolving fetal metabolic acidemia/ongoing hypoxic injury. Clinicians should consider all causes of tachycardia when evaluating this tracing.

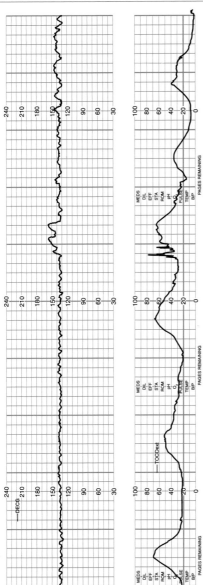

Fig. B-12

12. **Monitoring Mode:** US/TOCO
Baseline FHR: 135 bpm. **Baseline variability:** Moderate, although some clinicians may consider it minimal in the first minutes of the tracing. **Accelerations:** Present. **Decelerations:** Absent. **Uterine activity:** With six contractions in 10 minutes, this would be tachysystole. **Category:** This is a Category 1 tracing, unless the clinician believes the variability is minimal for the majority of the tracing, which would result in a Category 2 designation.

Interpretation
There is no evidence of interrupted oxygenation because there are no clinically significant decelerations. The possibility of evolving metabolic acidemia/ongoing hypoxic injury can be ruled out by the accelerations and the moderate variability. Remember, *either moderate variability or acceleration* of the FHR precludes the possibility of ongoing hypoxic injury.

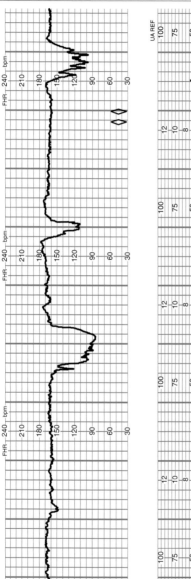

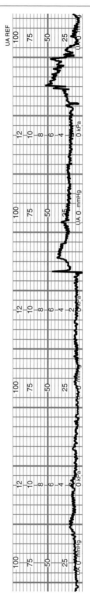

Fig. B-13

13. **Monitoring Mode:** IFE/TOCO
Baseline FHR: 160 bpm. Although portions of the tracing appear to have a baseline of 165, the majority of the baseline is at 160 bpm. **Baseline variability:** Minimal. **Accelerations:** Absent. **Decelerations:** Recurrent variable decelerations; note that the deceleration at approximately minute 4 has a gradual onset but cannot be identified as late or early because of a lack of contraction data. **Uterine activity:** Normal, but it appears toco may need to be adjusted. **Category:** This is a Category 2 tracing.
Interpretation
Variable decelerations reflect interruption of the oxygen pathway at one or more points; unable to rule out the possibility of evolving fetal metabolic acidemia because of the lack of either acceleration(s) or moderate variability.

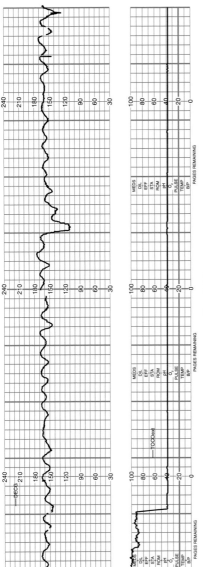

Fig. B-14

14. **Monitoring Mode:** IFE/TOCO
Baseline FHR: 155 or 160 bpm, sinusoidal. **Baseline variability:** Not applicable because of sinusoidal tracing. **Accelerations:** Absent. **Decelerations:** Variable deceleration noted. **Uterine activity:** N/A, toco was removed as patient was being prepped for cesarean delivery. **Category:** This is a Category 3 tracing.
Interpretation
The sinusoidal pattern is rare, and this fetus was born with severe anemia caused by a maternal–fetal hemorrhage, but the neonatal course went well after transfusion. Although the variable deceleration reflects interruption of the oxygen pathway at one or more points, the key finding here is the sinusoidal pattern.

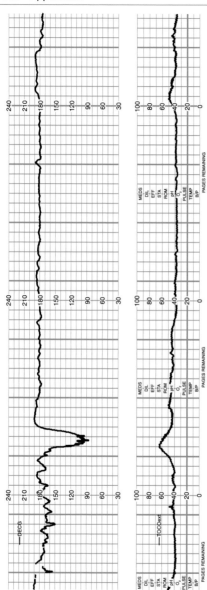

Fig. B-15

15. Monitoring Mode: IFE/TOCO

Baseline FHR: 180 bpm for the majority of the tracing. **Baseline variability:** Minimal for the majority of the tracing. **Accelerations:** Absent. **Decelerations:** Obvious variable deceleration at the beginning of the tracing; however, immediately before the variable, it is unclear whether there is a deceleration, and clinicians would need to evaluate the previous tracing portion to be certain. **Uterine activity:** Difficult to assess; the toco may need adjustment, and palpation should be used to assess for hypertonus and to evaluate the onset and offset of contractions because excessive contraction duration may be an issue at the beginning of the tracing. **Category:** This is a Category 2 tracing.

Interpretation

The variable deceleration reflects interruption of the oxygen pathway at one or more points; unable to rule out the possibility of evolving fetal metabolic acidemia because of the lack of either acceleration(s) or moderate variability. Additionally, tachycardia is noted.

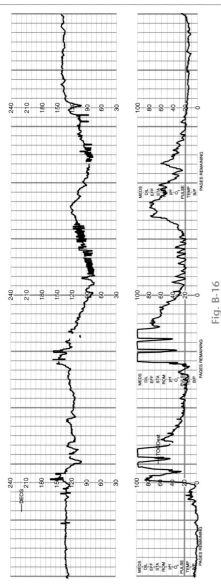

Fig. B-16

16. Monitoring Mode: IFE/TOCO

Baseline FHR: 130 or 135 bpm. **Baseline variability:** Minimal. **Accelerations:** Absent. **Decelerations:** Variable and prolonged decelerations. **Uterine activity:** Normal as to frequency; however, the contraction duration time may be excessive, resulting in inadequate relaxation time. **Category:** This is a Category 2 tracing.

Interpretation

The variable and prolonged decelerations reflect interruption of the oxygen pathway at one or more points; unable to rule out the possibility of evolving fetal metabolic acidemia/ongoing hypoxic injury because of the lack of either acceleration(s) or moderate variability. *Note the artifact during the prolonged deceleration. If this was persistent, it could represent an arrhythmia such as premature atrial contractions (PACs).*

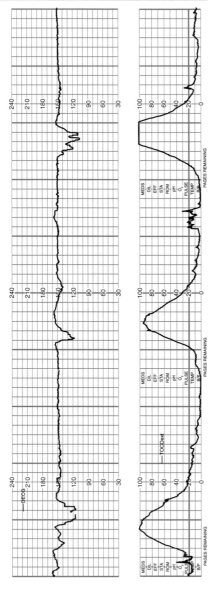

Fig. B-17

17. **Monitoring Mode:** IFE/IUPC
Baseline FHR: 150 bpm. **Baseline variability:** Minimal. **Accelerations:** Minimal. **Decelerations:** Absent. **Decelerations:** Variable decelerations. **Uterine activity:** Normal frequency, duration borders on excessive. **Category:** This is a Category 2 tracing.
Interpretation
The variable decelerations reflect interruption of the oxygen pathway at one or more points; unable to rule out the possibility of evolving fetal metabolic acidemia/ongoing hypoxic injury because of the lack of either acceleration(s) or moderate variability.

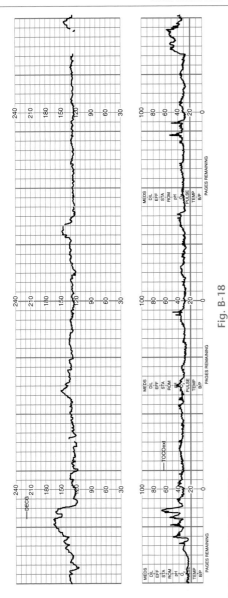

Fig. B-18

18. **Monitoring Mode:** US/TOCO

Baseline FHR: 125 bpm. **Baseline variability:** Minimal for the majority of the tracing, although some clinicians may tend to call it moderate at first glance because of the accelerations. **Accelerations:** Present. **Decelerations:** Absent. **Uterine activity:** Difficult to determine; toco needs to be adjusted and palpation used to evaluate uterine activity thoroughly. **Category:** This is a Category 2 tracing (because of the lack of moderate variability).

Interpretation

There is no interruption of the oxygen pathway; the accelerations rule out the possibility of evolving fetal metabolic acidemia/ongoing hypoxic injury.

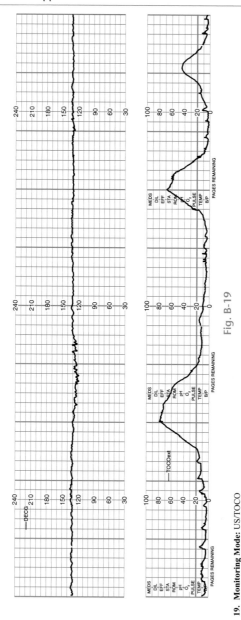

Fig. B-19

19. Monitoring Mode: US/TOCO

Baseline FHR: 130 bpm. **Baseline variability:** Minimal. **Accelerations:** Absent. **Decelerations:** Late deceleration. **Uterine activity:** Normal frequency; duration of contraction associated with late deceleration is excessive. **Category:** This is a Category 2 tracing.

Interpretation

The late deceleration reflects interruption of the oxygen pathway at one or more points; unable to rule out the possibility of evolving fetal metabolic acidemia/ongoing hypoxic injury because of the lack of either acceleration(s) or moderate variability.

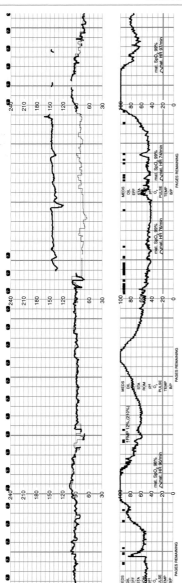

Fig. B-20

20. **Monitoring Mode:** US/TOCO

Baseline FHR: 145 bpm; note the limited segment (approximately 21½ minutes only) of FHR baseline caused by the pickup of MHR (initial 5 minutes of tracing). Question marks at the top of the tracing alert the clinician to the possibility of signal coincidence, and MHR of 90 bpm at the beginning of the tracing (see notation on lower portion of uterine activity panel) is consistent with the tracing showing a heart rate recorded in the 90s for the first 5 minutes of the tracing. **Baseline variability:** Moderate, but limited amount of FHR baseline to assess. **Accelerations:** Absent, but limited amount of tracing to assess. **Decelerations:** Absent, but limited amount of tracing to assess. **Uterine activity:** Probably normal, but toco needs to be adjusted and palpation used to assess contraction duration and uterine resting tone. **Category:** Of the limited portion of FHR available, it would fit into Category 1, but the majority of clinicians would wait for a clearer picture of FHR (adjust the Doppler and reassess) before committing to a category designation.

Interpretation

Most clinicians would not provide an interpretation of such a limited amount of tracing; the correct action here is to adjust the Doppler and reassess the tracing when signal coincidence has been resolved.

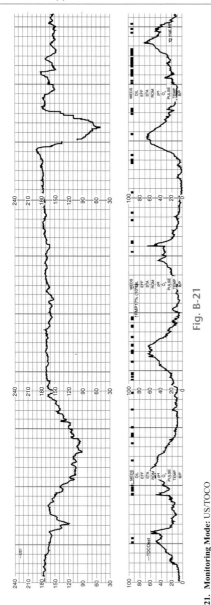

Fig. B-21

21. Monitoring Mode: US/TOCO

Baseline FHR: The beginning and middle portions of this tracing reveal an FHR baseline of 170 bpm; there may be a change in baseline near the end of the tracing, but this would require evaluation of the ongoing tracing to conclusively determine the change. **Baseline variability:** Minimal, for the portion of the tracing with a clearly identifiable baseline rate of 170 bpm. **Decelerations:** Present; a prolonged deceleration is seen at the beginning of the tracing, followed by a late deceleration in the middle of the tracing, and a variable deceleration is seen at the end of the tracing. This tracing clearly demonstrates that a variety of decelerations can be seen within a short period of time during labor. **Uterine activity:** Tachysystole, assuming this represents the average frequency over a 30-minute period. If this contraction pattern is new (<30 minutes), it would still qualify as excessive uterine activity because the relaxation time is not sufficient. During the first stage, relaxation time should be at least 60 seconds between contractions to avoid deterioration of fetal acid–base status. **Category:** This is a Category 2 tracing.

Interpretation

Three types of clinically significant decelerations (prolonged, late, and variable) reflect interruption of the oxygen pathway at one or more points; the possibility of evolving fetal metabolic acidemia cannot be ruled out because the tracing lacks either acceleration(s) or moderate variability.

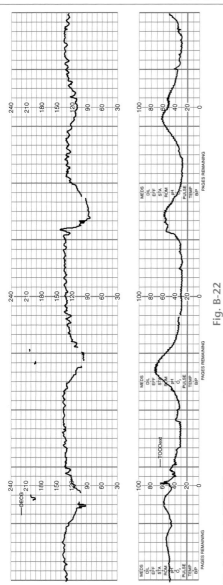

Fig. B-22

22. Monitoring Mode: US/TOCO

Baseline FHR: 130 bpm. **Baseline variability:** Minimal. **Accelerations:** Absent. **Decelerations:** Late and variable (third decel) decelerations. **Uterine activity:** Normal frequency, but there may be an issue with resting tone, and toco should be readjusted. **Category:** This is a Category 2 tracing.

Interpretation

The late and variable decelerations reflect interruption of the oxygen pathway at one or more points; unable to rule out the possibility of evolving fetal metabolic acidemia/ongoing hypoxic injury because of the lack of either acceleration(s) or moderate variability. *Note: maternal blood pressures were low (94–106/40–49 mm Hg) during this tracing and should have been corrected.*

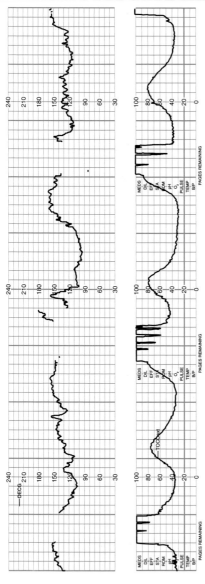

Fig. B-23

23. **Monitoring Mode:** US/TOCO

Baseline FHR: Indeterminate. **Baseline variability, Accelerations, and Decelerations:** Unable to assess because of the indeterminate baseline. **Uterine activity:** Tachysystole. **Category:** This is a Category 2 tracing.

Interpretation

The indeterminate baseline results in an inability to assess the FHR components; therefore no interpretation can be provided. Clinicians will need to look to other portions of this tracing to assist in assessment and interpretation, and correcting the tachysystole is crucial because there is a strong likelihood of significant decelerations of the FHR (given the overall characteristics of the tracing).

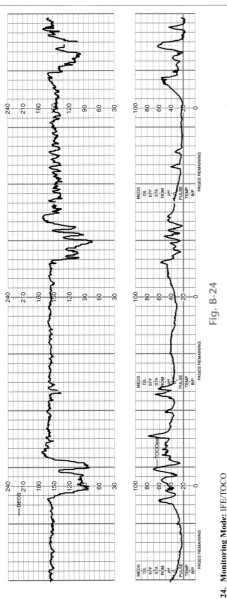

Fig. B-24

24. Monitoring Mode: IFE/TOCO
Baseline FHR: 155 bpm. **Baseline variability:** Moderate. **Accelerations:** Moderate. **Decelerations:** Absent. **Decelerations:** Variable decelerations. **Uterine activity:** Unable to accurately assess; toco should be readjusted. **Category:** This is a Category 2 tracing.
Interpretation
The variable decelerations reflect interruption of the oxygen pathway at one or more points; the moderate variability rules out the possibility of evolving fetal metabolic acidemia/ongoing hypoxic injury.

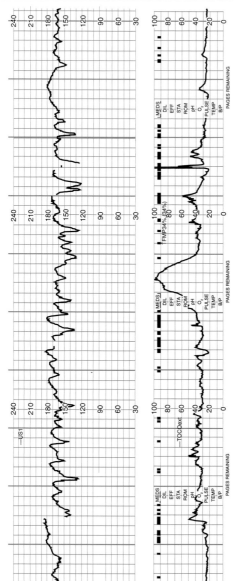

Fig. B-25

25 Monitoring Mode: US/TOCO

Baseline FHR: Indeterminate, because of the period of marked variability. **Baseline variability:** Marked. **Accelerations:** Unable to determine because of marked variability. **Decelerations:** None apparent but difficult to determine because of marked variability. **Uterine activity:** Appears normal, but toco may need to be adjusted and baseline resting tone should be evaluated by palpation. **Category:** This is a Category 2 tracing.

Interpretation

The significance (if any) of marked variability is unknown, and it is most frequently seen with fetal movement or fetal stimulation. Unlike moderate variability, it does not allow the clinician to rule out the possibility of evolving fetal metabolic acidemia/ongoing hypoxic injury.

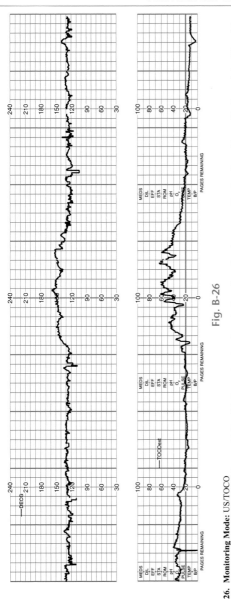

Fig. B-26

26. Monitoring Mode: US/TOCO
Baseline FHR: 130 bpm. **Baseline variability:** Moderate. **Accelerations:** Prolonged acceleration present. **Decelerations:** Absent. **Uterine activity:** Normal frequency, but contraction duration appears excessive. **Category:** This is a Category 1 tracing.
Interpretation
There is no interruption of the oxygen pathway; the prolonged acceleration rules out the possibility of evolving fetal metabolic acidemia/ongoing hypoxic injury.

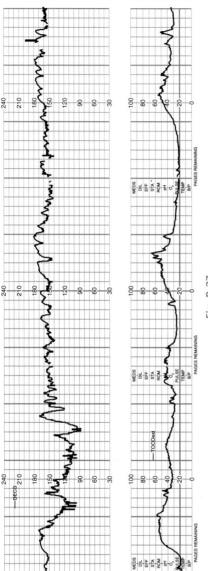

Fig. B-27

27. **Monitoring Mode:** IFE/TOCO

Baseline FHR: 155 bpm. **Baseline variability:** Moderate. **Accelerations:** Present. **Decelerations:** Prolonged deceleration. **Uterine activity:** Normal frequency (five contractions in 10 minutes), but uterine activity should be considered excessive because of lack of relaxation time. **Category:** This is a Category 2 tracing.

Interpretation

The prolonged deceleration reflects an interruption of the oxygen pathway; the prolonged accelerations and moderate variability rule out the possibility of evolving fetal metabolic acidemia/ongoing hypoxic injury.

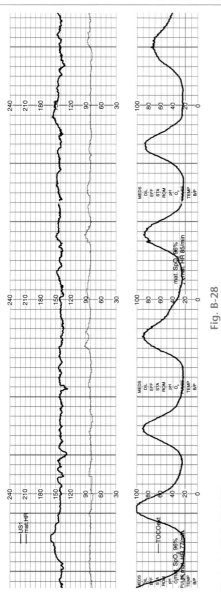

Fig. B-28

28. **Monitoring Mode:** US/TOCO
Baseline FHR: 140 bpm. **Baseline variability:** Moderate. **Accelerations:** Moderate. **Decelerations:** Absent. **Uterine activity:** Tachysystole. **Category:** This is a Category 1 tracing.
Interpretation
There is no evidence of interruption of the oxygen pathway; the possibility of evolving fetal metabolic acidemia can be ruled out by the presence of moderate variability and accelerations. Even though this is a Category 1 tracing, the tachysystole should be addressed to avoid deterioration of fetal acid–base status.

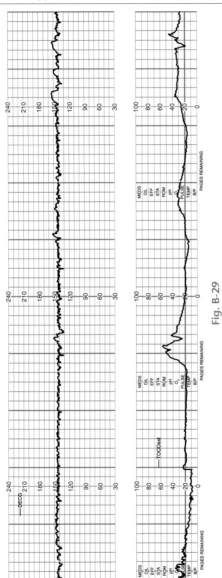

Fig. B-29

29. **Monitoring Mode:** IFE/TOCO
Baseline FHR: 140 bpm. **Baseline variability:** Minimal for majority of the tracing, changing to moderate near the end of the tracing. **Accelerations:** Absent.
Decelerations: Absent. **Uterine activity:** Unable to adequately assess; toco should be adjusted. **Category:** This is a Category 2 tracing.
Interpretation
Although there is no evidence of interruption of the oxygen pathway, the possibility of evolving fetal metabolic acidemia/ongoing hypoxic injury cannot be ruled out initially because of the lack of either accelerations or moderate variability . However, continued observation may reveal moderate variability as the tracing continues.

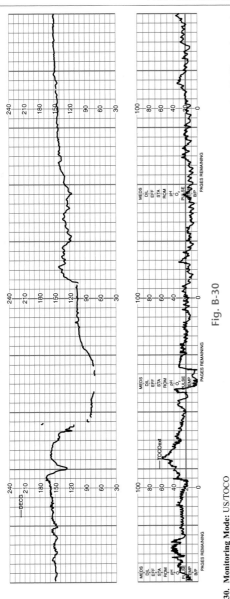

Fig. B-30

30. **Monitoring Mode:** US/TOCO

Baseline FHR: 150 bpm. **Baseline variability:** Minimal. **Accelerations:** Minimal. **Baseline variability:** Minimal. **Accelerations:** Minimal. **Decelerations:** Prolonged deceleration. **Uterine activity:** Unable to adequately assess; toco should be adjusted. **Category:** This is a Category 2 tracing.

Interpretation

The prolonged deceleration is evidence of interruption of the oxygen pathway; the possibility of evolving fetal metabolic acidemia/ongoing hypoxic injury cannot be ruled out because of the lack of either accelerations or moderate variability.

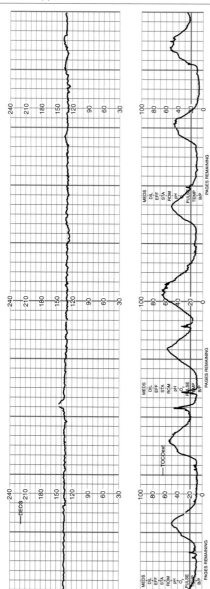

Fig. B-31

31. **Monitoring Mode:** US/TOCO
Baseline FHR: 130 bpm. **Baseline variability:** Minimal. **Accelerations:** Absent. **Decelerations:** Absent. **Uterine activity:** Tachysystole. **Category:** This is a Category 2 tracing.
Interpretation
There is no evidence of interruption of the oxygen pathway; however, the possibility of evolving fetal metabolic acidemia/ongoing hypoxic injury cannot be ruled out because of the lack of either accelerations or moderate variability.

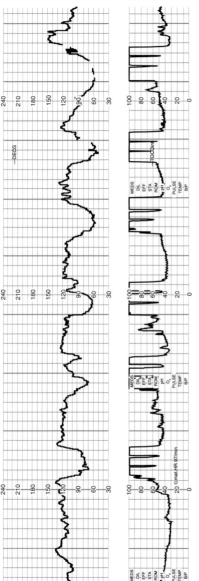

Fig. B-32

32. **Monitoring Mode:** IFE/IUPC
Baseline FHR: 120 bpm (**Note:** baseline may be decreasing near the end of the tracing). **Baseline variability:** Moderate. **Accelerations:** Absent. **Decelerations:** Recurrent variable decelerations for the majority of the tracing. **Uterine activity:** Tachysystole. Also note the hypertonus and the apparent use of closed glottis pushing.
Category: This is a Category 2 tracing.

Interpretation
The variable decelerations reflect interruption of the oxygen pathway at one or more points; the possibility of fetal metabolic acidemia/ongoing hypoxic injury can be ruled out because of the presence of moderate variability. Although this type of tracing is fairly common in second-stage labor, the moderate variability allows one to rule out evolving fetal metabolic acidemia, which may not continue to be the case unless clinicians intervene to decrease uterine activity and alter pushing technique.

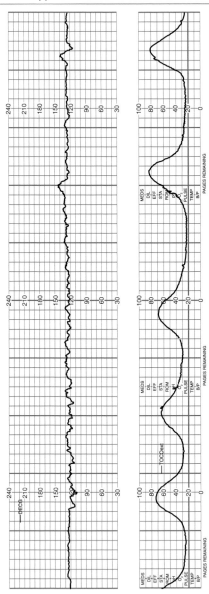

Fig. B-33

33. **Monitoring Mode:** US/IUPC

Baseline FHR: 125 bpm. **Baseline variability:** Moderate. **Accelerations:** Absent. **Decelerations:** Absent. **Uterine activity:** Tachysystole, with the possibility of hypertonus during initial portion of tracing. Note that total Montevideo units may be less than adequate, but without adequate relaxation time, steps to adjust uterine activity should be instituted. **Category:** This is a Category 1 tracing.

Interpretation

There is no evidence of interruption of the oxygen pathway; the possibility of fetal metabolic acidemia/ongoing hypoxic injury can be ruled out because of the presence of moderate variability.

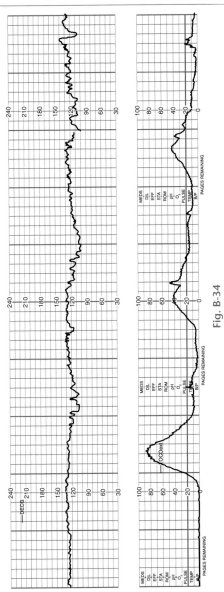

Fig. B-34

34. Monitoring Mode: US/TOCO
Baseline FHR: 130 bpm. **Baseline variability:** Moderate. **Accelerations:** Moderate. **Decelerations:** Absent. **Decelerations:** Late decelerations. **Uterine activity:** Normal, although toco may need adjustment. **Category:** This is a Category 2 tracing.

Interpretation
The late decelerations are evidence of interruption of the oxygen pathway; however, the possibility of fetal metabolic acidemia/ongoing hypoxic injury can be ruled out because of the presence of moderate variability.

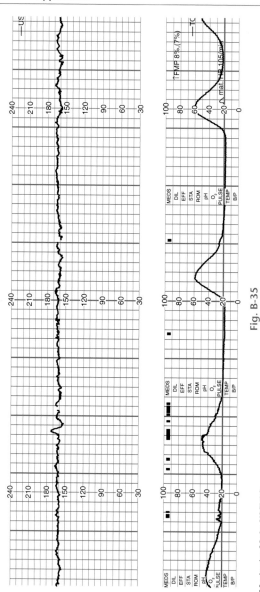

Fig. B-35

35. Monitoring Mode: US/IUPC

Baseline FHR: 160 bpm. **Baseline variability:** Minimal. **Accelerations:** Absent. **Decelerations:** Absent. **Uterine activity:** Normal. **Category:** This is a Category 2 tracing.

Interpretation

Although there is no evidence of interruption of the oxygen pathway, the possibility of evolving fetal metabolic acidemia/ongoing hypoxic injury cannot be ruled out because of the absence of moderate variability or accelerations. Although the baseline is not technically tachycardic for a term pregnancy, it should be evaluated as such because it is the high end of normal and not expected at term.

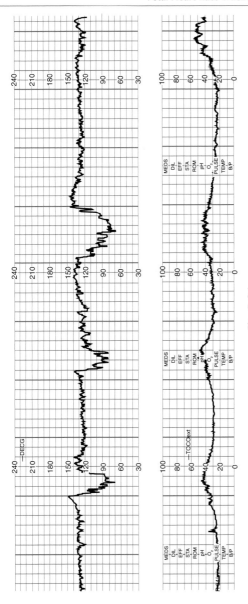

Fig. B-36

36. **Monitoring Mode:** IFE/TOCO
Baseline FHR: 130 bpm. **Baseline variability:** Moderate. **Accelerations:** Moderate. **Accelerations:** Absent. **Decelerations:** Recurrent variable decelerations. **Uterine activity:** Normal frequency, but palpation should be used to rule out hypertonus. **Category:** This is a Category 2 tracing.
Interpretation
The variable decelerations reflect interruption of the oxygen pathway; the possibility of evolving fetal metabolic acidemia/ongoing hypoxic injury can be ruled out because of the presence of moderate variability.

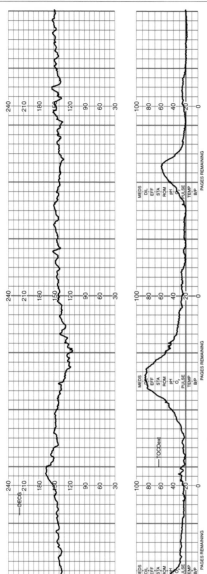

Fig. B-37

37. **Monitoring Mode:** IFE/TOCO
Baseline FHR: 145 bpm. **Baseline variability:** Moderate. **Accelerations:** Moderate. **Decelerations:** Prolonged deceleration. **Uterine activity:** Normal.
Category: This is a Category 2 tracing.
Interpretation
The prolonged deceleration reflects interruption of the oxygen pathway; the possibility of evolving fetal metabolic acidemia/ongoing hypoxic injury can be ruled out because of the presence of moderate variability. *Note: Some clinicians may believe there is an acceleration immediately preceding the prolonged deceleration, but it appears that the deceleration begins before a return to baseline. Although an argument can be made for either view; it does not alter the interpretation of the tracing because there is moderate variability.*

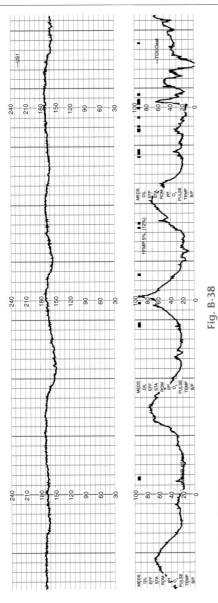

Fig. B-38

38. **Monitoring Mode:** US/TOCO
Baseline FHR: 170 bpm. **Baseline variability:** Absent (although some clinicians may believe this is minimal variability, most would consider this to be absent).
Accelerations: Absent. **Decelerations:** Recurrent late decelerations. **Uterine activity:** Although the uterine activity here may be considered normal rather than tachysystole based on frequency, it should be viewed as excessive because of the inadequate relaxation time between several of the contractions. **Category:** This is a Category 3 tracing if the clinician believes the variability is minimal. Regardless of category, the interpretation (as follows) will be the same.
Interpretation
The late decelerations reflect interruption of the oxygen pathway; the possibility of evolving fetal metabolic acidemia/ongoing hypoxic injury cannot be ruled out because of the absence of either moderate variability or accelerations.

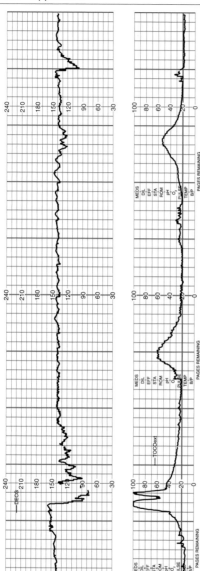

Fig. B-39

39. **Monitoring Mode:** IFE/TOCO
Baseline FHR: 140 bpm. **Baseline variability:** Moderate. **Accelerations:** Moderate. **Decelerations:** Absent. **Variable decelerations:** Variable decelerations. **Uterine activity:** Normal. **Category:** This is a Category 2 tracing.
Interpretation
The variable decelerations reflect interruption of the oxygen pathway; the possibility of evolving fetal metabolic acidemia/ongoing hypoxic injury can be excluded because of the presence of moderate variability.

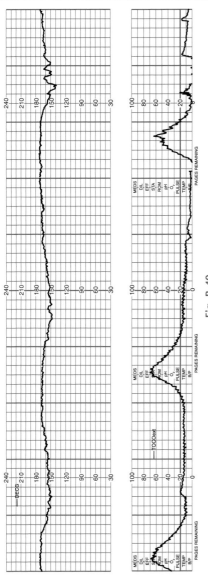

Fig. B-40

40. **Monitoring Mode:** US/TOCO
Baseline FHR: 170 bpm. **Baseline variability:** Minimal. **Accelerations:** Absent. **Decelerations:** Recurrent prolonged decelerations. *Note: Some clinicians may identify these as late decelerations, depending on the visual points identified as onset and offset.* **Uterine activity:** Normal. **Category:** This is a Category 2 tracing.

Interpretation

The prolonged (or late) decelerations reflect interruption of the oxygen pathway; the possibility of evolving fetal metabolic acidemia/ongoing hypoxic injury cannot be excluded because of the absence of either moderate variability or accelerations.

Self-Assessment

1. Prior to 32 weeks' gestation, a fetal heart rate (FHR) acceleration is defined as an increase in FHR that must be at least
   a. 15 bpm above the baseline and the acceleration must last at least 10 seconds.
   b. 10 bpm above the baseline and the acceleration must last at least 10 seconds.
   c. 10 bpm above the baseline and the acceleration must last at least 15 seconds.

2. FHR variability can be interpreted with an external monitor
   a. only after 32 weeks' gestation.
   b. but not as clearly as with an internal monitor.
   c. using a Doppler technology called *autocorrelation*.

3. Use of the terms "beat-to-beat" variability and "long-term" variability is not recommended by the National Institute of Child Health and Human Development (NICHD) because in actual practice, they are
   a. visually determined as a unit.
   b. not really very different from each other.
   c. of no consequence to management or outcome.

4. Variable deceleration of the FHR is defined as a visually apparent *abrupt* decrease in FHR. *Abrupt* is defined as an onset of the deceleration to the nadir (lowest point) that is less than
   a. 15 seconds.
   b. 20 seconds.
   c. 30 seconds.

5. According to NICHD definitions of FHR variability, which of the following is accurate?
   a. Range visually detectable but ≤5 bpm = reduced variability
   b. Range 6 to 25 bpm = average variability
   c. Range visually detectable but ≤5 bpm = minimal variability

6. According to standardized NICHD terminology, the normal FHR baseline range is
   a. 120 to 160 bpm regardless of gestational age.
   b. 110 to 160 bpm after 32 weeks of gestation.
   c. 110 to 160 bpm regardless of gestational age.

7. According to the 2008 NICHD consensus report, at the time it is observed, moderate FHR variability is highly predictive of the absence of fetal
   a. metabolic acidemia.
   b. respiratory acidemia.
   c. hypoxemia.

8. Late deceleration of the FHR is associated most specifically with
   a. transient fetal tissue hypoxia during a uterine contraction.
   b. transient fetal tissue metabolic acidosis during a uterine contraction.
   c. transient fetal hypoxemia during a uterine contraction.

9. Clinically significant FHR decelerations (late, variable, prolonged) are associated with interruption of the normal delivery of oxygen from the environment to the fetus along a pathway including
   a. lungs, heart, vasculature, kidneys, uterus, placenta, and umbilical cord.
   b. lungs, heart, vasculature, uterus, placenta, and umbilical cord.
   c. heart, vasculature, kidneys, uterus, and umbilical cord.

10. According to standardized NICHD nomenclature, decelerations that occur with at least 50% of uterine contractions in a 20-minute window are defined as:
    a. Repetitive
    b. Recurrent
    c. Persistent

11. Which setting is most appropriate for fetal vibroacoustic stimulation?
    a. 38 weeks, active labor, FHR baseline 140 bpm, minimal variability, no accelerations, no decelerations
    b. 40 weeks, active labor, FHR baseline 150 bpm, moderate variability, prolonged deceleration to 60 bpm for 8 minutes
    c. 39 weeks, active labor, FHR baseline 115 bpm, minimal variability, frequent accelerations, occasional late decelerations

12. An intrapartum FHR tracing demonstrates a baseline rate of 125 bpm, moderate variability, accelerations, and intermittent late and variable decelerations. Which of the following statements is most accurate?
    a. Moderate variability and accelerations are highly predictive of the absence of metabolic acidemia at the time they are observed.
    b. Late decelerations reflect transient fetal asphyxia during uterine contractions.
    c. Variable decelerations are caused by respiratory acidosis during cord compression.

13. According to the 2008 NICHD consensus report, a Category I FHR tracing requires which of the following?
    a. Baseline rate 120 to 160 bpm
    b. Moderate variability
    c. Accelerations
    d. All of the above
    e. a and b only

14. According to the 2008 NICHD consensus report, which of the following would be classified as a Category III FHR tracing:
    a. Baseline 180 bpm, absent variability, no accelerations, no decelerations
    b. Baseline 180 bpm, minimal variability, no accelerations, recurrent late decelerations
    c. Baseline rate 140 bpm, absent variability, recurrent late decelerations
    d. b and c
    e. a and c

15. According to the 2008 NICHD consensus report, the normal frequency of uterine contractions is
    a. ≤5 contractions in 10 minutes averaged over 30 minutes
    b. <5 contractions in 10 minutes averaged over 30 minutes
    c. <6 contractions in 10 minutes averaged over 30 minutes

16. Which of the following most closely approximates normal umbilical artery pH at term?
    a. 6.9–7.0
    b. 7.0–7.1
    c. 7.1–7.2
    d. 7.2–7.3
    e. 7.3–7.4

17. According to the 2008 NICHD consensus report, the "overshoot" FHR pattern is highly predictive of
    a. fetal asphyxia.
    b. fetal hypoxia.
    c. fetal cerebral ischemia.
    d. preexisting fetal neurologic injury.
    e. None of the above.

18. Which of the following statements is accurate regarding the FHR tracing?
    a. The absence of decelerations indicates the absence of interruption of fetal oxygenation.
    b. Accelerations and moderate variability reliably predict the absence of fetal metabolic acidemia.
    c. The absence of metabolic acidemia reliably excludes ongoing hypoxic injury.
    d. This is a Category I tracing.
    e. All of the above.

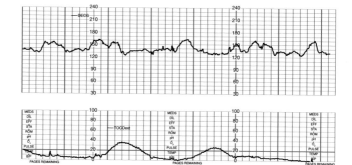

19. Which of the following statements is accurate regarding the FHR tracing?
    a. Decelerations reflect interruption of oxygen transfer from the environment to the fetus.
    b. Moderate variability reliably predicts the absence of fetal hypoxemia.
    c. The absence of accelerations predicts fetal hypoxemia and metabolic acidemia.
    d. Normal baseline FHR excludes chorioamnionitis.

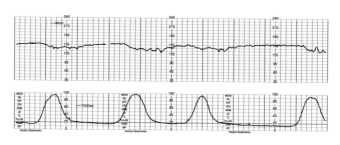

20. Which of the following is most accurate regarding the FHR tracing?
    a. Variable decelerations can be caused by umbilical cord compression.
    b. Variable decelerations reflect interruption of oxygen transfer from the environment to the fetus at one or more points.
    c. Variability is moderate.
    d. Accelerations are present.
    e. All of the above.
    f. Only a, b, and c.

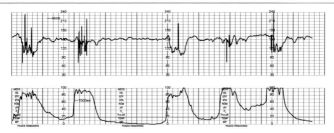

21. Appropriate management of the FHR pattern identified in the tracing includes all of the following except
    a. supplemental oxygenation.
    b. confirmation of maternal heart rate and blood pressure.
    c. maternal position changes.
    d. correct maternal hypotension if present.
    e. scalp stimulation.

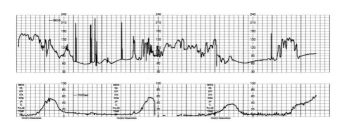

22. Which of the following statements most accurately interprets the change to the tracing?
    a. Baseline FHR 150 bpm
    b. Highly predictive of fetal metabolic acidemia
    c. Highly predictive of abnormal neurologic outcome
    d. Cannot exclude fetal metabolic acidemia at this time
    e. Subtle early decelerations present

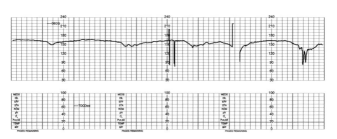

23. Umbilical vein pH is normally lower than umbilical artery pH:
    a. True
    b. False
    c. Only when late decelerations are present and recurrent

24. Fetal scalp stimulation is used to
    a. elicit FHR accelerations.
    b. correct prolonged decelerations.
    c. stimulate FHR variability during a prolonged deceleration.
    d. All of the above.

25. A key point regarding the occurrence of tachysystole is that
    a. it can occur in spontaneous or stimulated labor.
    b. it requires FHR decelerations to be clinically significant.
    c. it should be documented only if oxytocin is being used.

26. According to the algorithm for delivery decision-making authored by Clark and colleagues, the proper management of a patient with intermittent late decelerations and moderate variability in second-stage labor with normal progress is
    a. expedited delivery by operative vaginal delivery or cesarean delivery.
    b. performance of fetal scalp stimulation to rule out acidemia.
    c. continued observation.

27. Which of the following is true about electronic fetal monitoring (EFM) documentation?
    a. If something is not documented, it is legally considered not to have occurred.
    b. Documentation frequency should be every 5 minutes in the second stage if a patient has risk factors.
    c. Categories of the EFM tracing should be regularly documented.
    d. None of the above.
    e. All of the above.

28. The FHR dysrhythmia that can be associated with fetal hydrops is
    a. supraventricular tachycardia.
    b. atrioventricular heart block.
    c. persistent premature ventricular contractions.

29. Chemoreceptors are
    a. located in the aortic arch and carotid sinus.
    b. sensitive to changes in fetal blood pressure.
    c. sensitive to changes in fetal oxygenation.
    d. Both a and c.
    e. Both a and b.

30. When an FHR tracing is Category II, this means
    a. it requires further evaluation.
    b. it will progress to a Category III if no intervention.
    c. the fetus is at risk for acidemia.

ANSWER KEY FOR SELF-ASSESSMENT

1.	b	16.	d
2.	c	17.	e
3.	a	18.	e
4.	c	19.	a
5.	c	20.	f
6.	c	21.	e
7.	a	22.	d
8.	c	23.	b
9.	b	24.	a
10.	b	25.	a
11.	a	26.	c
12.	a	27.	d
13.	b	28.	a
14.	c	29.	d
15.	a	30.	a

INDEX

Note: Page numbers followed by *b* indicate boxes, *f* indicates figures, and *t* indicates tables.

A